Essentials of
Perioperative Nursing

The Pedagogy

Essentials of Perioperative Nursing, Fifth Edition drives comprehension through various strategies that meet the learning needs of students, while also generating enthusiasm about the topic. This interactive approach addresses different learning styles, making this the ideal text to ensure mastery of key concepts. The pedagogical aids that appear in most chapters include the following:

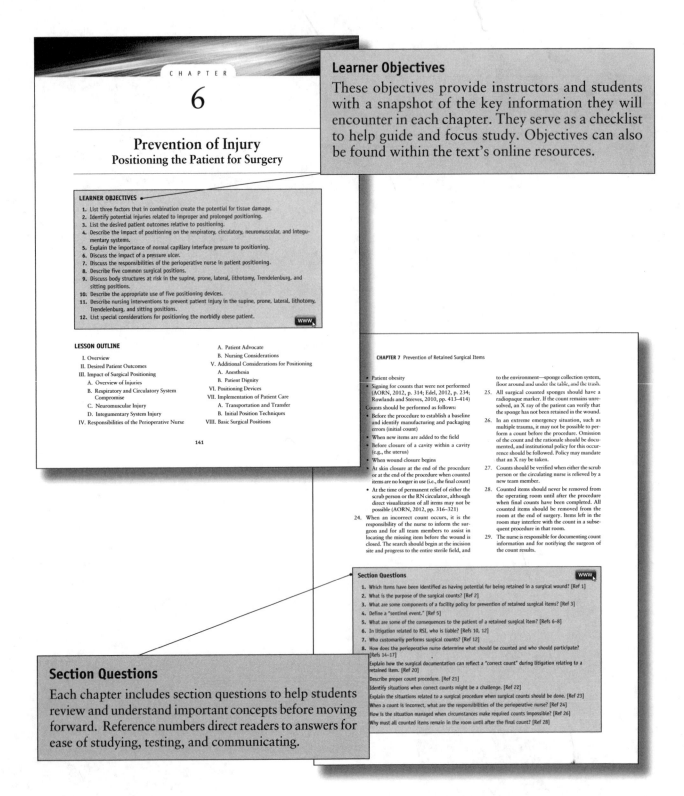

Learner Objectives

These objectives provide instructors and students with a snapshot of the key information they will encounter in each chapter. They serve as a checklist to help guide and focus study. Objectives can also be found within the text's online resources.

CHAPTER 6

Prevention of Injury
Positioning the Patient for Surgery

LEARNER OBJECTIVES

1. List three factors that in combination create the potential for tissue damage.
2. Identify potential injuries related to improper and prolonged positioning.
3. List the desired patient outcomes relative to positioning.
4. Describe the impact of positioning on the respiratory, circulatory, neuromuscular, and integumentary systems.
5. Explain the importance of normal capillary interface pressure to positioning.
6. Discuss the impact of a pressure ulcer.
7. Discuss the responsibilities of the perioperative nurse in patient positioning.
8. Describe five common surgical positions.
9. Discuss body structures at risk in the supine, prone, lateral, lithotomy, Trendelenburg, and sitting positions.
10. Describe the appropriate use of five positioning devices.
11. Describe nursing interventions to prevent patient injury in the supine, prone, lateral, lithotomy, Trendelenburg, and sitting positions.
12. List special considerations for positioning the morbidly obese patient.

LESSON OUTLINE

I. Overview
II. Desired Patient Outcomes
III. Impact of Surgical Positioning
  A. Overview of Injuries
  B. Respiratory and Circulatory System Compromise
  C. Neuromuscular Injury
  D. Integumentary System Injury
IV. Responsibilities of the Perioperative Nurse

  A. Patient Advocate
  B. Nursing Considerations
V. Additional Considerations for Positioning
  A. Anesthesia
  B. Patient Dignity
VI. Positioning Devices
VII. Implementation of Patient Care
  A. Transportation and Transfer
  B. Initial Position Techniques
VIII. Basic Surgical Positions

141

CHAPTER 7 Prevention of Retained Surgical Items

• Patient obesity
• Signing for counts that were not performed (AORN, 2012, p. 314; Edel, 2012, p. 234; Rowlands and Steeves, 2010, pp. 413–414)

Counts should be performed as follows:

• Before the procedure to establish a baseline and identify manufacturing and packaging errors (initial count)
• When new items are added to the field
• Before closure of a cavity within a cavity (e.g., the uterus)
• When wound closure begins
• At skin closure at the end of the procedure or at the end of the procedure when counted items are no longer in use (i.e., the final count)
  • At the time of permanent relief of either the scrub person or the RN circulator, although direct visualization of all items may not be possible (AORN, 2012, pp. 316–321)

24. When an incorrect count occurs, it is the responsibility of the nurse to inform the surgeon and for all team members to assist in locating the missing item before the wound is closed. The search should begin at the incision site and progress to the entire sterile field, and

to the environment—sponge collection system, floor around and under the table, and the trash.

25. All surgical counted sponges should have a radiopaque marker. If the count remains unresolved, an X ray of the patient can verify that the sponge has not been retained in the wound.

26. In an extreme emergency situation, such as multiple trauma, it may not be possible to perform a count before the procedure. Omission of the count and the rationale should be documented, and institutional policy for this occurrence should be followed. Policy may mandate that an X ray be taken.

27. Counts should be verified when either the scrub person or the circulating nurse is relieved by a new team member.

28. Counted items should never be removed from the operating room until after the procedure when final counts have been completed. All counted items should be removed from the room at the end of surgery. Items left in the room may interfere with the count in a subsequent procedure in that room.

29. The nurse is responsible for documenting count information and for notifying the surgeon of the count results.

Section Questions

1. Which items have been identified as having potential for being retained in a surgical wound? [Ref 1]
2. What is the purpose of the surgical counts? [Ref 2]
3. What are some components of a facility policy for prevention of retained surgical items? [Ref 3]
4. Define a "sentinel event." [Ref 5]
5. What are some of the consequences to the patient of a retained surgical item? [Refs 6–8]
6. In litigation related to RSI, who is liable? [Refs 10, 12]
7. Who customarily performs surgical counts? [Ref 12]
8. How does the perioperative nurse determine what should be counted and who should participate? [Refs 14–17]
Explain how the surgical documentation can reflect a "correct count" during litigation relating to a retained item. [Ref 20]
Describe proper count procedure. [Ref 21]
Identify situations when correct counts might be a challenge. [Ref 22]
Explain the situations related to a surgical procedure when surgical counts should be done. [Ref 23]
When a count is incorrect, what are the responsibilities of the perioperative nurse? [Ref 24]
How is the situation managed when circumstances make required counts impossible? [Ref 26]
Why must all counted items remain in the room until after the final count? [Ref 28]

Section Questions

Each chapter includes section questions to help students review and understand important concepts before moving forward. Reference numbers direct readers to answers for ease of studying, testing, and communicating.

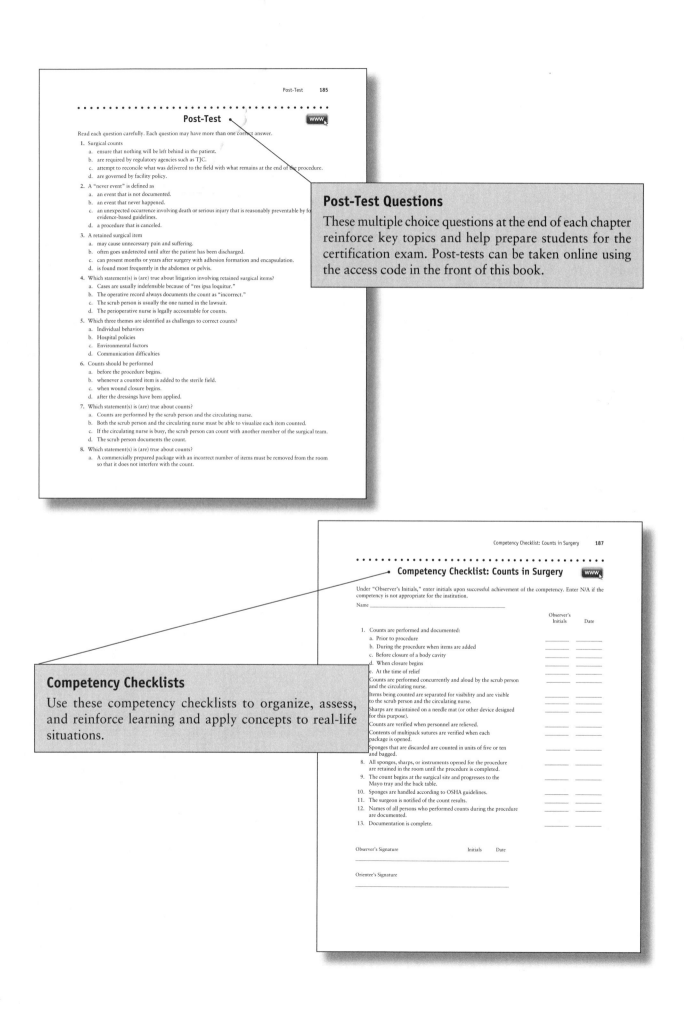

Post-Test

Read each question carefully. Each question may have more than one correct answer.

1. Surgical counts
   a. ensure that nothing will be left behind in the patient.
   b. are required by regulatory agencies such as TJC.
   c. attempt to reconcile what was delivered to the field with what remains at the end of the procedure.
   d. are governed by facility policy.

2. A "never event" is defined as
   a. an event that is not documented.
   b. an event that never happened.
   c. an unexpected occurrence involving death or serious injury that is reasonably preventable by fo
      evidence-based guidelines.
   d. a procedure that is canceled.

3. A retained surgical item
   a. may cause unnecessary pain and suffering.
   b. often goes undetected until after the patient has been discharged.
   c. can present months or years after surgery with adhesion formation and encapsulation.
   d. is found most frequently in the abdomen or pelvis.

4. Which statement(s) is (are) true about litigation involving retained surgical items?
   a. Cases are usually indefensible because of "res ipsa loquitur."
   b. The operative record always documents the count as "incorrect."
   c. The scrub person is usually the one named in the lawsuit.
   d. The perioperative nurse is legally accountable for counts.

5. Which three themes are identified as challenges to correct counts?
   a. Individual behaviors
   b. Hospital policies
   c. Environmental factors
   d. Communication difficulties

6. Counts should be performed
   a. before the procedure begins.
   b. whenever a counted item is added to the sterile field.
   c. when wound closure begins.
   d. after the dressings have been applied.

7. Which statement(s) is (are) true about counts?
   a. Counts are performed by the scrub person and the circulating nurse.
   b. Both the scrub person and the circulating nurse must be able to visualize each item counted.
   c. If the circulating nurse is busy, the scrub person can count with another member of the surgical team.
   d. The scrub person documents the count.

8. Which statement(s) is (are) true about counts?
   a. A commercially prepared package with an incorrect number of items must be removed from the room
      so that it does not interfere with the count.

Post-Test Questions

These multiple choice questions at the end of each chapter reinforce key topics and help prepare students for the certification exam. Post-tests can be taken online using the access code in the front of this book.

Competency Checklist: Counts in Surgery

Under "Observer's Initials," enter initials upon successful achievement of the competency. Enter N/A if the competency is not appropriate for the institution.

Name _____

	Observer's Initials	Date
1. Counts are performed and documented:		
a. Prior to procedure	_____	_____
b. During the procedure when items are added	_____	_____
c. Before closure of a body cavity	_____	_____
d. When closure begins	_____	_____
e. At the time of relief	_____	_____
Counts are performed concurrently and aloud by the scrub person and the circulating nurse.	_____	_____
Items being counted are separated for visibility and are visible to the scrub person and the circulating nurse.	_____	_____
Sharps are maintained on a needle mat (or other device designed for this purpose).	_____	_____
Counts are verified when personnel are relieved.	_____	_____
Contents of multipack sutures are verified when each package is opened.	_____	_____
Sponges that are discarded are counted in units of five or ten and bagged.	_____	_____
8. All sponges, sharps, or instruments opened for the procedure are retained in the room until the procedure is completed.	_____	_____
9. The count begins at the surgical site and progresses to the Mayo tray and the back table.	_____	_____
10. Sponges are handled according to OSHA guidelines.	_____	_____
11. The surgeon is notified of the count results.	_____	_____
12. Names of all persons who performed counts during the procedure are documented.	_____	_____
13. Documentation is complete.	_____	_____

Observer's Signature _____   Initials _____   Date _____

Orientee's Signature _____

Competency Checklists

Use these competency checklists to organize, assess, and reinforce learning and apply concepts to real-life situations.

Fifth Edition

Essentials of
Perioperative Nursing

Terri Goodman, PhD, RN, CNOR
Terri Goodman & Associates
Dallas, Texas

Cynthia Spry, MA, MS, RN, CNOR, CSIT
Independent Clinical Consultant
New York, New York

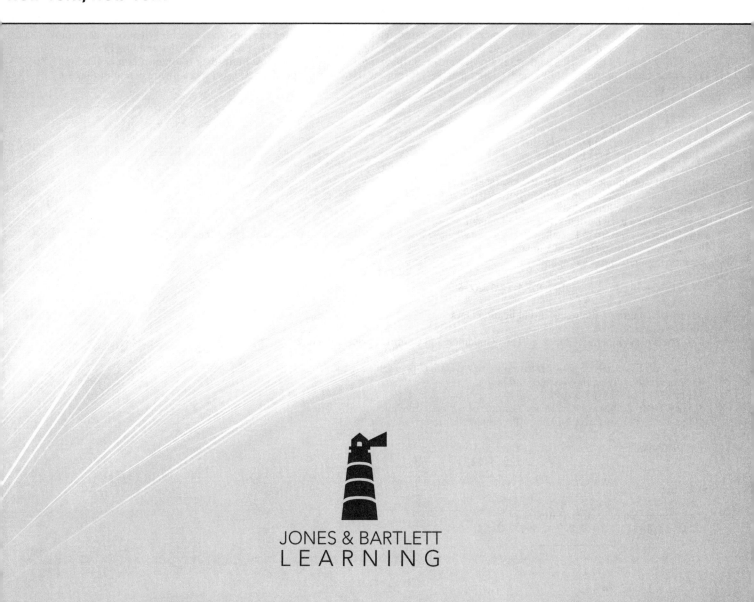

JONES & BARTLETT
LEARNING

World Headquarters
Jones & Bartlett Learning
5 Wall Street
Burlington, MA 01803
978-443-5000
info@jblearning.com
www.jblearning.com

Jones & Bartlett Learning books and products are available through most bookstores and online booksellers. To contact Jones & Bartlett Learning directly, call 800-832-0034, fax 978-443-8000, or visit our website, www.jblearning.com.

Substantial discounts on bulk quantities of Jones & Bartlett Learning publications are available to corporations, professional associations, and other qualified organizations. For details and specific discount information, contact the special sales department at Jones & Bartlett Learning via the above contact information or send an email to specialsales@jblearning.com.

Essentials of Perioperative Nursing, Fifth Edition is an independent publication and has not been authorized, sponsored, or otherwise approved by the owners of the trademarks or service marks referenced in this product.

The authors, editor, and publisher have made every effort to provide accurate information. However, they are not responsible for errors, omissions, or for any outcomes related to the use of the contents of this book and take no responsibility for the use of the products and procedures described. Treatments and side effects described in this book may not be applicable to all people; likewise, some people may require a dose or experience a side effect that is not described herein. Drugs and medical devices are discussed that may have limited availability controlled by the Food and Drug Administration (FDA) for use only in a research study or clinical trial. Research, clinical practice, and government regulations often change the accepted standard in this field. When consideration is being given to use of any drug in the clinical setting, the health care provider or reader is responsible for determining FDA status of the drug, reading the package insert, and reviewing prescribing information for the most up-to-date recommendations on dose, precautions, and contraindications, and determining the appropriate usage for the product. This is especially important in the case of drugs that are new or seldom used.

Production Credits
Executive Publisher: Kevin Sullivan
Acquisitions Editor: Amanda Harvey
Editorial Assistant: Sara Bempkins
Production Editor: Keith Henry
Marketing Communications Manager: Katie Hennessy
V.P., Manufacturing and Inventory Control: Therese Connell
Composition: Paw Print Media
Cover and Title Page Design: Michael O'Donnell
Cover Image: (bottom) © Excellent Backgrounds/ShutterStock, Inc., (top) © Sergii Teplov/Dreamstime.com
Printing and Binding: Courier Companies
Cover Printing: Courier Companies

To order this product, use ISBN: 978-1-4496-8806-6

Library of Congress Cataloging-in-Publication Data
Goodman, Terri.
  Essentials of perioperative nursing / Terri Goodman and Cynthia Spry.—5th ed.
    p. ; cm.
  Rev. ed. of: Essentials of perioperative nursing / Cynthia Spry. 4th ed. c2009.
  Includes bibliographical references and index.
  ISBN 978-1-4496-8762-5 (pbk.)
  I. Spry, Cynthia. II. Spry, Cynthia. Essentials of perioperative nursing. III. Title.
  [DNLM: 1. Perioperative Nursing—Programmed Instruction. WY 18.2]
  617.9'17—dc23
                    2012034462

6048

Printed in the United States of America
17 16 15 14 13   10 9 8 7 6 5 4 3 2 1

Contents

Introduction

Essentials of Perioperative Nursing provides the knowledge and skills required to navigate safely and effectively in an aseptic environment. It is a valuable text both for personnel working in a perioperative setting and as a basic academic nursing curriculum. The text provides the information and the skills that the perioperative nurse must master to function independently at an entry level. Many of these skills are also applicable to patient care outside of the perioperative setting, particularly with the focus in health care on preventing infection.

The competencies required to prevent infections apply to treating patients throughout the healthcare system. Creating and maintaining a sterile field requires the same knowledge, skills, and commitment to patient safety, whether that sterile field is created in the operating room for a surgical procedure, in interventional radiology, or for the insertion of a central line, a dressing change, or the insertion of a urinary catheter.

With the increase in the number and complexity of surgical procedures being undertaken in both inpatient and outpatient settings, managers and educators must orient a growing number of nurses to the perioperative arena quickly and efficiently. *Essentials of Perioperative Nursing* can be used by nurses independently or as an adjunct to the formal orientation process. The text can also be instrumental in preparing in-service programs for the entire perioperative nursing staff, for reference and review, and for preparing for the certification exam.

Essentials of Perioperative Nursing is an introductory text designed to teach and reinforce essential perioperative knowledge and skills. It does not cover all aspects of perioperative nursing, surgical specialties, or specific procedures. It does, however, prepare the new perioperative nurse to pursue competence in the wide variety of surgical specialties—a process that may take several years of exposure and hands-on experience.

Each chapter contains objectives, study questions, a post-test, and a competency checklist that the perioperative educator or the individual nurse can use to organize, assess, and reinforce learning. The companion website contains additional resources to augment each chapter and a bank of test questions.

Objectives

Following mastery of the content, the learner will be able to do the following:

- Describe essential elements of perioperative practice
- Discuss application of the Perioperative Nursing Data Set (PNDS)
- List nursing diagnoses commonly applicable to surgical patients
- Identify desired patient outcomes relative to surgical intervention
- Discuss the responsibility of the perioperative nurse in achieving desired patient outcomes
- Demonstrate understanding of basic principles and concepts of perioperative nursing by responding correctly to the section questions and post-test questions in each chapter
- Identify the behavioral skills necessary to demonstrate competency in essential perioperative practice

Assumptions about the Learner

The learner is assumed to have the following characteristics:

- Is a registered nurse
- May have no perioperative experience or may have varied clinical experience
- Is self-motivated
- Does not yet function at the expert level
- Views knowledge of perioperative nursing practice as desirable and useful
- Demonstrates competence in using the nursing practice

The first edition of *Essentials of Perioperative Nursing* was published in 1987, followed by revisions in 1997, 2005, and 2009. Although the basic principles have not changed markedly since the last edition, practice changes have occurred as the body of knowledge related to desired patient outcomes grows. Evidence-based practice continues to be a key phrase in the current literature, meaning that practice decisions should be supported by research or empirical evidence showing that the practice contributes to desired patient outcomes. This fifth edition has been revised to reflect the most current research findings, literature reviews, and the most recent Association of periOperative Registered Nursing (AORN) standards and recommended practices.

In addition, the section questions and post-test questions throughout the book are new. A companion website has been developed that provides additional and up-to-date resources to support the information in each chapter.

I am honored that the author of *Essentials of Perioperative Nursing*, Cynthia Spry, MSN, MA, RN, CNOR, requested that I edit the fifth edition. For more than 20 years, this text has been used by countless appreciative readers. It has been a valuable teaching tool, a source of reference and review, and an excellent resource for preparing for the certification exam. I hope that I will continue to hear "I use your book all the time," as Cynthia has over the years; then I will know that I have given her labor of love and her legacy to perioperative nursing continuing life.

Every surgical patient deserves the caring services of a registered nurse, whether the procedure is performed in an operating room, an ambulatory surgery facility, or an interventional site, or as a sterile procedure done at the bedside. I hope that *Essentials of Perioperative Nursing* will continue to be a premier text for perioperative nurses and for all nurses who will deliver aseptic care to patients regardless of the setting.

Terri Goodman

Acknowledgments

Cynthia Spry, MA, MS, RN, CNOR, CSIT
Independent Clinical Consultant
New York, New York

M. Ginny Baird, RN, BSN, CNOR
Nurse Clinician—Perioperative Education
The Methodist Hospital
Houston, Texas

Dru A. Beedle, RN, MN, CNOR, NE-BC
Perioperative Consultant and Educator
Lindenhurst, Illinois

Michelle J. Brents, MS, RN, CNOR
Perioperative RN IV/Clinical Leader
The Methodist Hospital
Houston, Texas

Vangie Dennis, BSN, RN, CNOR, CMLSO
Administrative Director
Spivey Station Surgery Center
Jonesboro, Georgia

Sandra Eversole, RN, CNOR(E)
Senior Analyst, Clinical Specialty
Cardinal Health
Houston, Texas

Karen B. Hammett, BSN, RN, CNOR
Perioperative Educator
Baylor University Medical Center
Dallas, Texas

Beverly A. Kirchner, BSN, RN, CNOR, CASC
Consultant
Genesee Associates, Inc.
Highland Village, Texas

Anita M. Mitchell, RN, CNOR
Staff Nurse
TexasHealth Arlington Memorial
Arlington, Texas

Joan Spear, MBA, RN, CNOR, CRCST
Group Director Clinical Services
Aesculap, Inc.
Center Valley, Pennsylvania

Margaret S. Tierney, MS, CRNA
Staff CRNA, Greater Houston Anesthesiology, PA
The Methodist Hospital
Houston, Texas

Introduction to Perioperative Nursing

LEARNER OBJECTIVES

1. Define the three phases of the surgical experience.
2. Describe the scope of perioperative nursing practice.
3. Identify members of the surgical team.
4. Discuss application of the Perioperative Nursing Data Set (PNDS).
5. Discuss the outcomes a patient can be expected to achieve following a surgical intervention.
6. Describe the roles of surgical team members.
7. Describe the responsibilities of the perioperative nurse in the circulating role.

www

LESSON OUTLINE

Phases of the Surgical Experience

1. The perioperative period begins when the patient is informed of the need for surgery, includes the surgical procedure and recovery, and continues until the patient resumes his or her usual activities. The surgical experience can be segregated into three phases: (1) preoperative, (2) intraoperative, and (3) postoperative. The word "perioperative" is used to encompass all three phases. The perioperative nurse provides nursing care during all three phases.

Preoperative

2. The preoperative phase begins when the patient, or someone acting on the patient's behalf, is informed of the need for surgery and makes the decision to have the procedure. This phase ends when the patient is transferred to the operating room bed.

3. The preoperative phase is the period that is used to physically and psychologically prepare

the patient for surgery. The length of the preoperative period varies. For the patient whose surgery is elective, the period may be lengthy. For the patient whose surgery is urgent, the period is brief; the patient may have no awareness of this period.

4. Diagnostic studies and medical regimens are initiated in the preoperative period. Information obtained from preoperative assessment and interview is used to prepare a plan of care for the patient.

5. Nursing activities in the preoperative phase are directed toward patient support, teaching, and preparation for the procedure.

Intraoperative

6. The intraoperative phase begins when the patient is transferred to the operating room bed and ends with transfer to the postanesthesia care unit (PACU) or another area where immediate postsurgical recovery care is given.

7. During the intraoperative period, the patient is monitored, anesthetized, prepped, and draped, and the procedure is performed.

8. Nursing activities in the intraoperative period center on patient safety, facilitation of the procedure, prevention of infection, and satisfactory physiologic response to anesthesia and surgical intervention.

Postoperative

9. The postoperative phase begins with the patient's transfer to the recovery unit and ends with the resolution of surgical sequelae. The postoperative period may be either brief or extensive, and most commonly ends outside the facility where the surgery was performed.

10. For patients who will remain in the hospital for an extended stay, the perioperative nurse may not provide care beyond patient transfer to the PACU, where postanesthesia care nurses assume responsibility for the patient. In an effort to better utilize nursing resources, many perioperative nurses, particularly in smaller hospitals, have been trained in postanesthesia care and are assuming responsibility for providing care in both the operating room and PACU. Care at home, if required, is delivered by home healthcare nurses.

11. The majority of operative procedures performed today are done on an outpatient basis.

For patients who undergo surgery in ambulatory surgery facilities, day surgery centers, or office-based surgical settings where the expectation is that they will return home on the same day they have surgery, it is not uncommon for the perioperative nurse to provide care for the patient during all three phases.

12. Nursing activities in the immediate postoperative phase center on support of the patient's physiologic systems. In the later stages of recovery, much of the focus is on reinforcing the essential information that the patient and other caregivers require in preparation for discharge.

Nursing Process Throughout the Perioperative Period

13. The words "perioperative" and "perioperative nursing" are accepted and utilized in nursing and medical literature. Perioperative nursing was formerly referred to as "operating room nursing," a term that historically referred to patient care provided in the intraoperative period and administered within the operating room itself. However, as the responsibilities of the operating room nurse expanded to include care in the preoperative and postoperative periods, the term "perioperative" was recognized as more appropriate. In 1999, the organization that represents perioperative nurses, once known as the Association of Operating Room Nurses (AORN), changed its name to the Association of periOperative Registered Nurses (AORN).

14. The perioperative nurse is a nurse who specializes in perioperative practice and who provides nursing care to the surgical patient throughout the continuum of care. The AORN Perioperative Patient-Focused Model identifies four specific domains—patient safety, physiologic response, behavioral responses, and the health system—that are the areas of concern for the perioperative nurse.

15. The domains of safety, physiologic response, and behavioral responses of patients reflect the nature of the surgical experience for the patient and serve as a guide for providing care.

16. The fourth domain represents other members of the healthcare team and the healthcare system. Perioperative nurses work collaboratively with other healthcare team members to formulate nursing diagnoses, identify desired outcomes,

and provide care within the context of the healthcare system so as to achieve desirable patient outcomes (AORN, 2012a, pp. 3–4).

17. Perioperative nurses provide patient care within the framework of the nursing process. They use the tools of patient assessment, care planning, intervention, and evaluation of patient outcomes to meet the needs of patients who are undergoing operative or other invasive procedures. Every patient is unique, and the plan of care is tailored to meet the patient's specific needs. The plan addresses physiological, psychological, sociocultural, and spiritual aspects of care.

18. Much of perioperative nursing involves technical expertise, including responsibility for equipment, instrumentation, and surgical techniques. Technical skills and responsibilities are purposeful within the nursing process during the implementation phase; however, the patient remains the focus of the perioperative nurse's activities.

19. The goal of perioperative nursing is to provide care to patients and support to their families, using the nursing process to assist patients and their families in making decisions and to meet and support the needs of patients undergoing surgical or other invasive procedures. The overall desired outcome is that the patient will achieve a level of wellness equal to or greater than the level prior to surgery.

20. Perioperative nursing care is provided in a variety of settings, including acute care facilities, ambulatory settings, and physician-based office settings. Perioperative nurses provide care to patients, their families, and others who support the patient. Three major activities of perioperative nurses are providing direct care, coordinating comprehensive care, and educating patients and their families.

Assessment

21. Nursing assessment of the patient may take place in a number of settings and time frames. Assessment may be performed a week or more before surgery or just prior to the procedure. It may occur in the patient's inpatient hospital unit, the surgeon's office, the preadmission testing unit of the surgical facility, or the same-day/ambulatory surgery unit.

22. In some instances, the assessment process is initiated in a telephone conversation with the patient prior to surgery, and completed on the day of surgery at the surgical facility. Often the initial nursing assessment is performed by a nurse who is not a perioperative nurse. It is more likely that the perioperative nurse's assessment of the patient will take place just prior to the patient's entry into the operating room. This assessment will include a brief interview, a quick physical inspection of the patient, and a review of the patient's record, including the results of diagnostic testing and assessment data obtained previously by other caregivers.

Nursing Diagnoses

23. Assessment data provide information that the perioperative nurse uses to formulate nursing diagnoses and identify desired outcomes. Several nursing diagnoses, such as knowledge deficit and high risk for infection, are typical for the surgical patient. Assessment data form the foundation for patient-specific nursing diagnoses and planning individualized care tailored to meet each patient's individual and unique needs.

Planning

24. The perioperative nurse uses knowledge of the patient, the proposed procedure, identified patient needs, related nursing diagnoses, and desired outcomes to plan care for each patient.

25. The perioperative nurse begins care planning before the patient is seen, based on knowledge of the planned procedure, the resources required, and the common nursing diagnoses related to surgical intervention. Knowledge of the individual patient obtained during the assessment process is combined with this previous planning to prepare for meeting the unique needs of the patient and providing care that is individually tailored to each patient.

Intervention

26. In the intervention stage of the nursing process, the perioperative nurse provides, coordinates, supervises, and documents care within the framework of accepted standards of nursing care, as identified by the AORN standards and recommended clinical practices (AORN, 2012).

Evaluation

27. In the final evaluation stage of the nursing process, the perioperative nurse evaluates the results of nursing care in relation to the extent that expected patient outcomes have been met.

Perioperative Nursing Data Set

28. In 2000, AORN published the first Perioperative Nursing Data Set (PNDS) (AORN, 2011). The PNDS is a controlled, structured nursing vocabulary that can be used to describe perioperative nursing practice. Following revisions, the PNDS, Third Edition, includes 40 nurse-sensitive patient outcomes, 44 nursing diagnoses, and 53 interventions. The PNDS may be used for the following purposes:

    - Provide a framework to standardize documentation.
    - Provide a universal language for perioperative nursing practice and education.
    - Assist in the measurement and evaluation of patient care outcomes.
    - Provide a foundation for perioperative nursing research and evaluation of patient outcomes.

29. A primary benefit in day-to-day practice is the use of a universal language for nursing diagnoses, interventions, and expected outcomes.

30. In some facilities, the PNDS has been entered into the documentation database, allowing nurses to access the common language via computer. Even when the documentation is not computerized, the perioperative nurse should refer to the PNDS when planning patient care. The PNDS is available through AORN.

31. Examples of nursing diagnoses using the PNDS include the following:

    - Risk of infection
    - Impaired transfer ability
    - Imbalanced nutrition: more than body requirement

32. Examples of desired patient outcomes include the following:

    - The patient is free of signs and symptoms of infection.
    - The patient is free of signs and symptoms of injury related to transfer/transport.
    - The patient demonstrates knowledge of nutritional requirements related to operative or other invasive procedures.

33. Examples of implementation include the following:

    - Implements aseptic technique, protects from cross-contamination
    - Evaluates for signs and symptoms of skin and tissue injury as a result of transfer or transport
    - Provides instruction regarding dietary needs

Patient Outcomes: Standards of Perioperative Care

34. Perioperative nursing is patient oriented, not task oriented. Perioperative nurses focus on

preventive practice rather than on the identification of problems (AORN, 2011, p. 4).
They must use knowledge, judgment, and skill
based on the principles of biological, physiological, behavioral, social, and nursing sciences to plan and implement care to achieve
desired patient outcomes. AORN has identified patient outcomes that describe the results
a patient can expect to achieve during surgical interventions. These standards reflect
the responsibilities of the perioperative nurse
and may serve as a framework with which
to evaluate patient response to perioperative
nursing interventions.

35. The PNDS describes 40 outcome relationships
    (AORN, 2011, pp. 139–391):
    - The patient is free from signs and symptoms
      of injury related to thermal sources.
    - The patient is free from unintended retained
      foreign objects.
    - The patient's surgery is performed on the
      correct site, side, and level.
    - The patient is free from signs and symptoms
      of injury caused by extraneous objects.
    - The patient's specimen(s) is (are) managed
      in the appropriate manner.
    - The patient's status is communicated
      throughout the continuum of care.
    - The patient is free from signs and symptoms
      of electrical injury.
    - The patient is free of signs and symptoms of
      injury related to positioning.
    - The patient is free from signs and symptoms
      of laser injury.
    - The patient is free from signs and symptoms
      of chemical injury.
    - The patient is free from signs and symptoms
      of radiation injury.
    - The patient is free from signs and symptoms
      of injury related to transfer/transport.
    - The patient receives appropriately adminis-
      tered medication(s).
    - The patient has wound perfusion consistent
      with or improved from baseline levels.
    - The patient has tissue perfusion consistent
      with or improved from baseline levels.
    - The patient's gastrointestinal status is main-
      tained at or improved from baseline levels.
    - The patient's genitourinary status is main-
      tained at or improved from baseline levels.
    - The patient's musculoskeletal status is main-
      tained at or improved from baseline levels.
    - The patient's endocrine status is maintained
      at or improved from baseline levels.
    - The patient is free from signs and symptoms
      of infection.
    - The patient is at or returning to normo-
      thermia at the conclusion of the immediate
      postoperative period.
    - The patient's fluid, electrolyte, and acid–
      base balances are maintained at or improved
      from baseline levels.
    - The patient's respiratory status is main-
      tained at or improved from baseline levels.
    - The patient's cardiovascular status is main-
      tained at or improved from baseline levels.
    - The patient demonstrates and/or reports
      adequate pain control.
    - The patient's neurological status is main-
      tained at or improved from baseline levels.
    - The patient or designated support person
      demonstrates knowledge of expected psy-
      chosocial responses to the procedure.
    - The patient or designated support person
      demonstrates knowledge of nutritional man-
      agement related to the operative or other
      invasive procedure.
    - The patient or designated support person
      demonstrates knowledge of medication
      management.
    - The patient or designated support person dem-
      onstrates knowledge of pain management.
    - The patient or designated support person
      demonstrates knowledge of wound
      management.
    - The patient or designated support person dem-
      onstrates knowledge of expected responses to
      the operative or invasive procedure.
    - The patient or designated support person
      participates in decisions affecting his or her
      perioperative plan of care.
    - The patient or designated support person
      participates in the rehabilitation process.
    - The patient's value system, lifestyle, eth-
      nicity, and culture are considered, respected,
      and incorporated in the perioperative plan
      of care.
    - The patient's care is consistent with the indi-
      vidualized perioperative plan of care.

- The patient's right to privacy is maintained.
- The patient is the recipient of competent and ethical care within legal standards of practice.
- The patient is the recipient of consistent and comparable care regardless of the setting.

36. Other desired patient outcomes not specifically listed in the AORN outcome standards may be identified by the perioperative nurse and included in the plan of care. New knowledge regarding patient responses to surgery and the effects of nursing interventions may lead to the identification of new desired patient outcomes that have implications for perioperative nursing practice. The perioperative nurse who plans patient care should be guided by, but not limited by, established patient outcome standards.

Roles of the Perioperative Nurse

37. Perioperative nurses function in various roles, including those of manager/director, clinical practitioner (e.g., scrub nurse, circulating nurse, clinical nurse specialist, registered nurse first assistant [RNFA]), educator, and researcher. In these roles, the perioperative nurse's responsibilities include, but are not limited to, the following:
- Patient assessment before, during, and after surgery
- Patient and family teaching
- Patient and family support and reassurance
- Patient advocacy
- Performing as scrub or circulating nurse during surgery
- Control of the environment
- Efficient provision of resources
- Coordination of activities related to patient care
- Communication, collaboration, and consultation with other healthcare team members

- Maintenance of asepsis
- Ongoing monitoring of the patient's physiological and psychological status
- Supervision of ancillary personnel

38. Additional responsibilities that promote personal and professional growth and contribute to the profession of perioperative nursing include, but are not limited to, the following:
- Participation in professional organization activities
- Participation in research activities that support the profession of perioperative nursing
- Exploration and validation of current and future practice
- Participation in continuing education programs to enhance personal knowledge and to promote the profession of perioperative nursing
- Functioning as a role model for nursing students and perioperative nursing colleagues
- Mentoring, precepting, and instructing other perioperative nurses

Expanded and Advanced Practice Roles

39. The RNFA is an expanded role of perioperative nursing. The RNFA practices under the direction of the surgeon and assists the surgeon during the intraoperative phase of the surgical experience. A more complete definition of the RNFA and the qualifications for this role are outlined in the revised *AORN Position Statement on RN First Assistants* (AORN, 2012b).

40. The perioperative nurse with a graduate degree may function in an advanced role. Examples of advanced practice roles include the clinical nurse specialist and nurse practitioner. Responsibilities and job descriptions may vary with employment settings and individual states' legislation.

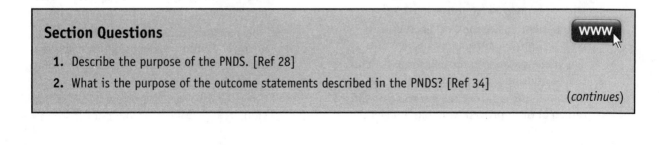

Section Questions

www

1. Describe the purpose of the PNDS. [Ref 28]
2. What is the purpose of the outcome statements described in the PNDS? [Ref 34]

(continues)

Practice Settings

41. Technological advances have resulted in dramatic changes in surgical technique. Many procedures that once required a hospital-based operating room, that necessitated a large incision, and that involved a hospital stay and an extended recovery can now be performed in same-day, outpatient, or ambulatory settings.

42. Minimally invasive surgical techniques encompass surgery performed through small puncture holes with specialized instruments and equipment. This surgical approach facilitates rapid recovery and same-day discharge. Innovations in technology are making this approach applicable to increasingly more complex procedures. Reimbursement guidelines also encourage same-day surgery and early discharge. As a result, many surgical procedures have moved into settings outside the acute care hospital-based operating room.

43. Many complex procedures are performed in freestanding surgical centers, satellite surgery facilities, mobile surgical units, surgeons' office-based operating rooms, and clinics. In addition, some procedures once performed exclusively in the operating room are now performed in the radiology unit using interventional techniques rather than open surgery. As long as reimbursement favors outpatient surgery and technological advances in instrumentation and procedures continue to emerge, the number and type of surgeries performed in the physician's offices will continue to increase.

44. The needs of the patient undergoing surgery transcend the setting in which the surgery takes place. In every setting, the perioperative nurse brings specialized skills, technical competence, knowledge, and caring that are essential to a successful surgical experience.

Members and Responsibilities of the Surgical Team

45. Safe and effective care of the surgical patient requires a team effort. Desired patient outcomes depend on the effective coordination of the unique skills of each member of the surgical team.

46. Team members may be categorized based on their responsibilities during the procedure. Sterile team members are those who scrub their hands and arms, don sterile attire, contact sterile instruments and supplies, and work within the sterile field (i.e., the area immediately surrounding the surgical site). They are referred to as the "scrubbed" members of the team.

47. Members of the sterile surgical team include the primary surgeon, assistants to the surgeon (i.e., other surgeons, residents, physician assistants, and RNFAs), and the scrub person who may be a registered nurse, a licensed practical nurse, or a surgical technologist.

48. Members of the nonsterile surgical team carry out their responsibilities outside the sterile field and do not wear sterile attire. Members of the nonsterile surgical team include the anesthesiologist, the nurse anesthetist, the anesthesia assistant, the circulating nurse, and others.

49. The primary surgeon is responsible for the preoperative diagnosis, selection of the procedure to be performed, and the actual performance of surgery.

50. The assistants work under the direction of the primary surgeon and are responsible for providing assistance during surgery, such as exposing the site, suctioning, handling tissue, and suturing. The nature of the surgery, the state in which the surgery is performed, the medical board and the board of nursing, the surgeon's preference, and hospital policies are factors that determine who may function as an assistant.

51. The scrub person works primarily with instruments and equipment. The scrub person has the following responsibilities:
    - Selecting instruments, equipment, and other supplies appropriate for the surgery
    - Preparing the sterile field and setting up the sterile table(s) with instruments and other sterile supplies needed for the procedure
    - Scrubbing, and then donning a gown and gloves
    - Maintaining the integrity and sterility of the sterile field throughout the procedure
    - Having knowledge of the procedure and anticipating the surgeon's needs throughout the procedure
    - Providing instruments, sutures, and supplies to the surgeon in an appropriate and timely manner
    - Preparing sterile dressings
    - Implementing procedures that contribute to patient safety (e.g., surgical counts for instruments, sponges, and sharps)
    - Cleaning and preparing instruments for terminal sterilization

52. Factors that determine the most appropriate scrub person include the nature of the surgery, the skills required for the procedure, the staffing skill mix, and hospital policy.

53. The anesthesiologist is responsible for assessing the patient prior to surgery and for administering anesthetic agents to facilitate surgery and provide pain relief. The anesthesia assistant administers anesthesia under the direct supervision of the anesthesiologist or, in some cases, the surgeon. In some cases, the certified registered nurse anesthetist (CRNA) also administers anesthesia under the direct supervision of the anesthesiologist or the surgeon.

54. Effective November 13, 2001, the Centers for Medicare and Medicaid Services (CMS) established an exemption for CRNAs from the physician supervision requirement. This exemption recognizes a governor's written request to CMS attesting that he or she is aware of the state's right to an exemption of the requirement and that it is in the best interests of the state's citizens to exercise this exemption.

55. As of October 2012, 16 states had chosen to opt out of the CRNA physician supervision regulation: Alaska, California, Colorado, Idaho, Iowa, Kansas, Minnesota, Montana, Nebraska, New Hampshire, New Mexico, North Dakota, Oregon, South Dakota, Washington, and Wisconsin (about.com Health Careers, 2012).

56. The perioperative nurse in the circulating role coordinates the care of the patient, serves as the patient's advocate throughout the intraoperative experience, and has responsibility for managing and implementing activities outside the sterile field. Activities are directed toward assuring patient safety and achieving desired patient outcomes. The nursing process is used as a framework for these activities. Examples of activities performed by the perioperative nurse in the circulating role include the following:
    - Providing emotional support to the patient prior to the induction of anesthesia
    - Performing ongoing patient assessment
    - Formulating a nursing diagnosis
    - Developing and implementing a plan of care
    - Documenting patient care
    - Evaluating patient outcomes
    - Teaching patient and family
    - Obtaining appropriate surgical supplies and equipment
    - Creating and maintaining a safe environment
    - Administering drugs
    - Implementing and enforcing policies and procedures that contribute to patient safety, such as surgical checklists, "time-out" protocols, surgical counts for instruments, sponges, and sharps, as well as performing equipment checks
    - Preparing and disposing of specimens
    - Communicating relevant information to other team members and to the patient's family

57. Perioperative nurse managers assume a variety of roles. In a very small facility, the perioperative nurse may serve as manager and also scrub or circulate on cases as needed. In very large facilities, it is common to have several clinical and administrative managers. Budgets for surgical care in excess of $20 million are not uncommon and are often administered by a dedicated business financial manager.

58. In addition to administrative department managers, other leadership/management positions include team leaders and managers

or coordinators who assume responsibility for a particular surgical specialty. Responsibilities may include assigning staff, managing and ensuring adequate inventory of specialty supplies, ensuring availability of supplies and equipment needed for scheduled surgeries, maintaining and updating preference cards that identify specific supplies and instruments needed by each surgeon for each procedure, creating preference cards for surgeons new to the service, periodically reviewing the contents of instrument trays for appropriateness, standardizing supplies and trays whenever possible, and promoting or providing education.

59. Scheduling coordinators may or may not be perioperative nurses. They "run the desk," which typically involves assigning surgeries to rooms, assigning staff to procedures, and making adjustments to keep the schedule moving throughout the day. An unanticipated emergency often requires quickly altering the daily schedule. The scheduling coordinator must have knowledge of patient acuity and the skill level of the staff, and be able to utilize resources appropriately.

60. Perfusionists, radiology and laboratory technicians, perioperative educators, pathologists, nurse's aides, clerks, and personnel from materials management, environmental services, and central service are among the nonsterile personnel necessary to ensure safe patient care and achieve desired patient outcomes. It is the perioperative nurse who coordinates the contributions of each of these team members.

Section Questions

1. Which factors have spurred the transition from inpatient surgery to same-day, outpatient, and ambulatory surgery? [Refs 41–42]

2. Describe the term "minimally invasive surgical techniques." [Ref 42]

3. Where, besides operating rooms, are invasive procedures performed? [Ref 43]

4. Identify members of the sterile and nonsterile components of the surgical team. [Refs 46–48]

5. What determines who may function as an assistant to the surgeon? [Ref 50]

6. Describe the responsibilities of the scrub person. [Ref 51]

7. Discuss the role of the circulating nurse. [Ref 56]

8. Describe the responsibilities of the circulating nurse. [Ref 56]

9. Which other roles do registered nurses fill in the perioperative setting? [Refs 57–58]

10. What are some of the positions of the nonsterile personnel who function within the operating room? [Ref 60]

● ● ● **References**

About.com Health Careers (2012). Which States Allow CRNAs to Practice Without Physician Supervision? Accessed online September, 2012: http://healthcareers.about.com/od/healthcareerissues/f/Which-States-Allow-Crnas-To-Practice-Independently-Without-Physician-Supervision.htm.

Association of periOperative Registered Nurses (AORN) (2012a). *Perioperative Standards and Recommended Practices.* Denver, CO: AORN.

Association of periOperative Registered Nurses (AORN) (2012b). *AORN Position Statement on RN First Assistants.* Accessed September, 2012: https://www.aorn.org/WorkArea/DownloadAsset.aspx?id=21931.

Association of periOperative Registered Nurses (AORN) (2011). *Perioperative Nursing Data Set* (PNDS). Denver, CO: AORN.

Post-Test

Read each question carefully. Each question may have more than one correct answer.

1. The perioperative period begins when the patient
   a. arrives in the holding area and ends in PACU.
   b. arrives in the hospital and ends with discharge.
   c. is informed of the need for surgery and ends with discharge from the hospital.
   d. is informed of the need for surgery and ends with the patient's return to his or her usual activities.

2. Which of the following is *not* a nursing focus during the preoperative period?
   a. patient teaching
   b. patient and family support
   c. diagnostic testing
   d. preparation for discharge

3. Intraoperative phase begins when
   a. the patient arrives at the hospital for surgery.
   b. the patient enters the operating room.
   c. the anesthesia provider induces the patient.
   d. the surgeon makes the initial incision.

4. Initial nursing focus in the postoperative period focuses on
   a. transferring the patient to the PACU.
   b. supporting the patient's physiological systems.
   c. preparing the patient for discharge.
   d. making arrangements for the patient to return to normal activity.

5. Why was the term "operating room nurse" changed to "perioperative nurse"?
   a. AORN decided it sounded more contemporary.
   b. To eliminate the "OR mystique" and encourage more nurses to join the specialty.
   c. The responsibilities of nurses in this specialty have expanded to support and care for the surgical patient through the continuum of care.
   d. Because PACU nurses wanted to be included.

6. AORN's Patient-Focused Model includes which of the following domains?
   a. patient safety, physiologic response, behavioral responses, the health system
   b. patient teaching, patient safety, behavioral responses, discharge planning
   c. patient safety, patient assessment, discharge planning, the health system
   d. patient assessment, plan of care, discharge planning, the health system

7. Perioperative nurses provide patient care
   a. in collaboration with the surgeon and the anesthesia provider.
   b. that primarily focuses on patient and family education and support.
   c. within the framework of the nursing process: assessment, planning, intervention, and evaluation of patient outcomes.
   d. that is focused primarily on the patient's surgical diagnosis.

8. The perioperative nursing assessment of the patient
    a. takes place in a number of settings and time frames.
    b. begins with a telephone call to the patient prior to surgery for teaching, support, and data gathering.
    c. is based on data collected by other healthcare professionals.
    d. usually takes place just prior to surgery and includes an interview, chart review, and physical inspection.

9. Typical nursing diagnoses for the surgical patient include
    a. knowledge deficit and high risk for infection.
    b. prevention of adverse outcomes and patient teaching.
    c. high risk for infection and support of patient and family.
    d. maintenance of normothermia and anatomical body alignment.

10. The perioperative nurses begins the patient's care plan
    a. prior to the procedure, based on information about the patient from the surgeon and other healthcare providers.
    b. in the holding area based on interview and assessment data.
    c. prior to the procedure based on knowledge of the planned procedure, typical related nursing diagnoses, and resources required.
    d. when the patient enters the operating room and all attention is focused on supporting the patient.

11. The framework for the intervention stage of perioperative patient is based on
    a. the surgeon's preferences related to the surgical procedure.
    b. the patient's medical diagnosis and comorbidities.
    c. the needs of the healthcare team participating in the surgical procedure.
    d. identified standards of clinical practice and professional performance.

12. The criteria upon which the final evaluation is made is the extent to which
    a. the goals of the surgical procedure were met and the patient was transferred to the appropriate recovery area.
    b. the desired patient outcomes have been achieved.
    c. hospital policy and professional standards were upheld.
    d. the patient and family express satisfaction with the entire surgical experience.

13. The *Perioperative Nursing Data Set* (PNDS) is
    a. standardized nursing vocabulary used to describe perioperative nursing practice.
    b. a collection of recommended practices to guide patient care.
    c. used by all electronic health record systems to standardize patient records.
    d. a set of evaluation tools to determine the extent to which patient care has been successful.

14. Perioperative nursing is
    a. task oriented and designed to care effectively for surgical patients.
    b. nursing science related to surgical patients.
    c. patient oriented, using knowledge, judgment, and skill.
    d. a framework to evaluate patients' responses to surgical and other invasive procedures.

15. Which of the following is not a standard of perioperative care?
    a. The patient is free from signs and symptoms of electrical injury.
    b. The patient receives appropriately administered medications.

    c. The patient's wound perfusion is consistent with or improved from baseline levels.

    d. The patient's comorbidities are managed effectively during the operative or other invasive procedure.

16. Which of the following facilitate(s) personal and professional growth?

    a. participating in research activities

    b. participating in professional organization activities

    c. mentoring and precepting other perioperative nurses

    d. all of the above

17. Which of the following is a true statement about the registered nurse first assistant (RNFA)?

    a. An RNFA is an advanced practice perioperative nurse, regardless of his or her academic level of preparation.

    b. The RNFA position is an expanded role in perioperative nursing.

    c. The RNFA practices under the license of the physician.

    d. The RNFA must have an advanced degree in nursing.

18. The transitioning of complex procedures from the traditional operating room to alternative settings is primarily the result of

    a. reimbursement guidelines.

    b. technological advances in surgical technique.

    c. patient preference.

    d. the nursing shortage.

19. Who may function in the scrub role? [Select *all* correct responses.]

    a. perioperative registered nurse

    b. licensed vocational or licensed practice nurse

    c. surgical technologist

    d. RNFA

20. Who or what determines who may function as an assistant to the surgeon during the procedure? [Select *all* correct responses.]

    a. surgeon

    b. facility policy

    c. state board of medicine

    d. state board of nursing

21. What is the primary focus of the perioperative nurse?

    a. managing the operating room environment

    b. patient safety and achieving the desired patient outcomes

    c. supervising the scrub person

    d. documenting intraoperative patient care

22. Which of the following roles is *not* part of the sterile surgical team?

    a. perfusionist

    b. RNFA

    c. first assistant

    d. surgical technologist

2

Preparing the Patient for Surgery

LEARNER OBJECTIVES

1. Identify desired patient outcomes related to the preoperative phase.
2. Describe the critical factors included in a preoperative patient assessment.
3. Recognize nursing diagnoses common to the surgical patient in the preoperative phase.
4. Describe interventions in the preoperative phase to achieve desired patient outcomes.
5. Identify at least eight factors that may contribute to wrong-site surgery.
6. Describe the three components of the Joint Commission protocol to prevent wrong-site surgery.
7. Discuss the content of preoperative patient teaching.

www

LESSON OUTLINE

Nursing Diagnoses

1. The perioperative nurse combines unique knowledge of the surgical procedure with patient assessment data and formulates nursing diagnoses that serve as the basis for the patient's plan of care.

2. The *Perioperative Nursing Data Set* (PNDS) developed by the Association of periOperative Registered Nurses (AORN) identifies 93 nursing diagnoses and 151 interventions relative to the patient undergoing a surgical or invasive procedure and 40 nurse-sensitive patient outcomes (AORN, 2011).

3. More than 70 nursing diagnoses and hundreds of nursing interventions have been identified through the North American Nursing Diagnosis Association (NANDA, 2012). These diagnoses and interventions are not mutually exclusive, and any one or more might be appropriate for an individual patient.

4. The plan of care is developed as the perioperative nurse identifies nursing interventions based on the patient's nursing diagnoses. Some nursing diagnoses will require interventions in all three phases of the surgical experience. For other nursing diagnoses, the interventions will be confined to a single period or after the patient has left the operating and recovery rooms.

5. Each plan of care must be customized based on specific individual patient needs. Nevertheless, several nursing diagnoses, desired outcomes, and interventions are common to all surgical patients.

Desired Patient Outcomes

6. A well-prepared patient will have an understanding of the events that can be anticipated in the preoperative and immediate postoperative periods. For example, one AORN expected patient outcome states, "The patient or designated support person demonstrates knowledge of the expected responses to the operative invasive procedure" (AORN, 2011, p. 114). This outcome includes knowledge of the procedure to be performed and an understanding of the risks delineated on the consent form.

7. The patient should also be prepared for discharge and should demonstrate understanding of the expectations of his or her participation in recovery and rehabilitation.

8. The patient should feel supported in the preoperative period and should be encouraged to express his or her feelings about the surgical experience.

9. The patient's level of anxiety or fear should be reduced to a minimum.

Preoperative Preparation

10. The patient is prepared psychologically and physiologically for surgery during the preoperative period. Interventions are directed toward treating or minimizing preexisting medical conditions, and providing information and support for the patient through the surgical experience.

11. Nursing activities are planned to achieve positive patient outcomes. Planning for the achievement of the desired patient outcomes begins with a patient assessment. The patient and family are included in these activities as much as possible. Assessing the patient's unique learning needs ensures that patient teaching will be relevant and delivered in a manner appropriate for the patient.

12. Providing appropriate information and support during the preoperative period addresses the desired outcome that the patient demonstrate knowledge of expected responses to the operative or invasive procedure.

13. Preoperative preparations focus on a variety of nursing activities, including data collection through patient assessment, patient/family teaching, emotional support, planning of care for the intraoperative and postoperative periods, and communication of patient information to healthcare team members.

14. The preoperative assessment provides information to address desired patient outcomes: freedom from infection, freedom from injury, skin integrity, electrolyte balance, and patient participation in the rehabilitation process. For example, assessment data that reveal limited range of motion in a shoulder would be used to plan positioning interventions to prevent further shoulder injury.

15. The body's defense against pathogens is directly related to tissue perfusion and oxygenation. Obese patients have decreased levels of tissue oxygen, which increases their risk for surgical-site infection (SSI) (Chopra et al., 2010). In addition, obese patients have an increased frequency of comorbid conditions, such as diabetes mellitus, that may increase their risk for SSIs.

16. The perioperative nurse may be responsible for administering antibiotics prior to surgery. Administration of antibiotics prior to the incision in certain types of surgery has been shown to significantly reduce the rate of surgical infection and has been incorporated into the Surgical Care Improvement Project (SCIP) sponsored by the Centers for Medicare & Medicaid Services (CMS) in collaboration with a number of other national partners, including the American Hospital Association (AHA), Centers for Disease Control and Prevention (CDC), Institute for Healthcare Improvement (IHI), and The Joint Commission (TJC).

17. Prophylactic antibiotics should be given far enough in advance of the start of surgery so that the level of antibiotic in the patient's serum and tissue is sufficient to destroy microorganisms that might be encountered during surgery. The ideal time frame is usually within 1 hour prior to incision (Alexander et al., 2011).

18. Until recently, prophylactic antibiotics were given just prior to the patient's transport to the operating room. However, delays in transport and preparations for surgery often result in delay of the surgical incision by more than 1 hour, in which case the antibiotics are not effective.

19. Most healthcare facilities have preoperative prophylactic antibiotic protocols that identify the type of surgery, the type of antibiotic, and the time frame in which the antibiotic should be given. Many facilities have determined that compliance with the 60-minute time frame is best achieved when the perioperative nurse assumes responsibility for antibiotic administration.

20. Body mass index (BMI), or percent body fat, has emerged as a major risk factor for postoperative SSIs on virtually all surgical services. Obese patients (BMI > 30 g/m^2) require a larger loading dose of antibiotic to provide consistent tissue concentrations over the duration of the surgical procedure. Prophylactic antibiotic protocols for morbidly obese patients often recommend twice the normal dose (Edmiston et al., 2011).

Preoperative Assessment and Interventions

Overview

21. The perioperative nurse is the patient's advocate during surgery. The patient, whose protective reflexes are compromised, is dependent on members of the healthcare team to advocate for his or her safety. Knowledge of the patient gained through assessment in the preoperative period provides the information that is necessary for advocacy responsibilities.

22. Typically, during the preoperative period the patient will interact with nurses other than the perioperative nurse. Only in small surgical centers where nurses practice in all three areas is it likely that the perioperative nurse will have the opportunity to perform a complete and thorough assessment of the patient a day or more prior to surgery. More commonly, preoperative testing is accomplished at another site, and the initial assessment is made by someone other than the nurse who will actually provide the intraoperative care.

Sources of Patient Information

23. The perioperative nurse most often encounters the patient for the first time in the holding area immediately prior to surgery. During this encounter, there is usually not enough time to carry out a comprehensive history and assessment. The perioperative nurse must, therefore, rely on the information gathered by others.

24. The nurse gathers assessment data from a combination of chart review, patient/family questionnaire and interview, patient observation, and communication with other healthcare providers. The patient's chart may include an assessment and preoperative checklist that was completed prior to transport to the holding area (Figures 2-1 and 2-2).

25. Transfer of care is an essential component of patient safety. Standardization in hand-off protocols is another effective way to promote patient safety (AORN, 2012, p. 467).

26. Several transfer protocols have been used successfully to share information comprehensively and concisely:

    - The SBAR (Situation, Background, Assessment, and Recommendation) technique is an example of a process that can be used for prompt and appropriate communication throughout the perioperative period, including during preoperative assessment, intraoperatively among caregivers, and during hand-off to the PACU. SBAR is modeled on naval military protocol and was adapted for use in health care by Kaiser Permanente (Figure 2-3).
    - I PASS the BATON (Introduction, Patient, Assessment, Situation, Safety concerns, Background, Actions, Timing, Ownership, Next) is a technique used in the Department of Defense's Patient Safety Program to provide a structure that improves communication during transitions in care. It should include opportunities to confirm receipt, ask questions, clarify information, and verify that the information is understood (Figure 2-4).

OR #: _____				PRE-OP VISIT			

PERSONAL PHYSICIAN	SURGEON	ANESTHESIOLOGIST	SEX ☐ M ☐ F	AGE	
DATE	TIME	PROCEDURE			NICKNAME
ALLERGIES			ISOLATION PRECAUTIONS ☐ TB ☐ Other		

MEDICAL & SURGICAL HISTORY:

	SKIN ASSESSMENT	MENTAL/ EMOTIONAL	VISION	PRE-OP TUBES	LABORATORY INFORMATION	PRE-OP:
HT:	COLOR:	☐ Oriented	☐ Adequate	☐ Foley		
WT:	☐ Pale	☐ Disoriented To:	☐ Decreased	☐ NG		TIME:
	☐ Flushed	☐ Time	☐ Blind	☐ Other:		
T:	☐ Dusky	☐ Place				
P:	☐ Cyanotic	☐ Person	☐ Rt ☐ Lt			ROUTINE MEDS:
	☐ Jaundice	☐ Lethargic	☐ Glasses	**CHART REQUIREMENTS**		
R:	☐ Normal	☐ Comatose	☐ Contacts	☐ Permit		
BP RANGE:	☐ Other:	☐ Dementia/ Alzheimers	**HEARING**	☐ H & P		
			☐ Adequate			
PERIPHERAL PERFUSION:	CONDITION:	☐ Protective Devices	☐ Decreased	**DENTURES**	☐ BLOOD GLUCOSE MONITORING	
	☐ No Problem		☐ Deaf	☐ Upper	SHA / OR / PACU INSTRUCTIONS:	
PULSES:	☐ Rash	☐ Calm	☐ Rt ☐ Lt	☐ Lower		
RR:	☐ Boney Area	☐ Apprehensive	☐ Hearing Aid	☐ Partial	X-RAYS:	
LR:	☐ Redness	☐ Emotional Disorders	COMMUNICATION BARRIERS:			
RP:	☐ Decubiti					
LP:	☐ Contusions/ Abrasions	UNITS OF BLOOD:			SCANS:	
SMOKES:		☐ T & C	CONSULTING PHYSICIANS/ SPECIALTY:			
☐ Yes	☐ Edema	Number of Units on Hand:			EKG:	
☐ No	☐ Other:					
☐ PPD _____						
☐ Quit _____					FAMILY ☐ FWA ☐ ICU FWA ☐ HOME ☐ OTHER:	

COMMENTS:

IVs: ☐ Central ☐ Peripheral DATE OF INSERTION: _____	Fluids: _____ Support Meds: Type _____ Rate _____ TPN & Rate: _____	☐ OR RN ☐ PACU RN Signature:

Figure 2-1 Preoperative Visit Assessment

Source: Pilot Draft form courtesy of St. Luke's Medical Center, Milwaukee, Wisconsin.

Operative Permit Complete ☐ Yes ☐ No	ID Bracelet ☐ Yes ☐ No	Glasses/Contact Lenses ☐ Yes ☐ No	Dentures ☐ Yes ☐ No	Hearing Aid ☐ Yes ☐ No
Chest X-ray on Chart ☐ Yes ☐ No	Allergy Bracelet ☐ Yes ☐ No	Blood Bracelet ☐ Yes ☐ No No. of Units	Preop Bath/Shower ☐ Yes ☐ No	

ECG on Chart ☐ Yes ☐ No	History and Physical ☐ Yes ☐ No	List any abnormalities, blindness, deafness, prosthesis, amputation, paralysis, etc. _____
Ordered Lab Work on Chart ☐ Yes ☐ No Abnormal Called to:		Isolation Required: ☐ Yes ☐ No Reason:

General Appearance: Flushed ☐ Yes ☐ No Diaphoretic ☐ Yes ☐ No Pale ☐ Yes ☐ No Skin Intact ☐ Yes ☐ No Cyanotic ☐ Yes ☐ No Other _____ Jaundice ☐ Yes ☐ No	Jewelry Removed ☐ N/A ☐ Yes ☐ No ☐ Rings Tape ☐ Given to Family, Who?_____ Hospital Gown ☐ Yes ☐ No Voided/Foley ☐ Yes ☐ No Time	Level of Consciousness: ☐ Alert ☐ Oriented x3 ☐ Drowsy ☐ Other _____ Patient's Emotional Status ☐ Accepting ☐ Apprehensive

NURSING INTERVENTION

For SAU Nurse Only		Patient Sent on O₂ Patient ECG Monitored ☐ Yes ☐ No
☐ Blood Pressure Cuff On	Antibiotic Hanging ☐ Yes ☐ No ☐ N/A	☐ Yes L/m _____ ☐ Nasal Cannula ☐ Mask ☐ Ambu Bag

Preop Medication/Dosage	Time	Int.		Time	Int.	Transporter's Initial:
1.			4.			
2.			5.			
3.			6.			

Beta Blocker Given: ☐ Yes ☐ No ☐ N/A Reason held _____

Sending RN	Initial	Receiving RN verifies above information	Initial

MARKING OF OPERATIVE SITE

OR SAU	OR SAU
☐ ☐ Patient identified using 2 indicators—Name, DOB ☐ ☐ Correct site verified w/OR schedule, H&P, patient & physician order	☐ ☐ Operative site marked "Yes"—Laterality identified ☐ N/A ☐ ☐ Site marked by ☐ Patient ☐ Nurse ☐ Physician ☐ Diagnostics available in OR suite for site verification

PATIENT ASSESSMENT BY OPERATING NURSE	Antibiotic Administration	Time	Int.
	☐ Ancef 1 gm IVPB		
	☐ Zinacef 1.5 gms		
☐ Lab Values Reviewes ☐ Chart Reviewed	☐ Vancomyacin 1 gm IVPB		
Allergies:	☐ Cefotan 2 gms IVPB		
Condition of skin:	☐ Ciproflaxin 400 mg IVPB		
Motor/Sensory impairment	☐ Claforan 2 gms IVPB		
Abnormalities	☐ Clindamyacin 600 mg IVPB		
Operative/Procedure confirmed ☐ Yes ☐ No	☐ Flagyl 500 mg IVPB		
Cardiovascular	☐ Unasyn 3 gms IVPB		
Respiratory	☐ Mefoxin 2 gms IVPB		
Additional Findings	☐ Other		

PATIENT/FAMILY EDUCATION

Relevant information on surgical procedure given to patient. ☐ Yes ☐ No Family Present ☐ Yes ☐ No
If no, why? _____

NURSING COMMENTS _____

_____ RN
Operating Room Nurse Signature   Date   Time

Figure 2-2 Preoperative Flowsheet

Source: Copyright © INTEGRIS Baptist Medical Center, Inc. The copyright has been assigned to Jones & Bartlett Learning in conjunction with this publication only.

SBAR Communication Technique

The SBAR communication technique can be adapted to hand-off documentation for patient transfer at any stage in the continuum of care. Specific content in each section should be customized for each facility.

Situation *(Why are we here?)*
- Introduce yourself
- Confirm correct
  - patient
  - surgeon
  - procedure
  - side
  - level

Background *(What brought us to this point?)*
- Pertinent medical information
  - primary diagnosis
  - age (if it is significant)
  - allergies
  - results of diagnostic testing available
  - comorbidities
  - X rays (if needed)

Assessment *(What issues have I identified that might alter the patient's plan of care?)*
- Current lab values outside of normal limits
- Allergies
- Medical/surgical history relevant to current procedure
- Where can patient's family be reached?
- Prosthestics (lenses/glasses/hearing aid/dentures/other)
- Missing information or documentation
- Comorbidities requiring attention

Recommendations *(How can we appropriately respond to the issues?)*
- Alert team to lab values outside normal limits
- Prevent allergic reaction
  - medication
  - latex
  - history suggesting at risk for malignant hyperthermia
- Disposition of personal items
- Positioning needs

This SBAR tool was developed by Kaiser Permanente. Please feel free to use and reproduce these materials in the spirit of patient safety, and please retain this footer in the spirit of appropriate recognition.

Figure 2-3 SBAR

Source: Kaiser Permanente.

"I PASS THE BATON"

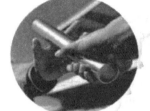

**Handoffs and Healthcare Transitions
with opportunities to ask
QUESTIONS, CLARIFY and CONFIRM**

I	**Introduction**	Introduce yourself and your role/job (include patient)
P	**Patient**	Name, identifiers, age, sex, location
A	**Assessment**	Presenting chief complaint, vital signs and symptoms and diagnosis
S	**Situation**	Current status, medications, circumstances, including code status, level of (un)certainty, recent changes, response to treatment
S	**SAFETY Concerns**	Critical lab values/reports, socio-economic factors, allergies, alerts (falls, isolation, etc.)
THE		
B	**Background**	Co-morbidities, previous episodes, past/home medications, family history
A	**Actions**	What actions were taken or are required AND provide brief rationale
T	**Timing**	Level of urgency and explicit timing, prioritization of actions
O	**Ownership**	Who is responsible (nurse/doctor/team) including patient/family responsibilities
N	**Next**	What will happen next? Anticipated changes? What is the <u>PLAN</u>? Contingency plans?

Figure 2-4 I PASS THE BATON

Source: Courtesy of Department of Defense Patient Safety Program. Used with permission.

Assessment Parameters

Physiologic

27. Critical physiological assessment data include the following:

   • Medical diagnosis, chronic diseases, and treatment

   • Medications, especially antibiotics; herbal medications; anticoagulants, including aspirin; diuretics that deplete potassium; over-the-counter medications; history of chemotherapy

   • Surgery to be performed and verification of the surgical site

   • Previous surgeries and any complications, including anesthesia complications

   • Vital signs, diagnostic data, and laboratory data as ordered—abnormalities
     – Hemoglobin and hematocrit
     – White blood count
     – Platelet count
     – Serum electrolytes
     – Urinalysis
     – Chest X ray
     – Diagnostic X rays pertinent to the surgical procedure
     – Electrocardiogram
     – Blood type and cross-match information and availability of replacement blood
     – Results of specific tests or studies specific to the planned procedure

   • Age—very young or very old

   • Substance abuse—smoking, alcohol, drugs

   • Skin condition—color, rashes, lesions

   • Allergies—medication and latex allergies are critical (Exhibit 2-1)

   • Nutrition and nothing-by-mouth (NPO) status

   • Sensory impairments—presence of lenses, hearing aids, dentures

   • Mobility impairments

   • Presence of prosthetic devices—orthopedic implants, pacemaker, vascular prosthesis

   • Weight/height/BMI—extreme underweight and overweight; height greater than length of the operating room table; implications for medication dosage

   • Preoperative medication as ordered has been given; timing of prophylactic antibiotics

Exhibit 2-1 Parma Community General Hospital Latex Allergy Patient Questionnaire

---

NOTE: These questions are not intended to be all-inclusive. Individuals who are potentially latex allergic should seek additional testing through their primary care physician. This questionnaire is merely a collection of relevant data to be passed onto your physician for further evaluation/testing for confirmation of allergy.

1. Have you ever been told that you have a latex allergy?   **Yes   No**
   If so, do you have documented laboratory tests to confirm this?   **Yes   No**

2. What specifically are you allergic to that contains latex?

   _____

3. Have you ever had any reaction to any of the following sources of latex?

Balloons	☐	Rubber gloves	☐	Rubber balls	☐	Rubber bands	☐
Adhesive tape	☐	Ace bandages	☐	Dental bite blocks	☐	Belts	☐
Brassieres	☐	Carpet backing	☐	Clothing with elastic	☐	Rubber cement	☐
Suspenders	☐	Teething rings	☐	Condoms	☐	Corsets	☐
Erasers	☐	Face masks	☐	Foam pillows	☐	Garden hoses	☐
Latex cuffs	☐	Ostomy bags	☐	Milking machines	☐	Tennis grips	☐
Dental masks	☐	Pacifiers	☐	Weather stripping	☐	IV tubing	☐
Golf grips	☐	Poinsettias	☐	Elastic bandages	☐	Other	☐

Exhibit 2-1 Parma Community General Hospital Latex Allergy Patient Questionnaire (continued)

4. Do you have a history of any symptoms as stated below, following the use of latex products as stated above?

"Contact dermatitis" (redness, itching, cracked skin)	Yes	No
Rhinitis/allergic rhinitis (nasal congestion, sneezing, runny nose)	Yes	No
Conjunctivitis (red swollen itchy/sore eyes)	Yes	No
Hay fever (sneezing)	Yes	No
Eczema (flaky, itchy, red skin)	Yes	No
Auto-immune disease	Yes	No
Asthma (wheezing-type breathing, difficulty with breathing)	Yes	No
Fatigue/drowsiness	Yes	No
Facial swelling/redness	Yes	No
Reactions to bandages/tape	Yes	No
Hives/unexplained rash	Yes	No
Sudden onset of bronchitis/sinusitis following contact with above products	Yes	No

Please describe

_____

_____

5. Do you have any food allergies?   Yes   No

   List: _____

   Are you allergic to any of the following?

Banana	Avocado	Potato	Milk	Kiwi	Chestnuts	Peaches
Tomato	Papaya	Passion fruit	Other tropical fruit			

   Describe your allergic reaction: _____

6. After handling any latex products have you experienced any of the following:

Chapping/cracking of skin on hands	Yes	No	Redness	Yes	No
Swelling	Yes	No	Hives	Yes	No
Runny nose or nasal congestion	Yes	No	Itching	Yes	No

7. Have you ever had previous surgery?   Yes   No
   If so how many surgical procedures: _____

   Types: _____

   _____

8. Do you suffer from any congenital abnormalities (e.g., spina bifida)?   Yes   No

   Name: _____

9. Does your occupation require you to have frequent contact with latex products?   Yes   No

   List: _____

10. Have you ever had an anaphylactic reaction to latex or latex-containing products?   Yes   No
    Explain/describe the circumstances:

    _____

    _____

Source: Questionnaire developed and provided by: Ruth Bakst RN CNOR RNFA. Perioperative and Emergency Room Clinical Instructor. Parma Community General Hospital. Parma, Ohio.

Psychosocial

28. Critical psychosocial assessment data include the following:

    - Understanding and perception of the procedure to be performed
    - Coping ability/support system
    - Ability to comprehend
    - Readiness to learn
    - Anxiety related to the surgical intervention or surgical outcome
    - Knowledge of perioperative routines
    - Cultural or spiritual beliefs relevant to the surgical intervention

---

Section Questions

www

1. What information can be found in the *Perioperative Nursing Data Set*? [Ref 2]
2. How does the perioperative nurse develop the patient's plan of care? [Ref 4]
3. Describe four desired outcomes that apply to all surgical patients. [Refs 6–9]
4. What is the first step in planning to achieve positive patient outcomes? [Ref 11]
5. In which ways does the perioperative nurse collect necessary data? [Ref 13]
6. Identify five desired postoperative outcomes that the perioperative nurse develops a plan to achieve. [Ref 14]
7. How does obesity affect the risk of adverse outcomes of surgery? [Ref 15]
8. What is the ideal time frame in which to provide most prophylactic antibiotics to ensure that the tissue and serum levels of the antibiotic are sufficient? [Ref 17]
9. Which steps have healthcare facilities taken to ensure that antibiotics are, in fact, administered within the appropriate time frame? [Refs 18–19]
10. How does obesity influence the effects of prophylactic antibiotics? [Ref 20]
11. Describe the impact on patient information of the perioperative nurse's role as patient advocate. [Refs 21–23]
12. From which sources does the perioperative nurse gather essential information about the patient? [Ref 24]
13. Describe two hand-off protocols that have been used successfully in the healthcare environment. [Ref 26]
14. Describe critical components of the perioperative nurse's physiologic assessment of the patient that have implications for tailoring the plan of care to the individual patient. [Ref 27]
15. Describe critical components of the psychosocial assessment that will help the perioperative nurse address the specific needs of the patient. [Ref 28]

Nursing Diagnoses and Interventions

Preoperative Period

29. The most common nursing diagnoses in the preoperative period are knowledge deficit and anxiety.

30. Knowledge deficit may be related to perioperative routines, surgical interventions, or outcome expectations.

31. Knowledge deficit may be the result of impaired communication ability, a language barrier, a patient's insufficient mental capacity, or a lack of information regarding the surgical procedure. Nursing interventions must be appropriate to the etiology of the patient's knowledge deficit and to the patient's learning needs.

32. Anxiety can range from mild to severe and may have a variety of etiologies. Some patients experience the greatest anxiety just prior to surgery. For others, anxiety is most acute at the time the decision to have surgery is made.

33. An increased heart and respiratory rate and an elevated blood pressure can be signs of anxiety. The patient may feel nervous or tense and may not be able to concentrate or retain information. Patients who are anxious, uneasy, or nervous cannot always identify the exact cause of their anxiety.

34. Anxiety is different from fear. Fear is marked by apprehension and dread of something specific; the fearful patient can identify the focus of his or her fear. Fear may be related to the surgical intervention, surgical outcome, anesthesia, impact of surgery on lifestyle, loss of control, pain, or death, among other things. It is more common for patients to be anxious than fearful.

35. The desired outcome related to anxiety is that anxiety and fear will be lessened through increased knowledge and the ability to express feelings about the surgical intervention. It is important to assess readiness to learn, because providing more information than the patient desires or can handle can exacerbate anxiety.

36. The following nursing interventions are ways to address anxiety and fear:

    - Attentive listening
    - Provision of information as needed and desired (Providing information that the patient does not wish can increase the patient's anxiety.)
    - Solicitation of the patient's expression of anxiety or fear
    - Provision of emotional support and reassurance

37. The desired outcome related to a knowledge deficit is that the patient will demonstrate knowledge of the physiological and psychological responses to surgery.

38. The following nursing interventions are ways to assess knowledge and address any knowledge deficits:

    - Confirmation of the patient's identity
    - Verification of the surgical site and procedure
    - Verification of consent
    - Solicitation of the patient's perception of planned surgery
    - Solicitation of questions related to surgery
    - Identification of teaching needs, readiness, and ability to learn
    - Explanation of surgical routines
    - Explanation of procedures that need to be followed postoperatively upon discharge (especially critical for patients who will be discharged on the day of their surgery, which limits the time available for teaching)
    - Provision of appropriate information with consideration for the patient's level of understanding, ability to comprehend, desired information, culture, and religious beliefs, as well as medical concerns referred to the surgeon
    - Solicitation of feedback regarding perioperative procedures

39. Criteria that can be used to evaluate the achievement of these outcomes include that the patient will (1) confirm the consent, (2) describe the expected sequence of events, (3) express feelings about the surgical experience, (4) indicate knowledge of expected surgical outcomes, and (5) confirm procedures to be followed upon discharge.

40. Another preoperative nursing diagnosis is anticipatory grieving related to possible changes in body image.

Section Questions   www

1. What are the two most common nursing diagnoses in the preoperative period? [Ref 29]

2. Describe the type of information that the perioperative nurse might share with the patient to address a knowledge deficit. [Ref 30]

3. Which factors might be involved in a patient's knowledge deficit that the perioperative nurse must assess and address? [Ref 31]

4. What are some signs that might suggest a patient is anxious? [Refs 32–33]

5. Contrast anxiety with fear. [Ref 34]

6. What impact should the patient's readiness to learn have when the perioperative nurse addresses the patient's knowledge deficit? [Ref 35]

(continues)

41. Each patient is unique, and some nursing diagnoses will apply to some patients but not to others. Nursing diagnoses must be identified through individual patient assessment, and interventions must be individualized for each patient.

Intraoperative Period

42. The intraoperative period begins when the patient enters the actual operating room.

43. During the intraoperative period, the patient is at high risk for injury related to the following factors:

    - Transport and transfer
    - Positioning
    - Equipment such as electrosurgery devices or a tourniquet
    - Chemical agents such as skin prep solutions
    - Use of X ray or laser
    - Fluid deficit
    - Impaired gas exchange related to general anesthesia
    - Retained objects such as a sponge inadvertently left in the wound

    Nursing interventions to prevent these injuries are presented in subsequent chapters.

44. The patient is also at high risk for infection as a result of surgical intervention.

Prevention of Wrong-Site Surgery

45. In 1999, the Institute of Medicine (IOM) issued a report, *To Err Is Human: Building a Safer Health System*, which reported that as many as 98,000 patients die in hospitals each year as a result of errors (IOM, 2000, p. 1). In response, healthcare facilities, professional organizations, the Centers for Medicare & Medicaid Services, the Centers for Disease Control and Prevention, and The Joint Commission have focused intently on initiatives to improve patient safety.

46. Wrong-site surgery, identified by TJC as a "never event," includes surgery on the wrong patient, body part, side, level, or site, or it may the wrong surgical procedure altogether.

47. The following factors contribute to wrong-site surgery (Center for Transforming Healthcare [CTH], 2011):

    - Unapproved abbreviations, cross-outs, and illegible handwriting
    - Missing consent, history, and physical examination, or surgeon's operative orders
    - Inconsistent use of site-marking protocol
    - Inconsistent or absent time-out process
    - Rushing during patient verification
    - Change of patient position
    - Inadequate patient verification by surgical team
    - Lack of intraoperative site verification when multiple procedures are performed by the same surgeon
    - Ineffective hand-off communication or briefing process
    - Site markings removed during prep or draping
    - Distractions and rushing during the time-out process
    - Time-out occurs before all staff are ready or before prep and drape
    - Time-out performed without full participation
    - Time-outs do not occur when there are multiple procedures performed by multiple surgeons in a single operative case

- Inconsistent organizational focus on patient safety
- Staff members are passive or not empowered to speak up
- Marketplace competition and pressure to increase surgical volume leading to shortcuts and variation in practice

48. Between 2004 and 2011, 782 cases of wrong-site surgery were submitted to the Joint Commission's Sentinel Event database. Reporting is voluntary, so actual numbers could be much higher (TJC, 2011).

49. The Joint Commission's 2012 National Patient Safety Goals include three protocols for preventing wrong-site, wrong-procedure, wrong-person surgery in a continuing effort to improve patient safety (TJC, 2012a):
    - Preprocedure verification
    - Mark the site
    - Time-out

50. In the preoperative period, the nurse performing the patient assessment should verify the patient's identity and the procedure. This should be done verbally with the patient and by checking the patient's name band.

51. Chart review should begin by ascertaining that the patient, the chart, and the name band refer to the same person. If the patient is unable to communicate, verification should be made with the family or authorized representative and through chart review.

52. Verification of the patient's identity and surgical procedure must be a priority for the perioperative nurse. A patient should never be transferred into the operating room suite without an identification band that has been verified for accuracy.

53. While the surgeon is responsible for determining the patient's need for surgery, identifying the procedure, and delineating the surgical site, verifying the patient's identity and verifying the correct surgical site are the responsibilities of all team members.

54. Most healthcare facilities have policies that identify how verification should occur, who is responsible for verification, and which documentation must be completed. Typically, the surgeon, the anesthesiologist, and the circulating nurse must all participate in verification.

55. TJC, AORN, and the American College of Surgeons (ACS) are among the organizations that have published guidelines regarding marking the surgical site. These guidelines specify what is marked, how it is marked, and by whom. They also provide guidelines for verifying the surgical site (ACS, 2002; AORN, 2010; CTH, 2011).

56. Individual institutional policies and procedures may vary; however, since July 2004, healthcare organizations must comply with the Joint Commission's universal protocol for preventing wrong-site surgery (TJC, 2012b). This protocol includes the following steps:
    - *Conduct a preprocedure verification process.* All documents and studies available prior to the procedure should be reviewed, and should consistent with each other, with the patient's expectations, and with the team's understanding of the intended patient, procedure, site, and, as applicable, any implants. Missing information or discrepancies must be addressed before starting the procedure.
    - *Mark the procedure site.* Unambiguously identify the intended site of incision or insertion (for all procedures involving right/left distinction or multiple structures such as fingers and multiple levels such as the spine).
    - *Perform a time-out.* The procedure is not started until all questions or concerns are resolved. During the time-out, all team members should verify the name of the patient, the procedure, and the site and should validate that the site is marked. Documentation should indicate that a time-out was performed in accordance with the healthcare facility's policy, and identify what was verified and who participated in the time-out.

57. Many facilities have developed forms to ensure that all steps are followed and to streamline documentation requirements (Figure 2-5). Facilities may also develop tools to collect data that will help them assess practices that promote safe and effective patient care (Figure 2-6).

Patient/Family Teaching

58. Patient/family teaching is especially critical in today's healthcare environment, where patients

---

Section Questions   www

1. Identify potential patient injuries during the intraoperative period. [Refs 43–44]

2. Which event triggered the current focus by healthcare facilities, government, and regulatory organizations on patient safety? [Ref 45]

3. Describe wrong-site surgery as defined by TJC. [Ref 46]

4. Identify factors that contribute to wrong-site surgery. [Ref 47]

5. What are the three protocols identified in the Joint Commission's National Patient Safety Goals for preventing wrong-site surgery? [Ref 49]

6. How does the perioperative nurse verify the patient's identity and surgical procedure? [Ref 50]

7. If the patient is unable to communicate, how can verification of identity be made? [Ref 51]

8. Who is responsible for verifying the patient's identity and correct surgical site? [Refs 53–54]

9. Which factors are included in guidelines regarding marking of surgical sites? [Ref 55]

10. Describe the three components of TJC's universal protocol for preventing wrong-site surgery. [Ref 56]

---

are often discharged shortly after surgery. Optimal surgical outcomes often depend on how completely the patient understands and complies with instructions for care in the postoperative period.

59. Often patient teaching begins where the prospect of surgery is first discussed—the physician's office or clinic. Whenever possible, the patient's family or support persons should be included in the teaching process.

60. Readiness to learn can be diminished in times of stress. When the patient first learns of the need for a surgical procedure, he or she might not assimilate information as readily as under normal circumstances. Important information may need to be repeated, and information pertaining to discharge and expected recovery should be reinforced with both the patient and the family in the postoperative period.

61. In addition to providing information to the patient, the perioperative nurse offers emotional support and reassurance. The perioperative nurse should encourage the patient to express feelings and concerns regarding the surgery.

62. Attentive listening, reassurance, and information delivered calmly and candidly can alleviate anxiety and fear. An attentive, caring attitude, accompanied by appropriate, reassuring touch, can comfort the patient. Reducing anxiety and fear is a first step in preparing the patient for teaching.

63. Patient teaching must be tailored to the patient's age, learning level, culture, and readiness to learn.

64. Elderly patients' short-term memory may be diminished, such that additional time and reinforcement may be necessary for them to comprehend and retain information. Additional time should be planned for instruction of these patients. Instructional materials and voice level should take possible sight and hearing deficits into consideration.

65. Written instructions, pamphlets, and videos related to preparation for surgery and rehabilitation can be good teaching tools. Teaching materials, however, need to meet the needs of the learner.

66. Printed instructional materials should take into account the patient's level of literacy as well as the patient's level of health literacy. Health literacy is defined as follows: "The degree to which individuals have the capacity to obtain, process, and understand basic health information and services needed to make appropriate health decisions" (National Network of Libraries of Medicine [NN/LM], 2012).

67. It is critical for the nurse to review printed material with the patient, to solicit feedback to determine whether the patient understands the material, and to provide further instructions as appropriate.

68. Patients who might require additional resources for learning include the elderly as

PREPROCEDURE: In Holding Area	SIGN-IN: Before Induction of Anesthesia	TIME-OUT: Before Skin Incision	SIGN-OUT: Before the patient leaves the O.R.
Patient Actively Confirms with Registered Nurse (RN): ☐ Patient Identity (Name) ☐ Birth Date ☐ Check Arm Band (Chart, Sticker) ☐ Allergies ☐ NPO Status ☐ Teeth, Loose, Dentures, Caps ☐ Verified with patient: Clothes, Jewelry/Body piercings, Metal inside (pacemaker, AICD, implants) Procedure: ☐ Correct Site ☐ Site Marked ☐ History and Physical ☐ Preanesthesia Assessment ☐ Pre-Moderate Sedation Assessment Consents: ☐ Surgical ☐ Anesthesia Pregnancy Test ☐ N/A ☐ Diagnostic Tests ☐ X-rays ☐ Blood Products Yes ☐ N/A ☐	**RN and Anesthesia Care Provider Confirm:** ☐ Procedure ☐ Procedure site and consents Site Marked ☐ Yes ☐ NA by person performing the procedure Patient Allergies ☐ Yes ☐ NKA Difficult Airway or Aspiration Risk ☐ No ☐ Yes (preparation confirmed) SCD Hose or Sequentials Applied ☐ DVT Protocol ☐ N/A ☐ Warm Blankets Applied **Briefing:** All members of the team have discussed care plan and addressed concerns ☐ Yes	**Initiated by designated team member** All other activities to be suspended (unless a life-threatening emergency) Introduction of team members ☐ Yes **All:** Confirmation of the following: Identity, procedure, incision site, consent(s) ☐ Yes ☐ No Site marked and visible ☐ Yes ☐ N/A Any equipment concerns: _____ **Anesthesia Provider:** Antibiotic prophylaxis within 1 hour before incision ☐ Yes ☐ N/A **Scrub and circulating nurse:** ☐ Sterilization indicators have been confirmed Additional concerns: _____ _____ _____	**RN Confirms** **Name of Operative Procedure** ☐ Completion of sponge, sharp, and instrument counts ☐ Yes ☐ N/A Specimens identified, numbered, and labeled ☐ Yes ☐ N/A **All Team Members:** Key concerns for recovery and management of the patient _____ _____ _____

Figure 2-5 Comprehensive Surgical Checklist

Definitions	Fire Risk 0-1	Fire Risk - 2
		Head, Neck, and Chest Guidelines
Oxygen delivery	**Standard Guidelines:**	☐ N/A
Open = Patient receiving oxygen via nasal cannula, face mask, or uncuffed endotracheal tube	☐ Sterile water or saline on field	☐ Verbal communication among team about fire risk in time-out
	☐ Alcohol base prep dried (at least 3 minutes)	☐ Use closed oxygen circuit when possible
Closed = Patient is intubated	☐ No pooling of prep solution	☐ Verbal communication of oxygen percentage
	☐ ESU holstered when not in use	☐ Oxygen concentration lowered to 30%
	☐ Laser safety precautions	☐ Barrier placed between ignition source and oxygen
	☐ Fiberoptic light cable safety	☐ Water soluble eye lubricant
	☐ NS used when using burrs and/or saw blade	☐ Use FDA laser safe ET Tube for airway surgery
		☐ Water or N/S on anesthesia machine
		☐ Suction to anesthesia to dissipate gasses
		☐ Coat facial hair with water soluble jelly.
		☐ Keep ESU settings as low as possible
		☐ Use wet sponges when in contact with ignition source (Airway fire)

Include in Preprocedure check-in as per institutional custom:
Beta blocker medication given (SCIP) ☐ Yes ☐ N/A
Venous thromboembolism prophylaxis ordered (SCIP) ☐ Yes ☐ N/A
Normothermia measures (SCIP) ☐ Yes ☐ N/A

Figure 2-5 Comprehensive Surgical Checklist (continued)
Source: Adapted from Spivey Station Surgery Center, Jonesboro, GA (with permission).

Determine if the patient is eligible for the measure by answering the question below.
Did the patient complete the registration process upon entry into the facility?   YES   NO
If **YES**, proceed to the next step.

Determine if the patient experienced the outcome described by this measure by answering the questions below.

Patient Burns:
Did the patient experience a burn prior to discharge?   YES   NO
If YES, the outcome should be reported.

Wrong Site, Wrong Side, Wrong Patient, Wrong Procedure, Wrong Implant:
Did the patient experience the wrong site, wrong side, wrong patient, wrong   YES   NO
procedure, or wrong implant event?

Prophylactic IV Antibiotic Timing:
Did the patient have a preoperative order for a prophylactic IV antibiotic?   YES   NO
Was the ordered IV antibiotic one of those listed below?   YES   NO
Ampicillin/Sulbactam, Aztreonam, Cefazolin, Cefmetazole, Cefotetan, Cefoxitin, Cefuroxime, Ciprofloxacin, Clindamycin, Ertapenem, Erythromycin, Gatifloxacin, Gentamicin, Levofloxacin, Metronidazole, Moxifloxacin, Meomycin, Vancomycin

Was the antibiotic *initiated* within 1 hour prior to the initial surgical incision or the beginning of the procedure (e.g., introduction of endoscope, insertion of needle, and inflation of tourniquet)? Or 2 hours prior if vancomycin or fluoroquinolones (ciprofloxacin, gatifloxacin, levofloxacin, moxifloxacin) was ordered?   YES   NO

Antibiotic Infusion Start Time: _____   Procedure Start Time:_____

Did the patient receive the antibiotic within the indicated time?   YES   NO

Appropriate Surgical Site Hair Removal:
Did the patient perform his/her own hair removal at the surgical site?   YES   NO
Did the patient use depilatory cream?   YES   NO
Did the patient use a razor?   YES   NO
Was hair removed at the surgical site performed with clippers in preop?   YES   NO

Hospital Transfer/Admission:
Was the patient directly transferred or admitted to a hospital or hospital emergency department on discharge from the facility?   YES   NO

Figure 2-6 Core Measure Data Collection
Source: Courtesy of Spivey Station Surgery Center, Jonesboro, GA.

well as patients who have low educational skill, low socioeconomic status, cultural barriers to health care, or limited proficiency in English.

69. Pediatric patients have special needs.
   - Toddlers are just beginning to gain autonomy, are active, and have short attention spans.

- Preschoolers are inquisitive and have active imaginations. They may feel that surgery is punishment for bad behavior.

- School-age children are capable of logic and reasoning and can benefit from learning the steps involved in the surgical process.

70. Patient teaching for pediatric patients may include an opportunity for them to handle simple items that they will encounter during surgery. The ability to touch and manipulate an anesthesia mask, for example, can provide the child with a feeling of control.

71. Patient teaching during a preadmission workup will be more extensive than teaching in the holding area just prior to surgery. Teaching should be directed toward preparation for surgery and participation in the postoperative rehabilitation process—for example, instruction on bowel cleansing in preparation for bowel surgery; teaching crutch-walking for the patient whose surgical outcome will be influenced by participation in postoperative rehabilitation.

72. Preoperative teaching content should include the following issues:

- The procedure, anticipated duration, and expected outcome

- Specific instructions such as whether to bathe or shower, whether to hold or take medications, and whether to maintain NPO status from a designated time onward

- An explanation of preoperative events such as diagnostic tests, skin preparation, intravenous (IV) line insertion, sedation, and transfer to holding area

- An explanation of intraoperative events such as function of the circulating nurse or case manager, application of monitoring equipment, administration of anesthesia, maintenance of privacy and dignity, staff communication with family members during the procedure, and transport to the PACU

- An explanation of postoperative events such as expected length of stay; coughing and deep breathing expectations; turning; presence of lines, drains, and indwelling catheters; pain control; and discharge to a step-down or other unit or to home

73. Teaching in the preoperative holding area will be abbreviated and will reinforce previous teaching. Teaching directed toward discharge will be reinforced in the postoperative period prior to discharge.

Communication of Relevant Patient Data

74. Assessment information with relevance to intraoperative and postoperative care must be communicated to other members of the healthcare team. Continuity of care and planning for appropriate therapeutic interventions depend on clear, concise, and complete communication of information.

75. Communication with other healthcare providers is critical. Written documentation and verbal communication of patient data and responses to interventions are essential components of safe and effective patient care.

76. Because a significant number of patient injuries are caused by poor communication or the absence of communication among caregivers, TJC made implementation of a standardized approach to hand-off communications, including the opportunity to ask and respond to questions, a standard in 2010 (TJC, 2012). The nurse providing care to the patient in the preoperative period must provide appropriate hand-off information to the nurse caring for the patient during the intraoperative period. (See Figures 2-3 and 2-4.)

77. Forms for documenting patient assessment and care in the preoperative period may be stand-alone forms or may be part of an integrated form that includes the assessment and patient care throughout the preoperative, intraoperative, and postoperative periods.

Section Questions   WWW

1. Describe the impact that a patient's knowledge and understanding can have on surgical outcomes. [Ref 58]

2. When does patient teaching begin? [Ref 59]

(continues)

Section Questions (continued)

3. Explain how teaching needs to be modified when readiness to learn is diminished by stress. [Ref 60]

4. How can the perioperative nurse address the patient's emotional concerns? [Refs 61–62]

5. Which factors may affect the perioperative nurse's approach to teaching? [Ref 63]

6. Which adjustments might be made when instructing an elderly patient? [Ref 64]

7. Explain some precautions related to printed materials and instruction sheets. [Refs 65–67]

8. Define "health literacy." [Ref 66]

9. Which patients might require additional resources for learning? [Ref 68]

10. Describe the learning characteristics of three groups of pediatric patients. [Ref 69]

11. What is the benefit of providing hands-on experience for pediatric patients? [Ref 70]

12. What are essential components of patient teaching that the perioperative nurse would address in the preoperative period? [Ref 72]

13. Describe the qualities of communication required for planning appropriate therapeutic interventions. [Ref 74]

14. Explain the importance of sharing information with other healthcare providers. [Refs 74–76]

15. What does TJC require in its standardized approach to hand-off communication? [Ref 76]

● ● ● **References**

Alexander JW, Solomkin JS, Edwards MJ (2011). Updated recommendations for control of surgical site infections: systemic prophylactic antibiotics. *Ann Surg*;253(6): 82–93. Available at: http://journals.lww.com/annalsofsurgery /Abstract/2011/06000/Updated_Recommendations_for _Control_of_Surgical.7.aspx. Accessed June 2012.

American College of Surgeons (ACS) (2002). Statement on ensuring correct patient, correct site, and correct procedure surgery. *Bull Am Coll Surg*;87(12): 22–23. Available at: www.facs.org/fellows_info/statements/st-4.html. Accessed September 2012.

Association of periOperative Registered Nurses (AORN) (2012). *Perioperative Standards and Recommended Practices*. Denver, CO: AORN.

Association of periOperative Registered Nurses (AORN) (2011). *Perioperative Nursing Data Set*, 3rd ed. Denver, CO: AORN.

Association of periOperative Registered Nurses (AORN) (2010). Preventing Wrong-Patient, Wrong-Site, Wrong-Procedure Events. Denver, CO: AORN. Available at: www.aorn.org/Clinical_Practice/Position_Statements /Position_Statements.aspx. Accessed September 2012.

Center for Transforming Healthcare (CTH) (2011). Reducing the risk of wrong site surgery. Available at: www .centerfortransforminghealthcare.org/assets/4/6/CTH_WSS _Storyboard_final_20 .pdf. Accessed September 2012.

Chopra T, Zhao J, Alangaden G, et al. (2010). Preventing surgical site infections after bariatric surgery: value of perioperative antibiotic regimens. *National Institutes of Health Public Access Author Manuscript*. June 2010. Available at: www.ncbi.nlm.nih.gov/pmc /articles/PMC2904239/. Accessed September 2012.

Edmiston C, Spencer M, Lewis B, et al. (2011). Reducing the risk of surgical site infections: did we really think SCIP was going to lead us to the promised land? *Surg Infect* 2011; 2(8): 69–77.

Institute of Medicine (IOM) (2000). *To Err Is Human: Building a Safer Health System*. Washington, DC: National Academy Press.

The Joint Commission (TJC) (2012a). 2012 critical access hospital national patient safety goals. Available at: www.jointcommission.org/assets/1/6/2012_NPSG_CAH .pdf. Accessed September 2012.

The Joint Commission (TJC) (2012b). The universal protocol for preventing wrong site, wrong procedure, and wrong person surgery: guidance for healthcare professionals (poster). Available at: www.jointcommission.org/assets /1/18/UP_Poster.pdf. Accessed September 2012.

The Joint Commission (TJC) (2011). Summary data of sentinel events reviewed by The Joint Commission. Available at: www.jointcommission.org/assets/1/18/3Q2011_SE _Stats_Summary.pdf. Accessed September 2012.

NANDA International (2011). *NANDA Nursing Diagnoses: Definitions and Classification, 2012–2014*. Hoboken, NJ: Wiley-Blackwell.

National Network of Libraries of Medicine (NN/LM) (2012). Health literacy. Available at: http://nnlm.gov/outreach /consumer/hlthlit.html. Accessed September 2012.

• •

Post-Test

WWW

Read each question carefully. Each question may have more than one correct answer.

1. What is the purpose of the nursing diagnoses identified by the PNDS?
   a. to serve as the basis for the plan of care developed by the perioperative nurse
   b. to increase NANDA's database of nursing diagnoses
   c. to eliminate the need for the perioperative nurse to develop an individualized plan of care
   d. to increase awareness of perioperative nursing

2. Preoperative preparation of the patient *does not* include
   a. clarifying expectations of the patient's participation in recovery and rehabilitation.
   b. reinforcing the patient's understanding of the risks delineated on the consent form.
   c. eliminating the patient's anxiety and fear.
   d. clarifying the events anticipated in the preoperative and immediate postoperative periods.

3. Preparing effectively for obese patients presents an additional challenge because they
   a. often have comorbid conditions.
   b. are at higher risk for surgical-site infection.
   d. do not respond well to antibiotics.
   d. are more fearful of surgery than nonobese patients.

4. The dose and timing of prophylactic antibiotic administration is determined by
   a. protocol, which states the dosage and specifies that it be given 1 hour before surgery.
   b. the attending surgeon.
   c. the anesthesia provider.
   d. the optimal level of antibiotic in the patient's serum and tissue at the time of surgery.

5. Communication protocols such as SBAR and I PASS THE BATON are important because they
   a. determine which information must be communicated.
   b. provide a framework for comprehensive and concise communication.
   c. are mandated by TJC's National Patient Safety Goals.
   d. become part of the patient's record.

6. The most common nursing diagnoses in the preoperative period are
   a. knowledge deficit and risk of injury.
   b. risk of injury and risk of infection.
   c. risk of infection and anxiety.
   d. knowledge deficit and anxiety.

7. Which of the following statements about anxiety and fear is true?
   a. The focus of fear is specific.
   b. The focus of anxiety is specific.
   c. It is more common for a patient to be fearful than anxious.
   d. It is more difficult to allay anxiety than fear.

8. Which of the following measures is effective in addressing the patient's anxiety?
   a. providing all of the information the patient should know
   b. reassuring the patient that there is nothing to worry about
   c. listening attentively and providing emotional support
   d. promising the patient that everything will go well

9. Which of the following is *not* a criterion for determining that the patient's knowledge deficit has been addressed ?
   a. The patient confirms the consent.
   b. The patient describes the expected sequence of events.
   c. The patient denies anxiety or fear.
   d. The patient confirms procedures to be followed upon discharge.

10. Anticipatory grieving is most frequently related to
    a. not waking up from anesthesia.
    b. waking up during the procedure.
    c. postoperative pain.
    d. possible changes in body image.

11. The intraoperative period begins when the patient
    a. leaves the preoperative holding area.
    b. enters the actual operating room.
    c. is transferred to the operating room table.
    d. is induced by the anesthesia provider.

12. Wrong-site surgery as defined by TJC includes surgery on the wrong
    a. side or wrong level.
    b. patient.
    c. procedure.
    d. patient, body part, side, level, or procedure.

13. Three protocols that TJC implements in an effort to prevent wrong-site surgery are
    a. site marking, time-out, and better documentation.
    b. time-out, better documentation, and consent form.
    c. preprocedure verification, site marking, and time-out.
    d. site marking, consent form, and time-out.

14. A priority for the perioperative nurse before bringing the patient into the operating room is
    a. verification of the patient's identity and surgical procedure.
    b. ensuring that the surgeon is in the room.
    c. ensuring the scrub person has completed setting up the sterile field.
    d. ensuring that family members are present in the waiting area.

15. Which techniques can the nurse use to alleviate anxiety and fear?
    a. telling the patient everything he or she needs to know
    b. attentive listening and reassuring touch
    c. giving information to the family instead of the patient
    d. postponing patient teaching until after the procedure

16. Which factors interfere with learning in the elderly?
    a. Elderly patients are more often frightened than anxious.
    b. They have difficulty with written materials.
    c. They do not need as much instruction because others will be caring for them.
    d. Their short-term memory may be impaired.

17. Which of the following statements is *true*?
    a. Toddlers may feel that surgery is punishment for bad behavior.
    b. School-age children have a short attention span.
    c. Becoming familiar with items they will encounter in surgery gives pediatric patients a sense of control.
    d. Preschoolers will benefit from discussing the steps involved in the procedure.

18. Which of the following statements is *false*?
    a. Adults learn best from printed materials.
    b. Printed materials must be tailored to the needs of the learner.
    c. The patient's literacy level and health literacy influence the value of printed teaching materials.
    d. The nurse should solicit feedback to determine the degree the patient's level of understanding of the printed material.

19. Health literacy is the patient's
    a. level of health and well-being.
    b. highest level of education.
    c. ability to assimilate information from printed literature.
    d. capacity to obtain, process, and understand health information.

20. TJC requires which of the following because patient injuries can result from poor communication among caregivers?
    a. written communication using the SBAR or I PASS THE BATON format
    b. a standardized hand-off protocol that includes the opportunity to ask and respond to questions
    c. a communication competency checklist to be completed by all healthcare providers
    d. the surgeon, perioperative nurse, and anesthesia provider to all be in the operating room before the patient can be brought in

• •

Competency Checklist: Preparing the Patient for Surgery

www

Under "Observer's Initials," enter initials upon successful achievement of competency. Enter N/A if competency is not appropriate for institution.

Name _____

	Observer's Initials	Date
1. Patient is identified.	_____	_____
2. Surgical procedure and operative site are verified with the patient.	_____	_____
3. Operative consent is verified with the patient.	_____	_____
4. Patient is assessed (or chart reviewed) for:		
a. Medical diagnosis	_____	_____
b. Medications (prescription, over-the-counter, herbal, prophylactic antibiotic)	_____	_____
c. Lab data (tests ordered, lab results, blood type and cross-match)	_____	_____
d. Previous surgeries	_____	_____
e. Anesthesia complications	_____	_____
f. Substance abuse	_____	_____
g. Skin condition	_____	_____
h. Allergies	_____	_____
i. Nutritional and NPO status	_____	_____
j. Sensory impairments	_____	_____
k. Dentures	_____	_____
l. Mobility impairments	_____	_____
m. Presence of prosthesis	_____	_____
n. Weight and height	_____	_____
o. Vital signs	_____	_____
p. Age	_____	_____
5. Patient is assessed for:		
a. Level of understanding	_____	_____
b. Ability to comprehend	_____	_____
c. Information desired	_____	_____
d. Cultural and religious beliefs	_____	_____
6. Patient is asked to verbalize understanding of the surgical experience.	_____	_____
7. Patient is encouraged to ask questions regarding the surgical procedure.	_____	_____
8. Patient is encouraged to verbalize concerns about the surgical experience.	_____	_____
9. Intraoperative routines that the patient should expect are explained.	_____	_____
10. Patient teaching takes patient's age and level of understanding into consideration.	_____	_____
11. Joint Commission universal protocol to prevent wrong-site surgery is implemented.	_____	_____
12. Chart is reviewed for preoperative antibiotic order and action taken as necessary.	_____	_____
13. Postoperative routines are explained to the patient.	_____	_____
14. The above information is communicated to the surgical team.	_____	_____

Observer's Signature   Initials   Date

_____

Orientee's Signature

_____

3

Prevention of Infection
Preparation of Instruments and Items Used in Surgery: Sterilization and Disinfection

---

LEARNER OBJECTIVES

1. Identify the critical factors that determine whether an item must be sterile or whether disinfection is sufficient.
2. Describe at least four methods of sterilization.
3. Discuss critical factors that determine selection of the appropriate sterilization method and cycle.
4. Discuss advantages and disadvantages of each method of sterilization.
5. Identify methods for monitoring sterilization and disinfection processes.

WWW

LESSON OUTLINE

I. Desired Patient Outcomes

II. Sterilization and Disinfection
  A. Critical, Semicritical, and Noncritical Items
  B. Sterility Assurance Level

III. Methods of Sterilization
  A. Overview
  B. Thermal Sterilization—Steam Under Pressure: Moist Heat
  C. Steam Sterilizers: Autoclaves
  D. Immediate-Use Steam Sterilization
  E. Chemical Sterilization: Low-Temperature Hydrogen Peroxide Gas Plasma
  F. Chemical Sterilization: Low-Temperature Vapor-Phase Hydrogen Peroxide
  G. Chemical Sterilization: Ethylene Oxide Gas
  H. Liquid Chemical Sterilant Processing System
  I. Chemical Sterilization: Low-Temperature Ozone/Hydrogen Peroxide

IV. Sterilization: Quality Control
  A. Overview
  B. Physical Monitors
  C. Chemical Indicators
  D. Biological Monitors
  E. Rapid-Readout Biological Monitors

V. Sterilization Documentation

VI. Disinfection
  A. Overview
  B. Levels of Disinfectants: Application

VII. Disinfection: Quality Control

VIII. Disinfection: Documentation

Desired Patient Outcomes

1. Freedom from infection is a critical desired patient outcome.
2. Postoperative wound infection/surgical-site infection (SSI) is a complication of surgery with

potentially dire consequences for the patient, including delayed recovery, increased length of stay and cost of care, increased pain and suffering, and even death. SSIs have also been shown to increase mortality, readmission rates, and length of stay (Institute for Healthcare Improvement [IHI], 2012).

3. Surgical-site infections are the second leading cause of hospital-associated infections, following urinary tract infections; they account for 17% of all hospital-acquired infections (Centers for Disease Control and Prevention [CDC], 2012). SSIs can double the cost of a surgical experience (Alexander et al., 2011). It is estimated that 750,000 to 1 million SSIs occur in the United States each year, requiring 3.7 million extra hospital days and costing more than $1.6 billion in excess hospital charges (Edmiston et al., 2011).

4. Skin is the body's first line of defense against infection. Surgical incisions interrupt skin integrity, providing a portal of entry for pathogenic microorganisms. Invasive drains, catheters, and monitors also alter skin integrity and contribute to the risk for infection.

5. Perioperative nursing activities are directed toward preventing infection, with the desired outcome that the patient will be free from infection following the operative procedure.

6. Pathogenic microorganisms are capable of causing disease when they invade human tissue. Invasive surgical procedures increase a patient's risk of getting an infection by giving bacteria a route into normally sterile areas of the body. Contaminated surgical instruments are a potential source of surgical-site infections (Linkin et al., 2005, pp. 1014–1015). Every effort must be made to remove microorganisms from articles and instruments that contact human tissue during surgical interventions.

7. Sterilization and disinfection—the cornerstones of infection control—are processes used to destroy microorganisms. Preventing infection requires the perioperative nurse to have an in-depth understanding of principles and practices of sterilization and disinfection.

8. Advances in surgical techniques have resulted in the proliferation and routine use of a wide variety of complex, sophisticated, and expensive surgical instrumentation. For example,

---

Definitions

Autoclave: A steam sterilizer.

Bioburden: A population of viable microorganisms on a product.

Biological indicator: A sterilization monitor, consisting of a known population of resistant spores, that is used to test a sterilizer's ability to kill microorganisms.

Bowie-Dick test: An air removal test designed to assure that the autoclave can remove air and noncondensable gases from the chamber and that steam can penetrate a specified pack.

Chemical indicator: A device used to monitor one or more process parameters in the sterilization cycle. The device responds with a chemical or physical change (usually a color change) to conditions within the sterilizer chamber. Chemical indicators are usually supplied as a paper strip, tape, or label that changes color when the parameter or parameters have been met.

Disinfectant: An antimicrobial agent used to destroy microorganisms on inanimate surfaces. The composition and concentration of the disinfectant and the amount of time an item is exposed to it determine the number and types of organisms that will be killed.

Disinfection: A process that kills all living microorganisms, with the exception of high numbers of spores.
- Low-level disinfection kills vegetative forms of bacteria, lipid viruses, and some fungi.
- Intermediate-level disinfection kills vegetative bacteria, mycobacteria, viruses, and fungi, but not spores.
- High-level disinfection kills vegetative bacteria, mycobacteria, viruses, fungi, and some spores.

Immediate-use steam sterilization (IUSS): A steam sterilization process for sterilizing heat and moisture-stable items that are needed immediately; previously known as "flash sterilization."

Spore: An inactive or dormant, but viable, state of a microorganism, which is notably difficult to kill. Sterilization methods are monitored by assessing their ability to kill a known population of highly resistant spores.

Sterile: Free of all viable microorganisms, including spores.

Sterility assurance level (SAL): The probability of a viable microorganism being present on an item after sterilization.

Sterilization: A process that kills all living microorganisms, including spores.

fiber-optic and robotic instruments costing many thousands of dollars are standard components of many procedures.

9. Cleaning, disinfection, and sterilization procedures are determined by the composition and configuration of the instrumentation, which dictate its compatibility with the disinfection and sterilization methods available within the healthcare facility. Manufacturers' instructions for processing of instruments and devices must be considered when purchasing and processing decisions are made.

10. Most instrument processing is performed by ancillary personnel; however, the perioperative nurse is a partner in this process and assumes varying degrees of responsibility for the care and preparation of instruments. Selecting the appropriate method of processing requires a broad knowledge of disinfection and sterilization principles and procedures.

11. When disinfection and sterilization are accomplished within the operating room department, it is often the perioperative nurse who is responsible for the process.

Sterilization and Disinfection

Critical, Semicritical, and Noncritical Items

12. How an instrument should be processed depends on its intended use. The Spaulding classification of devices, developed in 1968 by Earle Spaulding, was adopted by the Centers for Disease Control and Prevention (CDC). It categorizes devices as critical, semicritical, or noncritical (AORN, 2012, p. 473). This categorization is used today to determine whether an item must be sterilized or whether disinfection is sufficient.

Critical Items: Examples

13. Critical items come in contact with sterile tissue or the vascular system (i.e., devices introduced beneath a mucous membrane). These items must be sterile—that is, all living microorganisms, including spores, must be destroyed.

14. Critical items contaminated with microorganisms present a high risk of infection.

15. Examples of critical items include surgical instruments, orthopedic implants, sutures, and cardiac catheters.

Semicritical Items: Examples

16. Items that contact unbroken mucous membranes but do not penetrate them are considered semicritical items. Semicritical items may be sterile but must at least be high-level disinfected.

17. Examples of semicritical items include thermometers, cystoscopes, laryngoscope blades, and dental dams.

Noncritical Items: Examples

18. Noncritical items contact intact skin and require only low-level disinfection or cleaning.

19. Examples of noncritical items include crutches, blood pressure cuffs, and stethoscopes.

Sterility Assurance Level

20. The process of sterilization provides the greatest assurance that items are sterile (i.e., free of known and unsuspected microorganisms).

21. Devices sterilized for use in surgery must be sterilized with a sterility assurance level (SAL) of 10^{-6}. This mathematical expression means that there is equal to, or less than, one chance in 1 million that any viable microorganism will be present on an item after sterilization. This is a very high level of sterility assurance. For example, in some industries, a sterility assurance of 10^{-3} (one chance in 1000) might be acceptable.

22. In addition to the requirement for such a high level of sterility assurance, manufacturers of sterilizers must demonstrate that the sterilizer kills 1 million spores in half the programmed exposure time. For example, if the exposure phase in the sterilization cycle (the time within the cycle when the parameters required for sterilization are achieved) is programmed for 4 minutes, the sterilizer manufacturer must demonstrate that the kill is achieved in 2 minutes. In other words, a sterilizer must be capable of killing 1 million spores in half the time for which the sterilizer is programmed for hospital use (Favero & Bond, 2001, pp. 885–886).

23. Certain pathogenic bacteria such as *Clostridium tetani* (which produces tetanus), *Clostridium perfidens* (which results in gas gangrene), and *Clostridium difficile* are capable of developing spore forms. The environmental

conditions that facilitate spore formation are unknown; however, spores can remain alive for many years. When conditions are favorable for growth, such as when the spore is permitted entry into the body, the spore will germinate to produce a vegetative cell.

24. Spores are more resistant than other bacteria to heat, drying, and chemicals. In fact, they can survive even after long exposure to these processes.

25. Disinfection—a process that kills all living microorganisms, with the exception of high numbers of bacterial spores—does not provide the margin of safety associated with sterilization. Disinfectants vary in their ability to destroy microorganisms and are classified according to their cidal activity (i.e., their ability to kill microorganisms).

26. Only sterilization can render an item free of all microorganisms, including spores.

Section Questions   www

1. Which factors determine the appropriate processing method for an item? [Ref 12]

2. Define "critical items" according to the Spaulding classification. [Ref 13]

3. Give three examples of items that would be considered "critical" according to the Spaulding classification. [Ref 15]

4. Define "semicritical items" according to the Spaulding classification. [Ref 16]

5. Which level(s) of processing are appropriate for semicritical items? [Ref 16]

6. Give three examples of semicritical items. [Ref 17]

7. Define "noncritical items" according to the Spaulding classification. [Ref 18]

8. Which level of processing is appropriate for noncritical items? [Ref 18]

9. Give three examples of noncritical items. [Ref 19]

10. Explain the meaning of the sterility assurance level of 10^{-6} that is required for items sterilized for use in surgery. [Ref 21]

11. If a sterilization cycle in surgery is 4 minutes, at which point in the cycle must the manufacturer demonstrate that 1 million spores have been killed? [Ref 22]

12. Why can some pathogenic bacteria such as *Clostridium perfidens* and *Clostridium difficile* be particularly difficult to kill? [Ref 23]

13. Why are spores used to demonstrate the effectiveness of the sterilization process? [Ref 24]

14. What does "cidal activity" mean? [Ref 25]

15. What is the only level of processing for instruments that can render an item free of all microorganisms, including spores? [Ref 26]

Methods of Sterilization

Overview

27. The choice among methods of sterilization depends on the compatibility of the item to be sterilized with the sterilization process, the configuration of the item, the required equipment, cost, availability, safety factors, packaging of the item, and the length of time of the sterilization process.

28. Steam and ethylene oxide have been used in hospitals for sterilization for more than 50 years. Currently the most commonly used methods of in-house sterilization are steam and hydrogen peroxide gas plasma; the latter has replaced ethylene oxide (EtO) in many facilities. Hydrogen peroxide gas plasma was introduced in the 1990s; hydrogen peroxide vapor and ozone were introduced in the early 2000s. Each method has both advantages and disadvantages.

29. Steam is used for heat- and moisture-stable items. Hydrogen peroxide gas plasma, hydrogen peroxide vapor, O_2, and EtO are appropriate for items that cannot withstand moisture or high temperatures.

30. Two other accepted methods of sterilization are dry heat and ionizing radiation.

31. Because of equipment, safety, and cost considerations, ionizing radiation is confined to industrial settings and is used for bulk sterilization of commercially prepared items.

32. Dry heat is appropriate for powders, oils, and petroleum products that cannot be penetrated by steam or ethylene oxide or other sterilizing agents. Most of these products are supplied in sterile condition from the manufacturer; therefore, dry-heat sterilization is rarely used in hospitals in the United States.

Thermal Sterilization—Steam Under Pressure: Moist Heat

33. Moist heat in the form of saturated steam under pressure is an economical, safe, and effective method of sterilization used for the majority of surgical instruments. It is the most common sterilization method used within healthcare facilities. Sterilization by this method is accomplished in a steam sterilizer referred to as an autoclave.

34. For an item to be sterilized, steam must penetrate every fiber of the packaging and contact every surface of the item. In addition, the intended parameters of moisture, temperature, and time must be met.

35. Steam that is saturated (i.e., contains the greatest amount of water vapor possible) and is heated to a sufficient temperature is capable of destroying all living microorganisms, including spores, within a relatively short amount of time.

36. Saturated steam destroys microorganisms through a thermal process that causes denaturation and coagulation of proteins or the enzyme protein system contained within the microorganism's cell.

37. Steam at atmospheric pressure has a temperature of 212°F (100°C), which is inadequate for sterilization. The addition of pressure to increase the temperature of the steam is necessary for the destruction of microorganisms.

38. An increase in pressure of 15 to 17 pounds per square inch will increase steam temperature to 250°F–254°F (121°C–123°C). Twenty-seven pounds of pressure per square inch will increase steam temperature to 270°F (132°C).

39. The minimum generally accepted temperature required for sterilization to occur is 250°F (121°C) (Perkins, 1969, p. 161). Typical temperatures for the operation of steam sterilizers are in the range of 270°F–275°F (132°C–135°C), although 250°F (121°C) is also used (Association for the Advancement of Medical Instrumentation [AAMI], 2011, p. 63).

40. Steam sterilization is a function of time and temperature. Sterilization at 250°F (121°C) requires more time than sterilization at 270°F (132°C).

Advantages of Steam Sterilization

41. Steam sterilization has many advantages:
    - Steam is readily available (most often supplied from the healthcare facility boiler).
    - Steam is economical.
    - Steam sterilization is fast—destruction of most resistant spores occurs quickly.
    - Steam is compatible with most in-house packaging materials.
    - Steam leaves no toxic residue and is environmentally safe.
    - Steam sterilization is suitable for a wide range of surgical instrumentation. (The majority of items used for surgery can withstand repeated steam sterilization without sustaining damage.)

Disadvantages of Steam Sterilization

42. Steam sterilization is also associated with several disadvantages:
    - A variety of instruments and devices used in surgery cannot withstand moist heat at temperatures of 250°F (121°C) or higher.
    - Steam sterilization is prone to operator error with regard to preparation and packaging of items, cycle selection, setting of parameters, and loading of the autoclave.
    - Timing of the sterilization cycle must be adjusted based on the type of cycle, variances in materials, device configuration, and size of the load.
    - A temperature of 270°F cannot be used to sterilize all items. The temperature may need to be reduced from 270°F to 250°F to be

compatible with a specific item being sterilized, or the temperature may need to be increased to comply with the manufacturer's instructions.

43. Efficacy of steam sterilization depends on attention to detail. Improper preparation of items or improper placement within the autoclave can result in trapping of air, which can prevent steam contact with all surfaces and thereby cause inadequate sterilization. Items must be disassembled and thoroughly cleaned for steam to contact all surfaces.

Section Questions

www

1. Identify at least six factors that influence the choice of sterilization method for a particular item. [Ref 27]

2. What are the most common methods of sterilization at this time? [Ref 28]

3. For which types of items is steam the most appropriate sterilization modality? [Ref 29]

4. Which characteristics of surgical instruments and supplies make them appropriate for sterilization using hydrogen peroxide gas plasma, hydrogen peroxide vapor, ozone, and EtO? [Ref 31]

5. Why are dry-heat sterilization and ionizing radiation confined to industrial settings? [Refs 30–31]

6. Which items would be sterilized with dry heat? [Ref 32]

7. Why is dry-heat sterilization rarely found in hospitals in the United States? [Ref 32]

8. What is an autoclave? [Ref 33]

9. What is the importance of steam contact with every surface of an item to be sterilized? [Ref 34]

10. What are the three parameters involved in steam sterilization? [Ref 34]

11. What are the characteristics of steam required for it to be capable of killing all living microorganisms on an item, including spores? [Ref 35]

12. What is the process through which steam kills microorganisms? [Ref 36]

13. What must be done to increase the temperature of steam sufficiently to kill microorganisms? [Ref 37]

14. What is the minimum steam temperature required for sterilization to occur? [Ref 39]

15. What is the typical temperature used for steam sterilization? [Ref 39]

16. Besides temperature, which factor must be calculated to achieve sterilization? [Ref 40]

17. List the advantages of steam sterilization. [Ref 41]

18. List the disadvantages of steam sterilization. [Ref 42]

19. What are some aspects of steam sterilization prone to operator error? [Ref 42]

20. How does trapped air that can result from improper packaging or improper placement of items in an autoclave affect the sterilization process? [Ref 43]

Steam Sterilizers: Autoclaves

Overview

44. A steam sterilizer, referred to as an autoclave, generally consists of a rectangular metal chamber and a shell. Between the two is an enclosed space referred to as a jacket. When the autoclave is activated, steam and heat fill the jacket and are maintained at a constant pressure, keeping the autoclave in a heated, ready state (Figure 3-1).

45. Items are placed in the chamber, the door is shut tightly, and the sterilization cycle is initiated. Steam enters the chamber and displaces all the air from the chamber and from the contents of the load. As the pressure rises, steam penetrates the packaging and contacts all surfaces of the item(s) within. The steam forces the air out through a discharge port outlet at the bottom front of the autoclave.

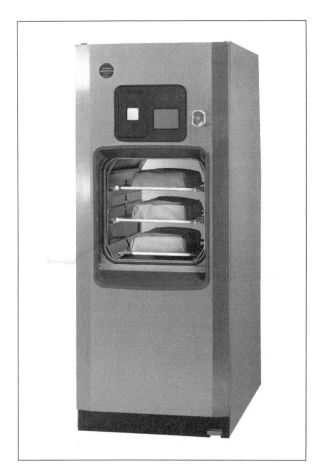

Figure 3-1 Steam sterilizer
Source: Courtesy of Steris Corporation, Mentor, OH.

46. It is essential that all the air in the chamber be displaced by steam. Air that is trapped will act as an insulator that interferes with heating and prevents moisture contact with every surface of every item, thereby compromising the sterilization process. Proper loading of the autoclave is critical. Items must be placed so that steam can circulate freely throughout the chamber and can contact all surfaces.

47. The discharge port outlet is the beginning of a filtered waste line. Beneath the filter is a thermometer. This is the coolest part of the autoclave.

48. The actual exposure or sterilization time does not begin until the thermometer senses that the steam has reached the necessary preset temperature.

49. If air is not trapped and the parameters of time, moisture, and temperature have been met, microbial destruction will occur.

50. Items such as cups or basins must be placed within the sterilizer so that water will not collect in them and compromise the sterilization process.

51. When the exposure time is complete, the steam is exhausted through the outlet port and, if desired, a drying cycle follows. A drying cycle must always be used for wrapped items.

52. Wrapped packages and instrument containers should be allowed to cool on the sterilizer rack. They should not be touched during this time. A minimum of 30 minutes is recommended, although some instrument sets may require as much as 2 hours to adequately cool (AAMI, 2011, p. 85).

53. Warm packages must not be placed on cool surfaces because condensate will form, causing the package to become damp. Microorganisms are capable of penetrating wet materials; therefore, moist packages that contact an unsterile surface must be considered contaminated.

54. Two types of steam sterilizers or autoclaves are used: gravity displacement and dynamic air removal (high vacuum, prevacuum, and pulse pressure). These autoclaves differ in how air is removed from the chamber during the sterilization process.

55. Sterilizers vary in terms of their design and performance characteristics. Some sterilizers offer both a gravity-displacement and a dynamic-air-removal cycle, and some offer only one type of cycle.

56. The nature of the items and the container in which they are sterilized determine the necessary time and temperature for sterilization. There is no single setting that is appropriate for all items. The manufacturers' instructions for use for the items and for the autoclave must be consulted to determine the correct cycle settings.

Gravity Displacement

57. In a gravity-displacement cycle or autoclave, steam replaces the air in the chamber by gravity.

58. As steam enters from a port located near the top and rear of the chamber, it is deflected upward. Air is heavier than steam; thus, by the force of gravity, the air is forced to the bottom while the steam rides on top of the air. The steam rapidly displaces the air under it and forces the air out through the discharge outlet port (Figure 3-2).

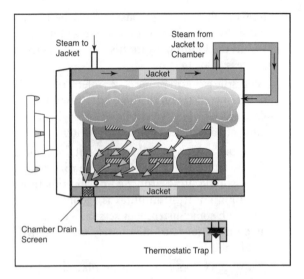

Figure 3-2 Steam sterilizer—steam entry and air removal
Source: Photo courtesy of AMSCO International Inc.

59. Most gravity-displacement autoclaves are operated at temperatures between 250°F and 274°F (121°C–134°C) with a 10- to 30-minute exposure time. For example, a wrapped instrument set requiring 30 minutes at 250°F (121°C) might require a 15-minute exposure at 270°F (134°C) (AAMI, 2011, p. 82). Certain powered equipment may require prolonged exposure times of as much as 55 minutes.

60. Sterilization at a higher temperature requires less time than at a lower temperature. A temperature of 270°F (132°C) will accomplish sterilization more rapidly than a temperature of 250°F (121°C). All recommended cycles achieve an SAL of 10^{-6}.

61. The disadvantages of a gravity-displacement process are the length of time required for sterilization and the dependence on gravity to remove air. A prevacuum or steam–flush–pressure–pulse cycle offers a greater margin of safety with regard to air removal.

62. Gravity-displacement cycles should not be used when a prevacuum or steam–flush–pressure–pulse cycle is available.

63. Gravity-displacement sterilizers are common in dentist and physician offices, clinics, and small surgicenters. Sterilizers that operate only with a gravity-displacement cycle can still be found in healthcare facilities; however, most sterilizers sold today for hospitals and large ambulatory surgery centers run dynamic-air-removal cycles (though they may offer gravity-displacement cycles as well).

64. A gravity-displacement cycle is most appropriate for liquids, although liquids are rarely sterilized within healthcare facilities. Liquids that must be sterile are generally supplied in sterile forms by the manufacturer. Some medical devices, because of their design, may require a gravity-displacement cycle. The device manufacturer's instructions should be consulted before selecting the cycle type, time, and temperature.

Dynamic Air Removal (Prevacuum Sterilizer)

65. The prevacuum autoclave is equipped with a vacuum pump that evacuates almost all air from the chamber prior to the injection of steam. The evacuation process, which takes approximately 5 minutes but may be longer, essentially creates a vacuum within the chamber. When the steam enters the chamber, the force of the vacuum causes instant steam contact with all surfaces of the contents. Steam will penetrate almost instantly to every surface without regard to the size of the package or load.

66. Following the prevacuum phase, an exposure time of 3 to 4 minutes at 270°F to 275°F (132°C to 135°C) is the usual recommended time and temperature for accomplishing sterilization (AAMI, 2011, p. 83).

67. It is imperative that the device manufacturer's instructions for use be consulted before selecting the cycle time and temperature.

Extended Cycles

68. Although a 4-minute exposure time is typically used, required exposure times of 5, 8, and 15 minutes are not uncommon. These cycles are commonly referred to as extended cycles. As the number and types of devices have proliferated, the variety in cycle times has likewise proliferated. Temperature requirements vary from 270°F to 275°F (132°C to 135°C). In other words, one cycle does not fit all devices. The manufacturer's instructions for sterilization of any instrument will determine the correct cycle. It should not be assumed that a 4-minute exposure at 270°F (132°C) is always appropriate.

69. If a device calls for an extended exposure or temperature variation, other devices that require less time should not be included in the load unless they have been validated by the device manufacturer for these extended cycles.

70. An extended cycle of 18 minutes at 270°F (134°C) minutes is also required for instruments exposed to prions (AAMI, 2011, p. 166).

71. A dynamic-air-removal (prevacuum sterilization) cycle has several advantages:
    - Incorrect placement of objects within the chamber will have less effect upon air removal than in a gravity-displacement cycle.
    - The entire load will heat rapidly and more uniformly than with a gravity-displacement autoclave; therefore, the exposure time is shorter.
    - The autoclave may be used to a maximum capacity, allowing more supplies to be sterilized within a given time.

72. The disadvantage of a dynamic-air-removal (prevacuum) sterilizer is that in the event of a leak, such as in the door seal, an air pocket can form and inhibit sterilization.

Bowie-Dick Test

73. To test whether air is effectively being eliminated from the chamber, dynamic-air-removal autoclaves are subjected to a Bowie-Dick test on a daily basis. A Bowie-Dick test verifies that air removal is sufficient to achieve steam penetration of a standard load.

74. The Association for the Advancement of Medical Instrumentation recommends this test be performed daily before the first processed load (AAMI, 2011, p. 119).

75. A commercially prepared sheet of paper with various patterns of heat-sensitive ink is used to perform a Bowie-Dick test. The sheet is placed in a specially constructed pack of towels or contained in a commercially prepared package, and is sterilized in an otherwise empty autoclave. A uniform color change indicates successful creation of a vacuum (Figure 3-3).

76. A daily air removal test is another commercially prepared test that may be used to test for air removal.

Steam–Flush–Pressure–Pulse Sterilizer

77. Instead of creating a vacuum to remove air from the chamber, a sterilizer may use a repeated sequence of steam, flush, and pressure pulses above atmospheric pressure. Because a vacuum is not drawn, a Bowie-Dick test or daily air removal test is not required for this type of sterilizer.

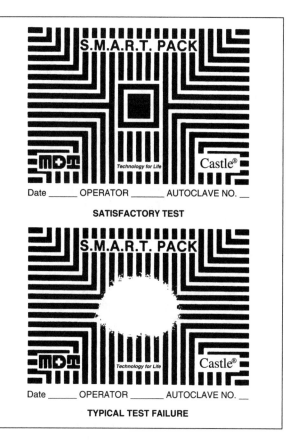

Figure 3-3 Air removal test
Source: Courtesy of MDT Biologic Company, Rochester, NY.

78. A variety of cycle times can be selected, based on the nature of the items to be sterilized.

79. The advantage to a steam–flush–pressure–pulse sterilizer is that sterilization is not affected in the event of an air leak into the sterilization chamber.

Immediate-Use Steam Sterilization

80. "Immediate use" means the shortest possible time between the removal of a sterilized item from the sterilizer and its aseptic transfer to the sterile field. Immediacy implies that a sterilized item is used during the procedure for which it was sterilized, in a manner that minimizes its exposure to air and other environmental contaminants. A sterilized item intended for immediate use is not stored for future use, nor held from one case to another (AAMI, 2011, p. 241).

81. Immediate-use steam sterilization (IUSS) has replaced the term "flash sterilization," which came from "sterilization in a flash," meaning it was a quick way to sterilize an unwrapped

item. "Just in time" sterilization is appropriate only for processing an item needed urgently, and for which there are no replacements immediately available, such as when an item is dropped during surgery and that item is necessary to complete the surgery.

82. IUSS should not be used for routine sterilization of instruments and was never intended for sterilizing whole sets of instruments.

83. IUSS should be used only in carefully selected, urgent clinical situations and should not be used to sterilize implantable devices (AORN, 2012, p. 550; Mangram et al., 1999). Use of IUSS is discouraged by a number of standards-setting organizations.

84. According to the CDC, IUSS is not intended to be used for convenience, as an alternative to purchasing additional instrument sets, or to save time (AORN, 2012, p. 500).

85. Items subject to IUSS have historically been sterilized unwrapped in an open tray. They should, however, be sterilized in containers specifically intended for IUSS. These containers facilitate aseptic delivery of the item to personnel at the sterile field; they are not intended, nor cleared by the US Food and Drug Administration (FDA), for storage of sterilized items for later use. Because there is little or no dry time with an IUSS cycle, items may be wet or moist at the end of the process.

86. Rigid containers not intended specifically for IUSS should not be used for this process. IUSS cannot be used for items to be terminally sterilized in packaging or containers intended for storage. The sterilization cycle includes dry time, and items may be stored and used at a later date.

87. IUSS may be done in a gravity-displacement or a dynamic-air-removal (prevacuum or steam–flush–pressure–pulse) sterilizer. The cycle for IUSS is preset by the sterilizer manufacturer according to the type of sterilizer and the load contents.

88. Exposure times for IUSS can vary by more than 30 minutes and are determined by factors such as the nature and configuration of the item, the type of sterilizer, and whether a dedicated container is available. For example, at 270°F (134°C), a 3-minute exposure is appropriate in both a gravity-displacement and a prevacuum sterilizer for most metal or nonporous or nonlumened items only. However, for metal items with a lumen, a 10-minute cycle

in a gravity-displacement sterilizer is required. In a prevacuum sterilizer, metal items with a lumen might require only 4 minutes (AORN, 2012, p. 552). If a dedicated container system is used, the exposure time and temperatures may vary further. For this reason, it is critical that sterilizer, container, and device manufacturer guidelines be followed.

89. When a device manufacturer does not provide instructions for IUSS, the item should not be sterilized in this manner. Perioperative nurses should always refer to the manufacturer's instructions for use when selecting the cycle type, time, and temperature. Inconsistencies between the device manufacturer's and the sterilizer manufacturer's instructions should be resolved before sterilization. If instructions are not available within the operating room, the perioperative nurse should consult with personnel from the sterile processing department. In the absence of instructions, the device should not be sterilized. It is important to refer to the most recent manufacturer's instructions for use, as instructions for sterilization continue to evolve.

90. Cleaning is absolutely critical to proper instrument processing, as inadequate cleaning will compromise the sterilization process. Instruments prepared for IUSS are often cleaned and prepared under less-than-ideal conditions. The processes and resources available in the sterile processing department (SPD) to clean instruments may not be available in the operating room. In addition, a separate decontamination area for cleaning instruments may not exist in the operating room. Regardless of where instruments are cleaned, the cleaning process should be consistent and in compliance with accepted standards. Appropriate personal protective equipment (PPE) is required for personnel, regardless of what is being cleaned or where cleaning is done. A scrub sink is not appropriate for cleaning instruments.

91. Although items that are sterilized via IUSS are usually sterilized in a "flash" container, a single wrapper may be used for certain types of instruments if sterilizer instructions indicate this approach is appropriate.

92. Another disadvantage of IUSS is that, following sterilization, transfer of the item from the autoclave to the sterile field may be difficult. Because the sterilizer may be located outside the actual operating room, there is a risk of contamination during transport.

Section Questions

www

1. What is the purpose of the jacket in an autoclave? [Ref 44]

2. How does every surface of an item to be sterilized come into contact with steam? [Refs 45–46]

3. When does the actual sterilization cycle begin? [Ref 48]

4. Which parameters must be met for sterilization to occur? [Ref 49]

5. Where should sterilized wrapped packages and instrument containers be left to cool? [Ref 52]

6. What is the danger of placing a warm package on a cool surface? [Ref 53]

7. Which process differentiates a gravity-displacement sterilizer from a dynamic-air-removal sterilizer? [Ref 54]

8. What determines the appropriate time and temperature for sterilizing items in an autoclave? [Ref 56]

9. What are the disadvantages of a gravity-displacement autoclave? [Ref 61]

10. For which items is a gravity-displacement cycle most appropriate? [Ref 64]

11. How does the prevacuum autoclave remove air from the chamber? [Ref 65]

12. How do you manage the sterilization of items with different time requirements for sterilization? [Refs 68–69]

13. What is the cycle time for sterilizing instruments that have been exposed to prions? [Ref 70]

14. Discuss the advantages and disadvantages of dynamic-air-removal sterilization. [Refs 71–72]

15. For what purpose is a Bowie-Dick test run? [Ref 73]

16. When does AAMI recommend that the Bowie-Dick test be run? [Ref 74]

17. When examining the Bowie-Dick results after the test has been run, what determines if the cycle was successful? [Ref 75]

18. How does a steam–flush–pressure–pulse sterilizer differ from a dynamic-air-removal sterilizer? [Ref 77]

19. What is the advantage of a steam–flush–pressure–pulse–sterilizer? [Ref 79]

20. What would you do with an item sterilized with IUSS if it is not used for the current procedure? [Ref 80]

21. When is it appropriate to use IUSS? [Refs 81–84]

22. How are items prepared for IUSS? [Ref 85]

23. Why should a container specifically intended for IUSS be used? [Ref 86]

24. How must instruments for IUSS be processed for sterilization? [Ref 90]

25. Discuss disadvantages of IUSS. [Ref 92]

---

93. Using the special containers designed for use with IUSS reduces the risk of contamination during transfer from the autoclave to the sterile field. Ideally, a sterilizer used for IUSS would open into the actual operating room. This configuration facilitates transport without contamination.

Chemical Sterilization: Low-Temperature Hydrogen Peroxide Gas Plasma

Description

94. Plasma is a state of matter that is produced through the action of a strong electric or magnetic field. In low-temperature hydrogen peroxide plasma sterilization, a plasma state is created by the action of radio-frequency or electrical energy on hydrogen peroxide vapor within a vacuum (Figure 3-4).

95. Items to be sterilized are placed in a sterilizing chamber, a vacuum is established, and liquid hydrogen peroxide is injected into a cap and enters the chamber in a vaporized or gas form. Hydrogen peroxide vapor is effective in killing microorganisms. The hydrogen peroxide gas is charged with radiofrequency energy that creates a plasma. The levels of residual hydrogen peroxide are removed, and at the end of the cycle the reactive species recombine to form oxygen and water vapor. The water vapor is in the form of humidity and cannot be felt.

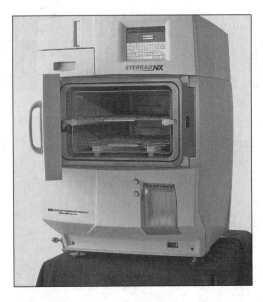

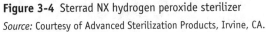

Figure 3-4 Sterrad NX hydrogen peroxide sterilizer
Source: Courtesy of Advanced Sterilization Products, Irvine, CA.

Packages are dry at the end of the cycle and may be used immediately or stored for future use.

Advantages

96. Advantages of low-temperature hydrogen peroxide gas plasma sterilization are as follows:

    • Gas plasma offers an efficient alternative to EtO sterilization; no toxic chemicals are retained, and no aeration is required. Because there are no toxic byproducts, personal protective equipment or monitoring of the environment is not required.

    • The sterilization cycle is short (approximately 30 minutes to more than 1 hour depending up the sterilizer model).

    • The sterilant is compatible with most metals and plastics.

    • The sterilizer is simple to operate. Cycle times are preset and temperature does not require adjustment.

    • There is no plumbing, no drain, nor other fixed requirements. Because the sterilizer connects to an electrical outlet, it can easily be relocated if the need arises.

Disadvantages

97. Disadvantages of low-temperature hydrogen peroxide gas plasma are as follows:

    • Hydrogen peroxide gas plasma is not compatible with powders, liquids, textiles, and other cellulose-containing items such as linen, gauze, and paper.

    • Packaging materials are limited to nonwoven polypropylene wraps, Tyvek and Mylar pouches, or specific container systems.

    • In some hydrogen peroxide gas plasma sterilizer models, lumen restrictions may prevent long, narrow-lumened devices, such as ureteroscopes, from being processed by this method.

Chemical Sterilization: Low-Temperature Vapor-Phase Hydrogen Peroxide

Description

98. In a vapor-phase hydrogen peroxide sterilizer, H_2O_2 is added to the sterilization chamber through a vaporizer under low pressure, creating a vapor that fills the sterilization chamber. As the hydrogen peroxide diffuses and contacts surfaces, an oxidative process inactivates microorganisms. Devices that are sterilized using this process do not require additional aeration beyond what is provided with the cycle, because the byproducts of the process are oxygen and water vapor in the form of humidity.

99. Three programmed cycles address specific parameters for sterilizing instruments of different types: instruments with and without lumens, and instruments with diffusion-restricted spaces (e.g., hinges, ratchets, box locks), and single- or dual-channel flexible endoscopes or other features.

100. All items to be sterilized must be thoroughly cleaned, rinsed, and dried before being packaged and loaded into the chamber.

101. Items should be arranged in a single layer with minimal overlap to ensure proper diffusion of sterilant vapor throughout the load.

102. Each of the three cycles has three phases:

    • Conditioning: Sterilant fills the reservoir and a vacuum pulse removes air and moisture from the chamber, filtered dry air is introduced, and the load is tested electronically for acceptable moisture content.

    • Sterilization: A series of four pulses create a vacuum and introduce sterilant vapor and filtered air into the chamber.

- Aeration: The sterilant vapor is evacuated from the chamber. When the aeration phase is complete, the chamber pressure is brought to atmospheric level and the chamber door unlocks.

103. Monitoring includes a special chemical indicator designed to change color in the presence of H_2O_2 and a biological indicator containing the spore *Geobacillus stearothermophilus*.

Advantages

104. Advantages of low-temperature hydrogen peroxide vapor sterilization are as follows:
   - Vaporized H_2O_2 offers an efficient alternative to EtO sterilization; there are no toxic byproducts, only water vapor and oxygen.
   - The sterilant is compatible with most metals and plastics, glass, and silicone.
   - The sterilizer is simple to operate. Cycle times are preset and temperature does not require adjustment.
   - There is no plumbing, no drain, nor other fixed requirements. The sterilizer connects to an electrical outlet and can be relocated easily if necessary.

Disadvantages

105. Disadvantages of vaporized hydrogen peroxide are as follows:
   - Hydrogen peroxide vapor is not compatible with liquids, linens, powders, and cellulose materials such as linen, gauze, and paper.
   - Packaging materials are limited to nonwoven polypropylene wraps, Tyvek and Mylar pouches, or specific container systems.

Chemical Sterilization: Ethylene Oxide Gas

Description

106. Ethylene oxide (EtO) is a toxic gas used to sterilize items that cannot tolerate the temperature and moisture of steam sterilization. Ethylene oxide achieves sterilization by interfering with protein metabolism and cell reproduction.

107. A wide variety of surgical items that cannot withstand moist heat without incurring damage may be sterilized with ethylene oxide gas. Commonly gas-sterilized items are flexible and rigid endoscopes, plastic goods, instruments with electrical components, and delicate instruments with sharp edges that will dull with exposure to repeated steam sterilization.

108. Because EtO is toxic, the sterilizers must be housed in a location that is closely monitored and vented. Even though EtO sterilizers are not found in the operating room, it is important to understand the technology and its associated responsibilities.

109. The essential parameters of gas sterilization are gas concentration, temperature, humidity, and exposure time.

110. Gas concentration varies with the size of the chamber, the temperature and humidity within the chamber, and the type of gas sterilizer used. Gas sterilizers operate at temperatures between 85°F (29°C) and 145°F (63°C). Optimal humidity levels are between 30% and 60%. Exposure times generally range from 3 to 7 hours. The sterilizer manufacturer's and the device manufacturer's recommendations must be followed carefully to determine exposure time. Items exposed to EtO must be thoroughly aerated to remove vestiges of the chemical from the packaging and the sterile items.

111. Ethylene oxide, which is supplied in a 100% concentration, is packaged in small unit-dose cartridges. Because this gas is flammable and explosive when supplied in large tanks, it is mixed with inert gases such as hydrochlorofluorocarbons (HCFCs) or carbon dioxide. The selection of 100% EtO or a mixture is determined by the sterilizer design.

112. In the EtO sterilization cycle, the air is evacuated from the chamber and its contents, the load is preheated, and humidity is introduced. This phase is termed the preconditioning phase. EtO is then released into the chamber, where it permeates and penetrates the load. EtO sterilization operates under negative pressure. The advantage to this approach is that if a leak occurs, the EtO will be drawn into the chamber rather than being vented to the outside work environment.

Advantages

113. Advantages of EtO sterilization:
   - EtO is effective against all types of microorganisms.

- EtO does not require high heat.
- EtO is noncorrosive.
- EtO effectively penetrates large bundles and permeates all porous items.

Disadvantages

114. Ethylene oxide is a toxic gas, and the sterilization process can be complex and potentially hazardous. Because of the toxic and hazardous nature of ethylene oxide sterilization, items that can tolerate steam sterilization should not be sterilized with EtO.

115. Other disadvantages:

- The sterilization cycle time is lengthy.
- EtO is highly flammable, and EtO cylinders and cartridges must be handled and stored carefully.
- The diluent HCFCs used in EtO sterilization are subject to strict local, state, and federal regulations and are being phased out because they deplete the ozone layer in the atmosphere.
- EtO sterilization is more expensive than steam sterilization.
- Toxic byproducts can form under certain conditions. For example, ethylene oxide combined with water yields the toxic byproduct ethylene glycol.
- Because a variety of materials can absorb EtO during the sterilization process, residual EtO must be removed from the load contents through an aeration or detoxification process following sterilization. Aeration times in a mechanical aerator may be as short as 8 hours or less or longer than 24 hours. The length of aeration time needed depends on the item, packaging, density of the load, type of sterilization and aeration system, and temperature in the aeration chamber. Items made from materials such as polyvinyl chloride require the most lengthy period of aeration. Sterilizer and device manufacturer guidelines for exposure and aeration must be followed. Items should never be removed from the aerator until the aeration cycle is complete.
- EtO is regarded as a human carcinogen by the Occupational Safety and Health Administration (OSHA). Personnel working with EtO must be provided with PPE and instruction in the hazards associated with EtO.
- EtO is also recognized as having the potential to cause adverse reproductive effects in humans. In areas where EtO is utilized, a sign must be posted that reads as follows: "Danger: ethylene oxide, cancer hazard and reproductive hazard. Authorized personnel only. Respirators and protective clothing may be required to be worn in this area" (OSHA, 2011).
- Exposure to EtO can cause eye irritation, nausea, dizziness, vomiting, nasal and throat irritation, shortness of breath, tissue burns, and hemolysis. Insufficiently aerated items may cause patient or personnel injury.
- Concentrations of EtO must be identified in the areas where EtO sterilization occurs. Monitoring devices that produce an alarm in the event of EtO exposure must be in place.
- The OSHA standard for exposure to EtO is an 8-hour time-weighted average (TWA) that limits personnel to one part EtO per million parts of air in 8 hours. OSHA requires a monitoring program to ensure compliance with this standard. Employees who work with EtO must periodically wear monitors that detect the amount of EtO in the work area.
- EtO gas must be vented to the outside to avoid personnel exposure. In addition, some states have abatement requirements that add to the cost of EtO processing. Abaters convert waste ethylene oxide into nontoxic gases that are then vented to the outside.

116. Because of safety issues and because prolonged aeration time means that instruments may be unavailable when needed, many healthcare facilities have significantly reduced or eliminated the use of EtO by switching to newer low-temperature sterilization methods that do not have the same safety issues, lengthy process, and aeration time as EtO.

Liquid Chemical Sterilant Processing System

Description

117. Peracetic acid solution contains acetic acid and hydrogen peroxide. Peracetic acid is acetic acid

plus an extra oxygen atom. It disrupts protein bonds and cell systems; the extra oxygen atom inactivates cell systems and causes immediate cell death.

118. Liquid peracetic acid is a low-temperature, nonterminal process that can be used to process reusable heat-sensitive devices such as endoscopes and their accessories that cannot be processed using steam.

119. The items to be processed are placed in a dedicated tray, then placed into the tabletop unit. The sterilant circulates through the tray, contacting all surfaces of the items. Items are then rinsed with filtered and UV-treated water.

120. Items with internal lumens are connected to irrigator adapters to ensure sterilant contact within the lumens. It is important to ensure that devices with lumens are fitted with the appropriate irrigator adaptors prior to processing. The manufacturer of each device should be consulted to determine if the device is validated for use in a liquid peracetic acid processing system. Both the device manufacturer and the liquid chemical sterilant processor manufacturer should be consulted to determine the appropriate irrigator adaptor(s).

121. Contact time is standardized at 12 minutes at a temperature of 50°C to 55°C (122°F to 131°F). A rinse period follows the contact period; the rinse time depends on the water temperature and fill time. An entire cycle takes less than 30 minutes.

122. Following processing, the circulating nurse opens the lid, retrieves the tray, transports it to the operating room, and opens it. The sterile scrub person removes the items (which are wet) from the tray and places them on the sterile field.

123. Processing using liquid chemical peracetic acid is a "just in time" process. Processed items must be used immediately; they cannot be packaged and stored for later use. Processed items that are not delivered to the sterile field are hand dried and returned to storage for future processing; these stored items are not considered sterile.

124. No biological indicator for this system is currently available. The system uses microprocessors to ensure that the required parameters are met.

Advantages

125. Advantages of liquid chemical peracetic acid processing include the following features:

- The cycle is less than 30 minutes and offers quick turnaround time.

- Peracetic acid is combined with anticorrosive and buffering agents that prevent corrosion of instruments and render the sterilant nontoxic to personnel and the environment.

- Liquid chemical peracetic acid processing is compatible with many materials that cannot withstand sterilization using existing sterilization technologies.

Disadvantages

126. Disadvantages of liquid chemical peracetic acid processing include the following features:

- The size of the tray used for processing does not permit large loads to be processed. Only one flexible scope can be processed at a time.

- Only immersible items that fit within the dedicated tray may be processed.

- Items are wet at the end of the cycle.

- Processed items must be used immediately. The nature of the process permits point-of-use processing but not storage. Processed items must be used immediately or dried and returned to storage for later processing; they cannot be left in the system to be used at a later time.

Chemical Sterilization: Low-Temperature Ozone/Hydrogen Peroxide

127. Ozone is an emerging low-temperature technology. Current technology combines ozone and hydrogen peroxide to form a powerful oxidizing agent. Highly reactive particles such as hydroxyl radicals (—OH) oxidize a variety of organic compounds. Ozone has an effect similar to plasma; however, ozone can penetrate lumens and hard-to-reach areas. At the end of the cycle, ozone and hydrogen peroxide are converted to nontoxic byproducts of oxygen and water. Cycle times for the currently available sterilizer are 46, 56, and 100 minutes.

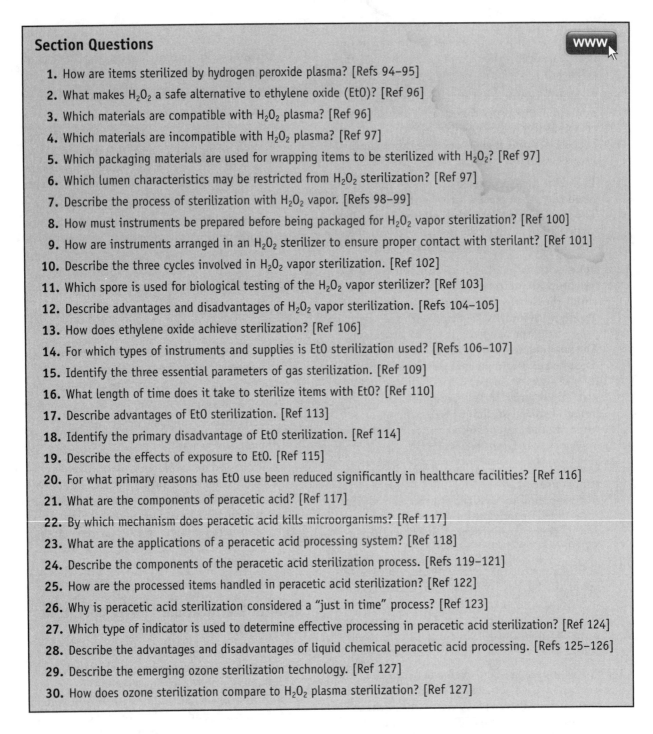

Section Questions

www

1. How are items sterilized by hydrogen peroxide plasma? [Refs 94–95]
2. What makes H_2O_2 a safe alternative to ethylene oxide (EtO)? [Ref 96]
3. Which materials are compatible with H_2O_2 plasma? [Ref 96]
4. Which materials are incompatible with H_2O_2 plasma? [Ref 97]
5. Which packaging materials are used for wrapping items to be sterilized with H_2O_2? [Ref 97]
6. Which lumen characteristics may be restricted from H_2O_2 sterilization? [Ref 97]
7. Describe the process of sterilization with H_2O_2 vapor. [Refs 98–99]
8. How must instruments be prepared before being packaged for H_2O_2 vapor sterilization? [Ref 100]
9. How are instruments arranged in an H_2O_2 sterilizer to ensure proper contact with sterilant? [Ref 101]
10. Describe the three cycles involved in H_2O_2 vapor sterilization. [Ref 102]
11. Which spore is used for biological testing of the H_2O_2 vapor sterilizer? [Ref 103]
12. Describe advantages and disadvantages of H_2O_2 vapor sterilization. [Refs 104–105]
13. How does ethylene oxide achieve sterilization? [Ref 106]
14. For which types of instruments and supplies is EtO sterilization used? [Refs 106–107]
15. Identify the three essential parameters of gas sterilization. [Ref 109]
16. What length of time does it take to sterilize items with EtO? [Ref 110]
17. Describe advantages of EtO sterilization. [Ref 113]
18. Identify the primary disadvantage of EtO sterilization. [Ref 114]
19. Describe the effects of exposure to EtO. [Ref 115]
20. For what primary reasons has EtO use been reduced significantly in healthcare facilities? [Ref 116]
21. What are the components of peracetic acid? [Ref 117]
22. By which mechanism does peracetic acid kills microorganisms? [Ref 117]
23. What are the applications of a peracetic acid processing system? [Ref 118]
24. Describe the components of the peracetic acid sterilization process. [Refs 119–121]
25. How are the processed items handled in peracetic acid sterilization? [Ref 122]
26. Why is peracetic acid sterilization considered a "just in time" process? [Ref 123]
27. Which type of indicator is used to determine effective processing in peracetic acid sterilization? [Ref 124]
28. Describe the advantages and disadvantages of liquid chemical peracetic acid processing. [Refs 125–126]
29. Describe the emerging ozone sterilization technology. [Ref 127]
30. How does ozone sterilization compare to H_2O_2 plasma sterilization? [Ref 127]

Sterilization: Quality Control

Overview

128. Before it can be assumed that a sterilizer is working properly and that an article can be considered sterile, certain parameters of time, humidity, pressure, and temperature must have been met. Chemical and mechanical process indicators and biological testing are used to monitor these parameters. Indicators provide an opportunity for a variety of personnel to check the process. The person removing the item from the sterilizer, the circulating nurse, and the scrub person all share responsibility for checking these monitors.

Physical Monitors

129. Physical monitors are graphs, temperature and pressure recorders, digital printouts, and gauges that record activities within the chamber during the sterilization cycle.
130. Historically, temperature graphs, using stylus and ink, indicated the temperature reached within the chamber and the length of time that this temperature was sustained, and provided information about the time of day during which the autoclave was used and the number of cycles run during a 24-hour period. Modern sterilizers employ a printout rather than a temperature graph.
131. A digital printout record correlates the exact times, temperatures, and pressures achieved during the conditioning, exposure, and exhaust phases of the sterilization cycle. The printout includes space for documentation items such as load identification and identity of the operator (Figure 3-5).
132. Gauges on the autoclave may register pressure and temperature within the jacket and the chamber. Gauges on the EtO sterilizer may register temperature, gas concentration, and humidity.
133. With liquid peracetic acid, a diagnostic cycle in which electricity supply, filters, temperature, pressure, and system integrity are checked is run at the beginning of each day, and a printout of the results is provided. A microprocessor system will abort the cycle if parameters are not met.

Chemical Indicators

134. Chemical indicators are impregnated with a dye or chemical that develops a visual or physical change when certain conditions have been achieved. Indicators are manufactured in the form of tapes, strips, or labels.
135. Chemical indicators referred to as integrators provide results that are based on the integration of some or all of the parameters that need to be met.
136. Chemical indicators should be placed both inside and outside of all packages. The chemical indicator on the outside of the package is inspected before the product is opened, and the ones inside are inspected after opening. It is possible that an outside indicator might indicate the proper conditions have been achieved, yet an inside indicator in the same product might fail. Improper packaging is one reason an inside indicator may fail while the outside one does not. Typically the circulating nurse, or whoever obtains the instruments for a procedure, will be the person in a position

```
========================
====== P R E V A C =====
========================
CYCLE START AT  8:43:23A
            ON  2/16/98

CYCLE COUNT           20
OPERATOR _____________
STERILIZER     VAC 00

    STER TEMP = 270.0F
 CONTROL TEMP = 273.0F
    STER TIME =  4 MIN
     DRY TIME = 20 MIN

                  V=inHg
- TIME       T= F P=psig
------------------------
C  8:43:35A 196.6     0P
C  8:44:35A 251.0    10P
C  8:45:42A 222.2    16V
C  8:46:13A 265.7    26P
C  8:47:31A 198.1    26V
C  8:47:57A 256.8    26P
C  8:49:13A 215.3    26V
C  8:49:40A 260.0    26P
C  8:50:57A 216.5    27V
S  8:51:33A 270.0    28P
S  8:52:33A 273.3    32P
S  8:53:33A 272.6    31P
S  8:54:33A 272.8    31P
S  8:55:33A 273.3    31P
E  8:55:33A 273.3    31P
E  8:55:54A 234.4     3P
E  9:15:55A 198.5    27V
Z  9:16:41A 200.1     2V

LOAD              021607

  TEMP MAX=273.9F
  TEMP MIN=270.0F

CONDITION    = 7:58
STERILIZE    = 4:00
EXHAUST      =21:08
TOTAL CYCLE  =33:06

PRINTOUT CHECKED BY:

------------------------

========================
=   READY TO UNLOAD    =
========================

* NOT READY    9:32:56A
DOOR OPEN
------------------------
```

Figure 3-5 Typical printout

Source: Copyright © Steris Corporation, Mentor, OH.

to inspect the outside indicator, and the scrub person will inspect the inside indicator.

137. Six classes of indicators are available:

- Class 1—Process indicator: Chemical indicator intended to demonstrate that the item has been exposed to the sterilization process. It typically consists of a tape or a paper strip that changes color and distinguishes between processed and unprocessed items. A Class 1 chemical indicator is an external indicator (Figure 3-6).
- Class 2—Bowie-Dick test indicator: Indicator designed to test the efficacy of air removal and steam penetration in dynamic-air-removal sterilizers.
- Class 3—Single-parameter indicator: Chemical indicator designed to react to one of the critical parameters of sterilization to indicate exposure to a sterilization cycle at a stated value of the chosen parameter.

- Class 4—Multiparameter indicator: Chemical indicator designed to react to two or more of the critical parameters of a sterilization cycle at stated values of the chosen parameters (Figure 3-7).
- Class 5—Integrating indicator: Chemical indicator designed to react to all critical parameters over a specified range of sterilization cycles and whose performance has been correlated to the performance of the stated test organism under the labeled conditions of use (AAMI, 2011, p. 103) (Figure 3-8).
- Class 6—Emulating indicator. A cycle-specific indicator that can be used only for the cycle specified in its instructions for use (Figure 3-9).

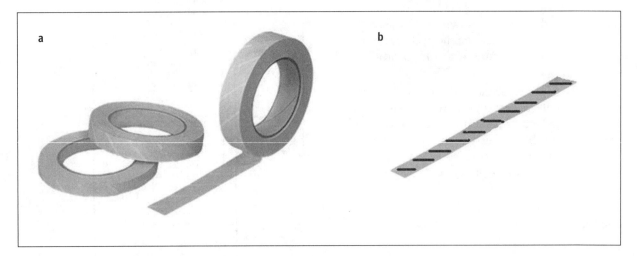

Figure 3-6 Class I process indicator (external) for steam sterilizer: a) before exposure b) after exposure

Source: Copyright © Steris Corporation, Mentor, OH.

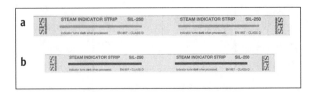

Figure 3-7 Class 4 multiparameter indicator for steam sterilizer: a) before exposure; b) after exposure

Source: Courtesy of SPSmedical, Rush, NY.

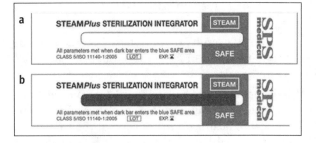

Figure 3-8 Class 5 integrating indicator: a) before exposure; b) after exposure

Source: Courtesy of SPSmedical, Rush, NY.

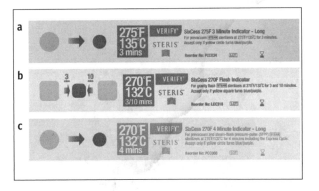

Figure 3-9 Class 6 emulating indicators for different steam sterilization cycles: a) 270°F/132°C 4 minute cycle; b) 275°F/135°C 3 minute cycle; c) IUSS 3 and 10 minute cycles

Source: Copyright © Steris Corporation, Mentor, OH.

138. Chemical indicators do not establish sterility. They are simply tools to determine whether conditions of sterilization have been met.

Biological Monitors

139. Biological monitoring is a process used to determine the efficacy of a sterilizer. It is the most accurate method of ensuring that the conditions necessary for sterilization have been achieved.

140. Biological indicators (BI) are available as capsules that contain a known, living, and highly resistant spore population; spore strips; and ampoules with spores suspended in the culture medium (Figures 3-10, 3-11, and 3-12).

141. *Geobacillus stearothermophilus* spores are used to test steam autoclaves and hydrogen peroxide sterilizers. Ethylene oxide sterilizers are tested with *Bacillus atrophaeus* spores. Both are highly resistant nonpathogenic microorganisms.

142. To routinely test the ability of the sterilizer to operate effectively, one or two strips, ampoules, or capsules containing the spores are placed at a specific location within the chamber, and the sterilizer is activated. For cycles used for terminal sterilization, the biological monitor should be contained within a process challenge device (PCD). A PCD is a device that constitutes a defined challenge to the sterilization process. It may be assembled by the user, but a commercially prepared PCD is commonly used. Commercially prepared PCDs are equivalent in performance to an AAMI BI test pack (Figure 3-13). For IUSS

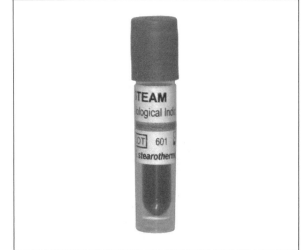

Figure 3-10 Self-contained biological indicators containing a known population of spores

Source: Courtesy of SPSmedical, Rush, NY.

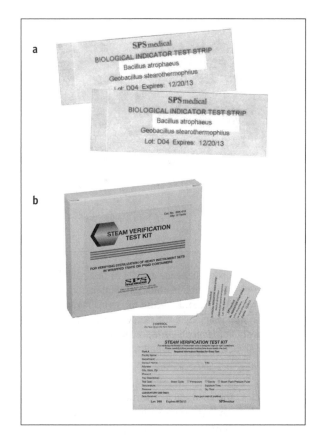

Figure 3-11 Biological indicator spore strips—dual (steam, EtO, dry heat, and chemical vapor): a) Hospitals sometimes send spore strips to an outside validation lab for third party verification; b) Clinics and office-based surgery often use a biological indicator mailing system.

Source: Courtesy of SPSmedical, Rush, NY.

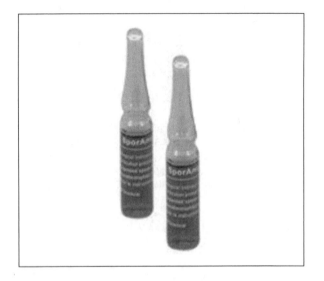

Figure 3-12 Spore ampoules—used primarily for monitoring liquid cycles in steam sterilizers

Source: Courtesy of SPSmedical, Rush, NY.

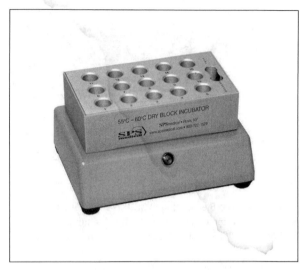

Figure 3-14 Self-contained biological incubator (note ampoule crusher to the right of the indicator wells…)

Source: Courtesy of SPSmedical, Rush, NY.

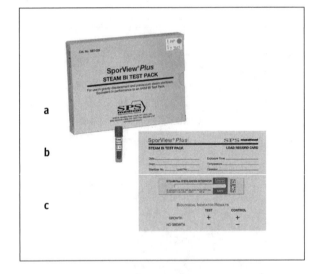
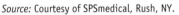

Figure 3-13 Process challenge device: a) test pack containing the self-contained biological indicator, an integrator, and a recording card for permanent documentation; b) ampoule with known quantity of *Geobacillus stearothermophilus*; c) recording card with integrator affixed to complete and file for documentation

Source: Courtesy of SPSmedical, Rush, NY.

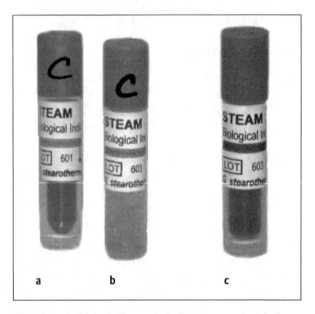

Figure 3-15 Biological capsule indicator control: a) before processing, marked clearly with a "C" for "control;" b) after incubation there is a change in color of ampoule contents indicating bacterial growth; c) biological capsule indicator that has been processed—there is a change in the color of the indicator strip compared to the control

Source: Courtesy of SPSmedical, Rush, NY.

cycles, the biological monitor is placed directly in the tray/container to be used, as the tray/container is considered to be the PCD.

143. Following the sterilization cycle, the spores are incubated. Capsules are crushed to expose spores to the culture medium. Spores in ampoules are already suspended in the culture medium. The length of their incubation varies according to the manufacturer's instructions. Growth is almost always visible within 24 hours; however, manufacturers are working to reduce biological incubation time (Figure 3-14).

144. A positive BI reading (demonstrating bacterial growth) indicates that sterilizing conditions have not been met; this indicates a "failed load" (Figure 3-15).

145. A positive BI should be reported immediately to the appropriate supervisor, the load quarantined, and the sterilizer taken out of service until the cause is determined.

146. In addition to sterilizer malfunction, a positive reading can indicate incorrect packaging, an incorrect cycle, items incompatible with the process, or incorrect placement within the sterilizer.

147. When the cause of the sterilizer failure can be immediately identified and the failure is confined to one load or one item within the load, corrective action is taken, the sterilizer is returned to service, and the load is reprocessed.

148. When the cause of failure is unknown, all items from the failed load must be recalled, as well as any items processed between that load and the last load with a negative BI.

149. The sterilizer is returned to service after repair and subsequent BI testing is negative

150. Identification of items to recall is made from the load/lot numbers, and SPD advises the operating room staff of those instruments and supplies to be recalled.

151. Because incubation of some biological indicators may be lengthy, because biological indicators may not be used with every load, and because sterilized items might be sent to the operating room prior to the receipt of biological testing results, a portion of the contents of the sterilizer may have been used.

152. It is essential that all of the items from the sterilizer be accounted for. Unused items are returned to the SPD for reprocessing; where items have been opened for procedures and patient exposure is known, facility policy determines the notification process, which usually involves the infection prevention staff and the operating surgeon.

153. Steam autoclaves should be tested at least weekly and preferably daily, and a BI should be run with every load containing an implant. EtO sterilizers should be tested with every load (AORN, 2012, p. 563). Hydrogen peroxide gas plasma and H_2O_2 vapor sterilizers should be tested daily.

154. Implants should not be implanted until the results of biological monitoring are known and are negative for growth.

Rapid-Readout Biological Monitors

155. A rapid-readout enzyme-based biological indicator is another type of monitor available for

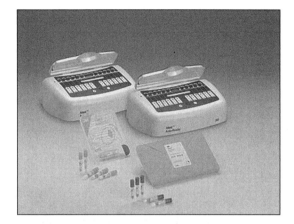

Figure 3-16 Rapid-readout biological monitor
Source: Courtesy of 3M Health Care, St. Paul, MN.

testing steam and ethylene oxide sterilizers (Figure 3-16).

156. Rapid-readout biological monitors for steam contain a standardized population of *Geobacillus stearothermophilus* spores. Ethylene oxide rapid-readout biological monitors contain a standardized population of *Bacillus atrophaeus* spores.

157. Fluorescence that occurs when an enzyme present within the *Geobacillus stearothermophilus* spores or *Bacillus atrophaeus* spores breaks down is noted by a color change that indicates that the conditions for sterilization have been achieved. The enzyme activity correlates to inactivation of the spores. Depending on the product used, a result is available within 1 to 3 hours after incubating. Because these monitors contain spores, it is possible, if desired, to incubate for a longer time to obtain spore testing results.

158. The benefit of a rapid-readout biological indicator is that monitoring results are available soon after testing. In the event that an emergency requires IUSS of an implant, a rapid-readout biological monitor should be used, as results can be obtained in 1 to 3 hours depending on which cycle is used.

159. Biological monitors are not interchangeable and must be selected according to the sterilizer type and the cycle being tested.

Sterilization: Documentation

160. The following records should be filed and kept as a permanent record:

- Results of Bowie-Dick/air evacuation test.
- Sterilizer graphs and printouts, which should be initialed by the operator for verification of cycle parameters. Everyone participating should initial the record (if one person puts in a load and another removes it, both persons should initial the document).

- Results of chemical and biological monitoring.
- Records indicating specific load contents and load control numbers used to designate which sterilizer was used for which items.
- Implantable biologic test results.
- Sterilizer failure results.

Section Questions

www

1. What are the parameters that must be assessed to ensure that a sterilizer is working properly? [Ref 128]
2. Who is responsible for checking to be sure that these parameters are met before introducing an item onto the sterile field? [Ref 128]
3. Which items are considered physical monitors? [Ref 129]
4. What is recorded on a digital printout? [Ref 131]
5. How is liquid peracetic processing monitored? [Ref 133]
6. How does a chemical indicator function? [Ref 134]
7. What is an integrator? [Ref 135]
8. Explain the purpose of using a chemical indicator both inside and outside of a package. [Ref 136]
9. Describe each of the six classes of indicators. [Ref 137]
10. In which type of sterilizer is the Class 2 (Bowie-Dick) indicator used? [Ref 137]
11. What is an emulating indicator (Class 6)? [Ref 137]
12. What is the purpose of a chemical indicator? [Ref 138]
13. What is the purpose of a biological monitor? [Ref 139]
14. Describe a biological monitor. [Ref 140]
15. Which spores are used to test steam, H_2O_2, and EtO sterilizers? [Ref 141]
16. What is a process challenge device? [Ref 142]
17. What is the implication of a positive BI? [Refs 144–145]
18. What might cause a BI to be positive? [Ref 146]
19. How is a positive BI managed? [Refs 147–152]
20. What is the minimum frequency for testing steam and EtO sterilizers with a BI? [Ref 153]
21. How is a BI used for implantable devices? [Ref 154]
22. How does a rapid-readout BI work? [Ref 157]
23. In what period of time can results be obtained from a rapid readout BI? [Ref 158]
24. How are BIs selected? [Ref 159]
25. What are the components of permanent documentation of sterilizer monitoring? [Ref 160]

161. IUSS records should be fully traceable to the patient on whom the instruments were used.

Disinfection

Overview

162. Disinfection is a process that destroys pathogenic microorganisms through the use of a liquid chemical germicide. A disinfectant is an agent that destroys vegetative forms of harmful microorganisms. Some disinfectants kill some spores; however, disinfectants do not kill high numbers of spores.

163. Chemicals used to destroy microorganisms on inanimate objects are identified as disinfectants. Chemicals used to destroy microorganisms on body surfaces are identified as antiseptics.

Levels of Disinfectants: Application

164. Disinfection is used to destroy pathogens on inanimate objects such as walls, tables, small equipment, and surgical instruments. Liquid chemicals are used for disinfection. Disinfectants must be selected according to their intended use. Disinfectants suitable for housekeeping purposes such as cleaning walls and surfaces are not suitable for disinfection of surgical instruments. Likewise, the most appropriate disinfecting agent for surgical instruments is not the most suitable for housekeeping.

165. Examples of disinfectants include alcohol, chlorine and chlorine compounds, formaldehyde, glutaraldehyde, hydrogen peroxide, iodophors, ortho-phthalaldehyde, phenolics, and quaternary ammonium compounds. Disinfectants vary in their ability to destroy microorganisms, and they are not interchangeable. Disinfectants are categorized as high level, intermediate level, and low level.

166. Factors that influence the efficacy of a disinfectant include the type of chemical, concentration and temperature of the chemical, amount and types of microorganisms present, configuration of the item to be disinfected, adequacy of prior cleaning, and exposure time.

167. High-level disinfectants kill all microorganisms, including vegetative bacteria forms, the tubercle bacilli, viruses, and fungi. They do not kill large numbers of spores, although some high-level disinfectants can achieve sterilization after prolonged exposure of 8 hours or more. Because waiting for such a long period of time is impractical and because a product that is intended for immediate use is needed, high-level disinfectants are not used for sterilizing instruments. Such disinfectants are used only for disinfecting instruments and medical devices; they are not used on environmental surfaces.

168. Intermediate-level disinfectants inactivate most vegetative bacteria, the tubercle bacillus, fungi, and viruses, but not necessarily bacterial spores. Low-level disinfectants kill most vegetative bacteria, some fungi, and some viruses; they do not kill the tubercle bacillus. Intermediate- and low-level disinfectants are formulated to be used on environmental surfaces and are never to be used on instruments and medical devices.

169. For instrument disinfection, only high-level disinfection is appropriate. The most frequently used high-level disinfectants are solutions of 2% to 3.2% alkaline glutaraldehyde or 0.55% ortho-phthalaldehyde.

170. Following exposure to the solution, the device must be thoroughly rinsed, preferably in sterile water. It is important to refer to the manufacturer's instructions, as some disinfectant products require as many as three separate rinses.

Glutaraldehyde

171. Glutaraldehyde is a commonly used high-level disinfectant. High-level disinfection is achieved in minutes, although the exact number of minutes varies with the concentration and temperature of the solution. The manufacturer's instructions and institutional policy should be consulted for the exact required immersion time.

172. Glutaraldehyde is irritating to mucous membranes and can irritate skin, eyes, throat, and nasal passages. It should be mixed in a well-ventilated room with a minimum of 10 air exchanges per hour. Local exhaust ventilation located at the level of the point of discharge is the preferred method of preventing vapor from escaping. Self-contained workstations with a fume hood should be installed where glutaraldehyde is used. Glutaraldehyde should always be stored in a closed container. Protective eyewear, nitrile gloves or a double set of latex gloves, a mask, and a repellent gown should be worn during use of glutaraldehyde. Exposure varies with the activity. Mixing and discarding the solution and immersing and retrieving items from the solution are the activities that pose the greatest risk of exposure.

173. Like all disinfectants, glutaraldehyde must be mixed and used strictly according to the manufacturer's instructions for use and the standards of practice. Information regarding mixing instructions, temperature, use, immersion time, toxicity, and length of effectiveness can be found on the product's label.

174. The current OSHA limit for exposure to glutaraldehyde is 0.2 part glutaraldehyde to 1 million parts air during any part of the work day. Monitoring of the work area and employee exposure is not required by OSHA; however, monitoring should be employed when high levels of exposure are suspected (OSHA, 2011).

175. Glutaraldehyde that is heated will achieve microbial killing faster than glutaraldehyde at

room temperature. Some automated systems are programmed to heat glutaraldehyde. However, when glutaraldehyde is heated, the vapor pressure is raised, which in turn increases the amount of vapor released into the air.

Ortho-phthalaldehyde

176. Ortho-phthalaldehyde (OPA) is a nonglutaraldehyde disinfectant widely used in operating rooms and endoscopy suites. Because it achieves disinfection faster than glutaraldehyde and does not release any irritating odors, OPA has replaced glutaraldehyde in many facilities.

177. Ortho-phthalaldehyde has a very low vapor pressure; as a result, it is rarely irritating to staff. There are no OSHA requirements and no monitoring requirements for OPA high-level disinfectants.

178. Ortho-phthalaldehyde will stain protein and items that are not thoroughly cleaned and rinsed prior to immersion. It will stain gray in spots where there are protein residuals.

Hydrogen Peroxide Vapor

179. Use of hydrogen peroxide vapor (HPV) to decontaminate healthcare spaces such as patient rooms or an operating room is an evolving technology that has recently been introduced in some facilities. Ozone hydrogen peroxide vapor is an advanced oxidative process providing a rapid and effective means of disinfecting healthcare spaces with numerous surface types and poorly accessible areas such as rooms vacated by patients with highly infectious pathogens (Zoutman et al., 2011, p. 873).

180. The advantages of vaporized biodecontamination compared to liquid cleaning agents include effective antimicrobial activity, wide dispersal, lack of residue, material compatibility, safety, and rapid turnaround time with limited disruption to the area under treatment (Galvin et al., 2012, p. 67). Application of this technology to operating rooms is fairly recent.

Disinfection: Quality Control

181. To avoid dilution of the disinfectant and compromise of the disinfection process, all items to be disinfected should be thoroughly cleaned, rinsed, and dried prior to immersion.

182. Disinfectant solutions have an expiration date that represents the length of anticipated effectiveness, as indicated on the label. Date of mixing and expiration date should be indicated on the container in which the disinfectant is stored.

183. A disinfectant can lose its minimum effective concentration before the expiration date. The number of times the solution is used, the amount of debris introduced into the solution, and any dilution that occurs when items are washed, rinsed, and not dried before immersion can all affect the minimum concentration and cause a solution to fail. One should never rely entirely on the label for proof of the expiration of the solution.

184. The minimum effective concentration (MEC) of disinfectant solutions should be monitored before each use with indicators designed for this purpose. These indicators are usually supplied in the form of paper or plastic strips that are dipped into the solution and then observed for appropriate color change as indicated on the label. Indicators are not interchangeable, and only those supplied with a particular product should be used to test that product.

185. Chemical properties and appropriate hazard warnings should be posted.

Disinfection: Documentation

186. When liquid chemical germicides are used for high-level disinfection, the following should be documented:
    - Results of quality control testing—performed according to the manufacturer's instructions
    - Results of testing for minimum effective concentration
    - Date solution is mixed/activated/opened/prepared
    - Expiration date—should be visible on the container
    - Person responsible for mixing
    - Item disinfected
    - Patient for whom disinfected item was used

Section Questions

1. Describe disinfection. [Refs 162, 164]

2. Differentiate between a disinfectant and an antiseptic. [Ref 163]

3. Identify some disinfectant chemicals. [Ref 165]

4. Explain the factors that that influence the efficacy of disinfection. [Ref 166]

5. Differentiate among high-, intermediate-, and low-level disinfection. [Refs 167–168]

6. Why are high-level disinfectants not often used to sterilize instruments? [Ref 167]

7. Which level of disinfection is used for surgical instruments? [Ref 169]

8. How is a high-level disinfected instrument prepared for patient use? [Ref 170]

9. Which factors affect the length of time it takes to disinfect an item with glutaraldehyde? [Ref 171]

10. Describe the responsibilities associated with using glutaraldehyde. [Refs 172–173]

11. What is the impact of heat on glutaraldehyde? [Ref 175]

12. Compare ortho-phthalaldehyde with glutaraldehyde. [Ref 176]

13. Describe the characteristics of OPA. [Refs 177–178]

14. How is hydrogen peroxide vapor used as a disinfectant? [Ref 179]

15. What are the advantages of HPV? [Ref 180]

16. Describe the importance of cleaning, rinsing, and drying items before beginning the process of disinfection. [Ref 181]

17. Discuss the implications of the expiration date on prepared disinfectant solutions. [Refs 182–183]

18. How is the minimum effective concentration of disinfectants determined? [Ref 184]

19. How should the environment in which chemical disinfectants are used be managed? [Ref 185]

20. Discuss documentation related to liquid chemical disinfection. [Ref 186]

● ● ● **References**

Alexander JW, Solomkin JS, Edwards MJ (2011). Updated recommendations for control of surgical site infections: systemic prophylactic antibiotics. *Ann Surg*;253(6):1082–1093. © 2011 Lippincott Williams & Wilkins. Available at: www.medscape.com/viewarticle/742992_11. Accessed September 2012.

Association for the Advancement of Medical Instrumentation (AAMI) (2011). *Comprehensive Guide to Steam Sterilization and Sterility Assurance in Health Care Facilities* (ANSI/AAMI ST79:2006). Arlington, VA: AAMI.

Association of periOperative Registered Nurses (AORN) (2012). *Perioperative Standards and Recommended Practices*. Denver, CO: AORN.

Centers for Disease Control and Prevention (CDC) (2012). Procedure-associated events: surgical site infection (SSI) event. Available at: www.cdc.gov/nhsn/PDFs/pscManual /9pscSSIcurrent.pdf. Accessed September 2012.

Edmiston C, Spencer M, Lewis B, et al. (2011). Reducing the risk of surgical site infections: did we really think SCIP was going to lead us to the promised land? *Surg Infect*;12(8):169–177.

Favero M, Bond W (2001). Chemical disinfection of medical and surgical materials. In Block SS, ed. *Disinfection, Sterilization, and Preservation,* 5th ed. Philadelphia: Lippincott Williams & Wilkins; 881–915.

Galvin S, Boyle M, Russell R, et al. (2012). Evaluation of a vaporized hydrogen peroxide, Citrox and pH neutral Ecasol for decontamination of an enclosed area: a pilot study. *J Hosp Infect*;80:67–70.

Institute for Healthcare Improvement (IHI) (2012). *How-to Guide: Prevent Surgical Site Infections*. Cambridge, MA: Institute for Healthcare Improvement. (Available at www .ihi.org). Accessed September 2012.

Linkin D, Sausman C, Santos L, et al. (2005). Applicability of healthcare failure mode and effects analysis to healthcare epidemiology: evaluation of the sterilization and use of surgical instruments. *Clin Infect Dis*;41(7):1014–1019. Available at: http://cid.oxfordjournals.org/content/41/7/1014.long. Accessed September 2012.

Mangram A, Horan T, Pearson M, et al. (1999). Guideline for prevention of surgical site infection. *Infect Control Hosp Epidemiol*;20(4):261.

Occupational Safety and Health Administration (OSHA) (2011). *Toxic and Hazardous Substances: Ethylene Oxide.: Occupation Safety and Health Standards*. Regulations and Standards 29CFR. 1910.1047. Washington, DC: OSHA. Available at: www.osha.gov/pls/oshaweb/owadisp.show_document?p_table=standards&p_id=10070. Accessed September 2012.

Perkins JJ (1969). *Principles and Methods of Sterilization*. Springfield, IL: Charles C. Thomas.

Rizzo T, Culvert L (2004). Hospital-acquired infections. In *The Gale Encyclopedia of Surgery: A Guide for Patients and Caregivers*. Farmington Hills, MI: The Gale Group Inc.

Zoutman D, Shannon M, Mandel A (2011). Effectiveness of a novel ozone-based system for the rapid high-level disinfection of health are spaces and surfaces. *Am J Infect Control*;39(10): 873–879.

Post-Test

Read each question carefully. A question may have more than one correct answer.

1. Disinfection differs from sterilization in what way?
    a. High-level disinfection and sterilization are the same.
    b. Sterilization kills all spores; disinfection does not.
    c. High-level disinfection kills vegetative bacteria; sterilization does not.
    d. Disinfection and sterilization both kill microorganisms, but only sterilization may be used for all medical devices

2. Which of the following definitions are correct? (More than one definition may be correct.)
    a. Bioburden represents the population of viable organisms on an item.
    b. A Bowie-Dick test demonstrates that air and noncondensable gases are adequately removed from the chamber of a steam sterilizer.
    c. An autoclave is another term for gravity-displacement steam sterilizer.
    d. A chemical indicator is a sterilization monitor with a known population of resistant spores.

3. Which statement(s) is (are) true?
    a. Surgical-site infections are the second leading cause of hospital-acquired infection.
    b. Contaminated surgical instruments are a potential source of infection.
    c. Perioperative nursing activities are directed at preventing infection.
    d. Sterilization and disinfection are cornerstones of infection prevention.

4. If instruments are processed outside of the operating room, why does the perioperative nurse need to know about sterilization and disinfection?
    a. Perioperative nurses rotate through the SPD and need to be prepared.
    b. Perioperative nurses must have a frame of reference when they are complaining to the SPD about instruments.
    c. The perioperative nurse is a partner in the process and assumes varying degrees of responsibility for the care and preparation of instruments.
    d. Instrument processing is a core competency in most operating rooms.

5. Critical items
    a. contact sterile tissue and the vascular system.
    b. must undergo high-level disinfection.
    c. do not penetrate mucous membranes.
    d. include thermometers, crutches, and blood pressure cuffs.

6. Semicritical items include
    a. surgical instruments.
    b. cystoscopes and laryngoscopes.
    c. blood pressure cuffs and crutches.
    d. thermometers and sequential compression devices.

7. The sterility assurance level is
    a. the number of organisms killed during sterilization.
    b. the amount of time it takes to kill 1 million organisms.
    c. a mathematical expression of the time, temperature, and pressure needed to kill microorganisms.
    d. a mathematical expression of the probability of a viable microorganism being present on an item after sterilization.

8. Spores are used to test for sterility because they are
    a. more resistant than any other bacteria to heat, drying, and chemicals.
    b. easier to process, incubate, and analyze.
    c. larger than bacteria and easier to see.
    d. a form of bacteria that is also representative of viruses and fungi.

9. The choice of sterilization method depends on
    a. what is most convenient for the facility.
    b. what is least expensive and readily available.
    c. the compatibility of the item with the sterilization process.
    d. the type of wrapping that must be used for sterilization.

10. For an item to be sterilized,
    a. it must be sequentially wrapped and placed upright in the sterilizer.
    b. steam must penetrate the packaging completely and the intended parameters of moisture, temperature, and time must be met.
    c. it must be subjected to unsaturated steam for the appropriate amount of time and under the correct amount of pressure.
    d. the temperature must remain at 250°F at atmospheric pressure for the proper amount of time.

11. Which statement(s) is (are) true about steam sterilization?
    a. Moist heat under pressure is economical.
    b. Steam sterilization denatures and coagulates protein.
    c. Steam sterilization occurs at atmospheric pressure.
    d. Steam sterilization is a function of time and temperature.

12. What are some advantages of steam sterilization?
    a. One cycle time is appropriate for all items.
    b. Cycles are preprogrammed to prevent operator error.
    c. It is inexpensive and sterilization is achieved quickly.
    d. It is suitable for all surgical instruments.

13. Which statement(s) is (are) true about autoclaves?
    a. Air trapped in the chamber will interfere with sterilization.
    b. Sterilization begins only when the correct temperature has been reached.
    c. Cups and basins must be placed so that water will collect in them and form steam.
    d. Wrapped packages should be removed from the sterilizer immediately and allowed to cool for 2 hours.

14. How might trapping of air in a steam autoclave interfere with sterilization?
    a. The presence of air forces the temperature above the target range.
    b. Air in the chamber prevents the sterilizer from reaching the target pressure.
    c. Air interferes with the humidity level in the chamber.
    d. Air pockets prevent steam from contacting all surfaces of an item, compromising the sterilization process.

15. Which statement(s) is (are) true about steam sterilizers?
    a. A Bowie-Dick test is done once each day in all gravity-displacement sterilizers.
    b. A prevacuum sterilizer is more efficient and preferred over a gravity-displacement sterilizer.
    c. Prevacuum sterilizers are used for liquids.
    d. Prevacuum sterilizers are less affected by incorrect arrangement of objects in the chamber.

16. Which statement(s) is (are) true about immediate-use steam sterilization?
    a. IUSS is not intended for sterilizing sets of instruments.
    b. Items sterilized with IUSS cannot be stored or held for use on a future case.
    c. Drying time is the same in IUSS as with regular sterilization.
    d. In an emergency, items can be rinsed in the scrub sink and sterilized with IUSS.

17. Which statement(s) is (are) true about immediate-use steam sterilization?
    a. IUSS is perfect for implants that arrive immediately before a procedure.
    b. IUSS is appropriate only in urgent clinical situations.
    c. IUSS is appropriate when there is only one specialty set of instruments.
    d. IUSS can be done only in a prevacuum sterilizer.

18. Which statement(s) is (are) true about immediate-use steam sterilization?
    a. Only devices with manufacturer's instructions for IUSS should be sterilized in this manner.
    b. There is risk of contamination during transport following IUSS.
    c. Items for IUSS cannot be wrapped.
    d. A rigid container should be used for IUSS.

19. What are some advantages of H_2O_2 sterilization?
    a. Items to be sterilized can be wrapped in any material.
    b. There is a single cycle for all items.
    c. The process is an efficient alternative to EtO sterilization.
    d. Cycle times are preset and the sterilizer is easy to operate.

20. The spore used to monitor H_2O_2 sterilization is
    a. *Bacilllus atrophaeus.*
    b. *Geobacillis atrophaeus.*
    c. *Geobacillus stearothermophilus.*
    d. *Bacillus subtilis.*

21. Which packaging materials can be used for H_2O_2 sterilization?
    a. muslin wrappers
    b. Tyvek pouches
    c. polypropylene wraps
    d. Mylar pouches

22. Which statement(s) is (are) true about EtO sterilization?
    a. EtO is a toxic gas that must be managed according to strict regulations.
    b. EtO is appropriate for items that cannot tolerate the temperature and moisture of steam sterilization.
    c. The essential parameters of EtO sterilization are gas concentration, temperature, humidity, and exposure time.
    d. Aeration must be done for all loads sterilized using EtO.

23. What are some advantages of EtO sterilization?
    a. The process is rapid.
    b. The process is safe for items that cannot tolerate high heat and humidity.
    c. EtO is noncorrosive.
    d. EtO effectively penetrates large bundles and permeates all porous items.

24. Which statement(s) is (are) true about liquid chemical processing?
    a. It is a low-temperature, nonterminal process.
    b. Items must be used immediately following processing; they cannot be packaged or stored for later use.
    c. Only one flexible endoscope can be processed at a time.
    d. Peracetic acid disrupts protein bonds and cell systems, causing immediate cell death.

25. Which statement(s) is (are) true about sterilization monitoring?
    a. Physical monitors record activities within the sterilizer chamber.
    b. Chemical indicators exhibit a visual or physical change when sterilization has been achieved.
    c. A chemical indicator should be placed both on the inside and on the outside of each package.
    d. The nurse relies on the outside indicator to determine whether the contents of a sterilized package are sterile.

26. A Class 5 indicator is
    a. A process indicator that demonstrates an item has been exposed to the sterilization process.
    b. A single-parameter indicator designed to react to one of the critical parameters of the sterilization process.
    c. An integrator that reacts to all of the critical parameters of the sterilization process.
    d. A multiparameter indicator that reacts to two or more parameters of the sterilization process.

27. Which statement(s) is (are) true about biological indicators?
    a. A biological indicator is the most accurate method of establishing that the conditions of sterilization have been met.
    b. A biological indicator contains a known quantity of a highly resistant virus.
    c. A biological indicator must be incubated before it can be read.
    d. A biological indicator should be contained within a process challenge device (PCD) for cycles used for terminal sterilization.

28. Which statement(s) is (are) true about a "failed load"?
    a. It should be reported immediately, the load quarantined, and the cause of failure researched.
    b. Failure can be caused by incorrect packaging, incorrect cycle, items incompatible with the process, or incorrect placement within the sterilizer.
    c. In any instance, all items from the failed load must be located and recalled for reprocessing.
    d. Items from a failed load that have already been used in or for a patient must be reported to TJC.

29. Which statement(s) is (are) true about biological monitors?
    a. Rapid-readout enzyme-based biological indicators are available for steam and EtO sterilizers.
    b. Rapid-readout monitors rely on fluorescence, which occurs when an enzyme present within the bacterial spore breaks down, to determine that the conditions for sterilization have been met.
    c. Rapid readouts show results within 30 minutes.
    d. A rapid readout can be used if an implant must be sterilized using IUSS.

30. Documentation of sterilization should include
    a. a supervisor's signature for every sterilizer load.
    b. records indicating which sterilizer was used for which items.
    c. an indication that biological tests were run in every sterilizer twice a day.
    d. Bowie-Dick test results for gravity-displacement sterilizers.

Competency Checklist: Sterilization and Disinfection

Under "Observer's Initials," enter initials upon successful achievement of the competency. Enter N/A if the competency is not appropriate for the institution.

Name _____

	Observer's Initials	Date
1. Identifies appropriate method of sterilization for item to be sterilized.	_____	_____
2. Steam sterilization		
a. Sets appropriate cycle	_____	_____
b. Sets appropriate time	_____	_____
c. Sets appropriate temperature	_____	_____
d. Places appropriate chemical indicator inside and outside of package	_____	_____
e. Selects tray compatible with sterilization method	_____	_____
f. Packages correctly	_____	_____
g. Loads correctly—sterilant can exit and enter packages	_____	_____
h. Documents required information	_____	_____
i. Operates sterilizer according to the manufacturer's instructions	_____	_____
j. Observes printout/indicator for parameters	_____	_____
k. (IUSS) Transports without contamination following sterilization	_____	_____
l. (Wrapped) Allows package to cool before removing from autoclave	_____	_____
3. Biological monitor—steam		
a. Selects appropriate monitor	_____	_____
b. Documents date, autoclave, and operator	_____	_____
c. Places biological indicator correctly within the chamber (follows the manufacturer's instructions for placement)	_____	_____
d. Sets appropriate cycle, time, and temperature	_____	_____
e. Incubates processed biological monitor and control according to the manufacturer's instructions	_____	_____
4. Hydrogen peroxide gas plasma sterilization	_____	_____
a. Places appropriate indicator outside and inside of package	_____	_____
b. Selects tray or container appropriate for sterilization process	_____	_____
c. Packages correctly	_____	_____
d. Loads correctly	_____	_____
e. Operates sterilizer according to the manufacturer's instructions	_____	_____
f. Documents required information	_____	_____
5. Biological monitor—hydrogen peroxide gas plasma		
a. Selects appropriate monitor	_____	_____
b. Documents date, sterilizer, and operator	_____	_____
c. Correctly places within chamber (follows the manufacturer's instructions for placement)	_____	_____
d. Incubates processed biological monitor and control according to the manufacturer's instructions	_____	_____

Observer's
Initials   Date

6. Disinfection
   a. Identifies items appropriate for high-level disinfection   _____   _____
   b. Prepares disinfectant according to the manufacturer's instructions   _____   _____
   c. Wears appropriate personal protective equipment during preparation
      of disinfectant and use   _____   _____
   d. Performs the MEC test and documents results   _____   _____
   e. Documents required information   _____   _____
7. Items are:
   a. Appropriately washed and dried before being disinfected   _____   _____
   b. Rinsed after being disinfected and before use
   c. Handled so as to prevent contamination

Observer's Signature   Initials   Date

_____

Orientee's Signature

_____

4

Prevention of Infection
Preparation of Instruments and Items Used in Surgery: Cleaning, Packaging, and Storage

---

LEARNER OBJECTIVES

1. Discuss the relationship of cleaning, packaging, and storage of sterile supplies to patient outcomes of freedom from infection and freedom from injury.
2. Describe the responsibilities of the registered nurse in relation to cleaning, packaging, and storage of sterile supplies.
3. Discuss the decontamination process for surgical instruments, including instruments exposed to prions.
4. Explain the role of ultrasonic cleaning in instrument decontamination.
5. List six criteria for packaging materials.
6. Discuss four principles of packaging.
7. Compare use, advantages, and disadvantages of packing materials.
8. Explain shelf life.
9. Discuss reuse of single-use devices.

www

LESSON OUTLINE

Nursing Diagnosis: Desired Patient Outcomes

1. The nursing diagnoses of "increased risk for infection" and "free from injury" are appropriate for patients undergoing invasive procedures. Infection may result from contact with

contaminated instruments, and instrumentation that fails to function properly can result in patient injury. The desired outcome is that the patient will be free from infection and free from injury following the procedure. Many perioperative nursing activities contribute to the achievement of these outcomes. Among these are cleaning, inspection, packaging, and storage of sterile instruments and supplies (e.g., surgical instruments, diagnostic devices, and other reusable patient care items).

Nursing Responsibilities

2. The perioperative nurse assumes varying levels of responsibility for cleaning, packaging, and storage of sterile supplies. There is no single cleaning or packaging process that is appropriate for all supplies. The processes involved require judgment based on comprehensive knowledge of scientific principles of cleaning, inspection, packaging, sterilization, and storage of sterile instruments and supplies.

3. Most instrument preparation and processing is accomplished in a separate sterile processing department (SPD) or area. Although the perioperative nurse may not make a hands-on contribution to these processes, the nurse must be a resource for those who do. More importantly, the perioperative nurse must be able to identify that specified requirements of cleaning, inspection, packaging, sterilization, and storage of

supplies or instruments have been met. The perioperative nurse makes the final decision as to whether an item is fit to be delivered to the sterile field for use on a patient.

4. In the event that immediate-use steam sterilization (IUSS) or high-level disinfection is required, the perioperative nurse may assume total responsibility for cleaning, inspection, and packaging, as well as for the sterilization or disinfection process.

5. As an advocate for the patient, with the goals of freedom from infection and injury, the perioperative nurse must be able to ensure that all instruments used in surgery have been appropriately prepared and processed and are in good working order. Improperly prepared or processed instruments and supplies that harbor microorganisms and items that fail to function as intended can result in infection or injury.

Preparation of Items and Instruments for Sterilization

Cleaning

6. All instruments and devices intended to penetrate a mucous membrane must be subject to a sterilization process. All instruments and devices intended to contact but not penetrate an intact mucous membrane must be at least high-level disinfected.

Definitions

Biofilm: A collection of microscopic organisms that exist in a polysaccharide matrix that adheres to a surface and prevents antimicrobial agents such as sterilants, disinfectants, and antibiotics from reaching the cells.

Cavitation: In an ultrasonic washer, the process by which high-intensity sound waves generate tiny bubbles that expand until they collapse or implode, causing a negative pressure on the surfaces of the instruments that dislodges soil.

Contaminated: (1) In the operating room environment, a term referring to items that are not sterile. Items soiled or potentially soiled with microorganisms are considered to be contaminated. Items that were opened for surgery, whether or not they were actually used during surgery and whether or not they are known to contain microorganisms, are also considered to be contaminated. (2) In the regulatory arena, a term referring to an item that has been in contact with an infectious agent.

Decontamination: The process that renders a contaminated item safe for handling. Decontamination may be accomplished manually or with an automated system.

Event-related sterility: A sterile item remains sterile until an event happens to render that package unsterile.

Washer-disinfector, washer-decontaminator: Automated processing units used to decontaminate instruments. Cycles within these machines vary but include washing and rinsing and may include ultrasonic cleaning. A chemical or thermal phase within the cycle destroys specific microorganisms.

7. The first and most important step in instrument decontamination is cleaning.

8. Effective sterilization and disinfection depend on proper decontamination. An instrument can be clean but not sterile, but no instrument can be sterile if it has not first been properly cleaned.

Intraoperative Cleaning

9. Contaminated instruments, including all instruments opened for a surgical procedure in an invasive procedure room, whether or not they are used, should be washed as soon as possible after use to prevent blood and other debris from drying in crevices or on instrument surfaces. Dried-on debris can interfere with the sterilization or disinfection processes by preventing the sterilizing or disinfecting agent from contacting every surface of every item.

10. During the surgical procedure, instruments should be periodically wiped and/or rinsed with a moist lap sponge or immersed in sterile water to remove large particles and to prevent debris from lodging in serrations and other crevices. Instrument lumens should be kept free of debris by immersing the device so as to fill the lumen with sterile water or by irrigating the channels using a syringe filled with sterile water. Irrigation should take place below the surface of the water to prevent aerosolization of particles.

11. Sterile water, not saline, should be used for cleaning items during surgery. Blood and body fluids as well as saline are highly corrosive, and can cause rusting and pitting (AORN, 2012, p. 515).

12. All instruments opened for a procedure are considered contaminated whether or not they are actually used. Used instruments should be returned to their sets, and instruments sets should be intact when they arrive in the SPD for processing.

Postoperative Cleaning

13. Instruments should be subject to a cleaning process as soon after surgery as possible. They should be transported to the dedicated decontamination area in a leak-proof container. The purpose of containment is to prevent personnel from contacting contaminated items during transfer (AAMI, 2011, p. 48). Place contaminated materials that are to be decontaminated at a site away from the work in a durable, leak-proof, labeled or color-coded container that is closed before being removed from the work area [OSHA, 29CFR 1910.1030 (e) (2) (ii) (B), 2012].

14. No instruments—even a single instrument intended for IUSS—should be washed in the scrub sink.

15. To prevent debris from drying on instruments, a damp towel may be used to cover them during transport. An enzymatic soak solution, spray, or gel may also be used before transport. These activities facilitate effective cleaning in the SPD and help prevent corrosion, rusting, and pitting that can occur when blood and debris are allowed to dry on instruments.

16. Instruments should not remain in water for lengthy periods of time, as biofilms may form, particularly within lumens. Once formed, a biofilm can be removed only by mechanical means. Biofilms can pose a serious threat to health. In addition to compromising the disinfection and sterilization processes, biofilm can break free from the surface of a device inside the patient's body, resulting in a massive infusion of bacteria that can cause an infection that is difficult to treat. Because the biofilm lives within a self-made protective glycocalyx, it may be 50 to 500 times more resistant to antibiotics (Center for Biofilm Engineering, 2011).

17. Before instruments are cleaned, the following steps should be taken:
    - Blades should be removed before instruments and/or equipment are placed in a containment device for transport.
    - Drill bits should be removed.
    - Sharp instruments, such as scissors and osteotomes, should be segregated from general instruments.
    - Box locks and other joints should be opened.
    - Before transport, heavy instruments should be placed in the bottom of the tray, with lighter ones on top.
    - Before decontamination, devices with multiple components should be disassembled; the parts should remain together.

Manual Cleaning

18. In the absence of an automated washer, instruments may be manually cleaned. Mechanical cleaning in an automated system is preferable

because the process is consistent. Nevertheless, manual cleaning can be equally effective if performed correctly.

19. Additionally, some powered surgical instruments and some heat-sensitive, delicate, or specialty items cannot tolerate immersion or mechanical washing. These items should be cleaned separately according to the device manufacturer's written guidelines.

20. When instruments are manually cleaned, regardless of whether they are cleaned in the decontamination section of the SPD or in a decontamination area within the operating room, it is important for the process to be standardized. Regardless of the location, the following supplies and equipment should be readily available:

    - Enzymatic detergent
    - Soft-bristle brushes of various sizes
    - Syringes for irrigation of lumens
    - Adaptors and accessories for specific devices as required by the manufacturer's instructions
    - An eyewash station
    - Compressed air
    - Personal protective equipment (PPE)

21. In addition, the decontamination area should have negative air pressure, with a minimum of 10 air exchanges occurring per hour (AAMI, 2011, p. 28; AORN, 2012, p. 221).

22. Before washing with a detergent, instruments should be rinsed in cold water to remove gross debris. Hot water coagulates protein and makes the cleaning process more difficult.

23. The detergent should be specific for instrument cleaning and should be used strictly according to the manufacturer's instructions. For example, mixing detergents to a higher concentration because of heavy debris is not appropriate and may, in fact, impede rinsing, thereby interfering with the sterilization or disinfection process. Detergents for instrument cleaning usually contain one or more enzymes.

24. During manual cleaning, personnel should wear PPE (i.e., a liquid-resistant covering, long-cuffed utility gloves, a mask, and eye protection [goggles or full-face shield]) (AAMI, 2011, p. 57).

25. Immersible items should be cleaned below the surface of the water to prevent aerosolization of debris. Lumens and cannulas should be flushed while submerged. Items that cannot be immersed should be cleaned in a manner that prevents aerosolization of debris. Soft-bristle brushes or pipe cleaners may be used to remove soil from hard-to-reach places such as hinges and serrations. Abrasive cleaners, scouring pads, metal brushes, or steel wool should not be used on surgical instruments.

Mechanical Cleaning

26. Instruments cleaned in an automated system are placed in trays with a wire open-mesh bottom. Trays are then placed in a washer-disinfector/decontaminator, where mechanical cleaning occurs.

27. Washer-sterilizers have a tendency to bake organic debris onto instruments that might not have been adequately cleaned; for this reason, decontamination is usually accomplished in a washer-disinfector/decontaminator that does not have a sterilization phase. Most facilities no longer use a washer-sterilizer, but instead use a washer-disinfector/decontaminator.

28. A washer-disinfector/decontaminator may have a variety of cycles. Phases in the cycle may include cool water rinse, enzymatic soak or rinse, detergent wash, ultrasonic cleaning, hot water rinse ($180°F–195°F$ [$70°C–76°C$]), demineralized water rinse, and drying.

29. Instruments that have been processed in a washer-disinfector/decontaminator or are manually washed are considered safe to handle, but are not ready for immediate patient use and are not considered sterile.

Special Protocols
Eye Instruments

30. Sometimes the perioperative nurse might be responsible for cleaning and sterilizing eye instruments within the operating room. Proper cleaning protocol must be followed to prevent patient injury.

31. Although the principles for cleaning are similar for all instruments, eye instruments require special attention. These instruments are delicate and for the most part cannot be cleaned in automated systems. Manual cleaning methods

are not as controlled as mechanical methods; hence, special care must be taken to ensure adequate cleaning.

32. Inadequately cleaned eye instruments can cause toxic anterior segment syndrome (TASS), a noninfectious inflammation of the anterior segment of the eye that can result in blindness. Most cases of TASS result from the introduction into the anterior chamber of the eye of foreign material that was not removed during cleaning and sterilization. Endotoxins from gram-negative bacteria in ultrasonic cleaners, viscoelastic solution used during eye surgery, and detergent and disinfectant residue have been associated with TASS and the processing of intraocular surgical instruments (AAMI, 2011, p. 229).

33. It is essential to clean eye instruments in accordance with the manufacturer's instructions. Eye instruments are delicate and have extremely small lumens. Thorough cleaning of lumens immediately following use is essential to ensure removal of debris that may be responsible for TASS.

34. Several organizations have established guidelines that should be referenced for detailed instructions on processing ophthalmic instruments.

    - Association of periOperative Registered Nurses (AORN): "Recommended Practices for Cleaning and Care of Instruments and Powered Instruments"
    - American Society of Cataract and Refractive Surgery (ASCRS) and the American Society of Ophthalmic Registered Nurses guidelines (ASORN): "Care and Handling of Ophthalmic Microsurgical Instruments"

Instruments Exposed to Prions (ANSI/AAMI, 2011)

35. A prion is an infectious protein particle. Prions are responsible for transmissible spongiform encephalopathies such as Creutzfeldt-Jakob disease (CJD), a rare and always fatal disease of the central nervous system. Unlike bacteria, viruses, and fungi, prions are resistant to routine sterilization and disinfection procedures. Instruments that have, or are suspected to have, come in contact with prions should be cleaned and sterilized according to special protocols.

36. Information and protocols regarding prions is evolving. The Centers for Disease Control and Prevention (CDC) and AORN are two agencies that should be consulted when determining protocols for instruments exposed to prions.

37. The brain, spinal cord, and dura mater are considered high-risk tissue for transmission of prion disease (AORN, 2012, p. 528). Instruments exposed to these tissues in patients known or suspected to be infected with a prion disease require special consideration with regard to decontamination. As a guideline, the following steps should be taken for decontaminating instruments exposed, or suspected to have been exposed, to prions:

    - Keep instruments moist until cleaned or decontaminated.
    - Clean the instruments as soon as possible to minimize drying of tissue, blood, and body fluids on the instruments.
    - At the point of use, avoid mixing instruments exposed to high-risk tissue (e.g., brain, dura mater, spinal cord, eye) with instruments used on other tissue.

38. Instruments exposed to high-risk tissue must be decontaminated using the following protocols:

    - For instruments that are easily cleaned, steam autoclave them, after thorough cleaning, at 272°F (134°C) for 18 minutes in a prevacuum sterilizer or at 250°F (121°C) for 60 minutes in a gravity-displacement autoclave/cycle.
    - For instruments that are difficult to clean or have small lumens:
        - Discard the instruments.
          Or
        - Immerse the instruments in a container filled with liquid (e.g., saline, water, or phenolic solution) to retard adherence of material to the device. Drain the liquid, and then initially decontaminate by steam sterilization at 272°F (134°C) for 18 minutes in a prevacuum sterilization cycle or at 250°F (121°C) for 1 hour in a gravity cycle.
          Or
        - Soak for 60 minutes, as recommended by the World Health Organization (WHO) in 1 normal sodium hydroxide (1N NaOH). This method can create dangerous vapors and damage instruments.

    Follow either of the preceding two steps with conventional cleaning, wrapping, and sterilizing (AAMI, 2011, Annex C; Rutala and Weber, 2010, pp. 113–114).

39. The perioperative nurse should follow institutional policies and procedures, and conduct a patient assessment to identify those patients who are at high risk for prion disease and to identify those procedures with the potential to expose instruments to tissue contaminated with prions.

Flexible Endoscopes

40. Flexible endoscopes are complex instruments, and cleaning them is a multistep process. Cleaning and disinfection or sterilization of flexible endoscopes is beyond the scope of this text. Personnel responsible for cleaning and disinfecting these devices should refer to the Multi-Society Guidelines for Reprocessing Flexible Gastrointestinal Endoscopes (AORN, 2012, pp. 499–512; Society of Gastroenterology Nurses and Associates [SGNA], 2009, pp. 4–23). The endoscope manufacturer's guidelines for cleaning and disinfection or sterilization must be followed, and personnel responsible for endoscope reprocessing should have demonstrated competence for this complex task.

Robotic Instruments

41. Robotic instruments are complex instruments with lumens and difficult-to-clean components. Special attention should be given to cleaning the ports and articulating areas on these instruments. Ports should be flushed while the articulating component of the device is rotated through its full range of motion. Ports should be flushed until the water runs clear. Failure to do so may result in incomplete removal of debris, which might then dry and harden—making cleaning more difficult and impeding effective sterilization. The device manufacturer's instructions for cleaning and checking for function must be followed.

Ultrasonic Cleaning

42. The purpose of ultrasonic cleaning is to dislodge and remove tenacious debris. With this method, high-intensity sound waves generate tiny bubbles that expand until they collapse or implode (cavitation). Implosion creates a negative pressure on the surfaces of the instruments, dislodging soil that might have remained in hard-to-reach crevices. Ultrasonic cleaning is especially beneficial for items with box locks, serrations, lumens, and crevices. It is not suitable for lensed instruments, powered instruments, or instruments that are chrome plated or made of plastic or rubber.

43. The instrument manufacturer's guidelines should be followed to determine whether ultrasonic cleaning is compatible with the instrument. If instruments of dissimilar metal are combined in the ultrasonic cleaner, etching and pitting may occur as a result of the ion transfer caused by the cleaning process.

44. When a detergent is added to the water in the ultrasonic cleaner, it is important that both the detergent manufacturer's and the ultrasonic manufacturer's guidelines are followed. The solution should be changed at least daily, whenever the detergent solution is visibly soiled, or more frequently if the manufacturer's guidelines so indicate.

45. To prevent aerosolization of contaminants, the lid on the ultrasonic cleaner should remain closed during use.

46. Ultrasonic cleaning is not a decontamination method. It is intended to be used in conjunction with manual or automated decontamination.

47. Most facilities use an ultrasonic cleaner prior to mechanical cleaning. Some facilities use this type of cleaning for most instruments, whereas others use it only for specialty or difficult-to-clean instruments.

48. Instruments should be rinsed until they are free of gross soil and placed in specially designed instrument baskets or trays before being put into an ultrasonic cleaner. Adaptors that flush cleaning solution through the lumens of cannulated instruments should be attached.

49. Instruments should not rest on the bottom of the unit because that will prevent cavitation on the part of the instrument not in contact with water.

50. If an automated rinse phase is not included in the ultrasonic cycle, and instruments are not placed in an automated washer, instruments should be manually rinsed with demineralized water.

Lubrication

51. Instruments with movable parts should be lubricated with an antimicrobial, water-soluble

lubricant that protects against rusting and staining. The lubricant must be water soluble to allow penetration of the sterilizing agent. Oils must not be used because they prevent penetration of the sterilant.

Inspection

52. Instruments should be inspected for cleanliness, integrity, alignment, sharpness of edges, and function. Semi-critical instruments and items intended for disinfection immediately prior to use should be dried and stored in a clean, dry area.

53. Items that do not function as intended should be removed. This is a critical requirement. The opportunity to check an instrument for function immediately prior to an emergency surgery situation is limited, so it is imperative that careful inspection and checking for function occur prior to packaging. Whether an instrument functions properly or fails in surgery can be the determining factor regarding patient injury.

Section Questions

1. Which perioperative nursing activities contribute to achieving the desired outcome that the patient will be free from infection and free from injury following the procedure? [Ref 1]

2. Even though instruments are usually processed in the SPD, why is it essential for the perioperative nurse to have comprehensive knowledge of cleaning, inspection, packaging, sterilization, and storage of sterile instruments and supplies? [Refs 2–5]

3. Differentiate the need for sterilization versus high-level disinfection. [Ref 6]

4. What is the most important step in the process of decontamination of instruments? [Refs 7–8]

5. What is the primary reason that instruments should be washed as soon as possible after use? [Ref 9]

6. When cleaning instruments on the field, how can the scrub person prevent aerosolization of particles? [Ref 10]

7. What is the rationale for choosing sterile water to clean instruments on the sterile field? [Ref 11]

8. How should used and unused instruments be returned to the SPD? [Ref 12]

9. How does OSHA require that contaminated materials be transported to a decontamination site away from the work area? [Ref 13]

10. Under which circumstances can instruments be washed in the scrub sink? [Ref 14]

11. What are some techniques for preventing debris from drying on instruments during transport to a decontamination area? [Ref 15]

12. Identify several reasons for preventing the formation of biofilm on instruments waiting for decontamination. [Ref 16]

13. Describe at least five steps in preparing contaminated instruments for transport to the SPD. [Ref 17]

14. Which supplies should be present wherever instruments are decontaminated? [Ref 20]

15. How many air exchanges per hour are required in the decontamination area? [Ref 21]

16. Why is hot water not used to rinse contaminated instruments? [Ref 22]

17. How can mixing detergents in a higher concentration than recommended interfere with sterilization? [Ref 23]

18. Which type of PPE is required when decontaminating instruments? [Ref 24]

19. Why is it preferable to use a washer-decontaminator and avoid washer-sterilizers when cleaning and decontaminating instruments? [Ref 27]

20. Which kind of special attention is needed for eye instruments? [Ref 31]

21. What is TASS? [Ref 32]

(continues)

Section Questions (continued)

22. Explain how TASS occurs. [Ref 32]

23. What is a prion and why is it a special challenge for surgical patients? [Ref 35]

24. Which tissues are considered to pose a high risk for transmission of prion disease? [Ref 37]

25. Which options are available for managing hard-to-clean instruments that have been exposed to prions? [Ref 38]

26. What is important to consider about ports and articulating areas on robotic instruments? [Ref 41]

27. Describe cavitation and identify the items for which an ultrasonic cleaner is most beneficial. [Ref 42]

28. Why must instruments not rest on the bottom of an ultrasonic washer? [Ref 49]

29. Describe the characteristics of lubricants appropriate for instruments. [Ref 51]

30. How are nonfunctioning items handled during the decontamination process? [Ref 53]

Packaging Materials: Barriers

Selection Criteria

54. Packaging materials and systems are intended to maintain the sterility of items up until their intended use.

55. Packaging material must be compatible with the sterilization process and the device manufacturer's recommendations. Certain materials are not compatible with every sterilization process; however, all materials must meet the following standard criteria:

    - Permit penetration and exit of the sterilant.
    - Allow for adequate air removal.
    - Permit identification of the contents.
    - Permit complete and secure enclosure of the contents.
    - Be fluid resistant.
    - Be intact.
    - Resist tears, punctures, and abrasions.
    - Be free of toxic ingredients and non-fast dyes.
    - Provide a barrier to microorganisms.
    - Provide adequate seal integrity.
    - Allow for aseptic delivery of contents to the sterile field.
    - Permit labeling to identify contents.
    - Be large enough to evenly distribute the contained mass.
    - Maintain sterility of items until package is opened (AAMI, 2011, p.54; AORN, 2012, pp. 537–546).

Types of Packaging

Overview

56. Types of packaging systems:
    - Woven fabrics
    - Nonwoven materials
    - Paper
    - Plastic and paper pouches
    - Plastic and Tyvek pouches
    - Rigid container systems made from various materials

Woven Fabric

57. Muslin was the standard woven, reusable wrapping material for many years. It is a reusable cotton suitable for steam and ethylene oxide (EtO) sterilization. To prevent the penetration of dust and airborne microorganisms, muslin wrappers with a minimum of 140 threads per square inch and consisting of two double layers (four thicknesses) were used.

    Although muslin permits entry and exit of the sterilant, it does not provide a tortuous path for microorganisms and does not provide a protective barrier against moisture. For these reasons, muslin has been replaced by cotton and polyester-blend fabrics that have been treated to be water resistant.

58. Packages are traditionally wrapped in two layers. In one technique, the two wrappers are folded sequentially to create a package within a package. The purpose of this technique is to provide a second sterile barrier. Newer woven fabrics have been developed that provide a

sufficient tortuous path and barrier without double sequential wrapping, and packages may be wrapped using a simultaneous double-wrapping technique. The policy for wrapping must be driven by the ability of the wrap to maintain items in a sterile state. Institutional policy may or not require double sequential wrapping.

59. Packages are secured with pressure-sensitive tape that also serves as a process indicator. Select process indicator tape that is specific to the intended sterilization method.

60. Woven wrappers do not exhibit "memory," a characteristic that causes material edges, when the package is opened, to return to their original folded position.

61. Woven fabrics may produce lint.

62. Woven fabrics should be laundered between uses to prevent superheating and deterioration of the fabric. They should be maintained for a minimum of 2 hours at room temperature (i.e., 68°F–73°F [20°C–23°C]) and at a relative humidity of 30% to 60% (AAMI, 2011, p. 67).

63. Woven wrappers are compatible with steam and EtO sterilization but may not be used with hydrogen peroxide gas plasma or ozone.

64. A process should be in place to determine and monitor the useful life of woven fabrics:

    - They must be inspected between uses for pinholes and tears that must be repaired with heat-sealed patches.
    - Woven fabrics lose their water-resistant properties over time and must be retreated or discarded.

Nonwoven Materials

65. Nonwoven wrappers are made of a combination of cellulose and/or other synthetic materials. Nonwoven wrappers are single use, disposable, almost entirely lint free, and tear resistant; they provide an excellent barrier protection against dust, airborne microorganisms, and moisture.

66. Items wrapped in nonwoven material are wrapped according to the manufacturer's recommendations. Some nonwoven wraps require two layers and sequential wrap; others require only a single wrap that is equivalent to a sequential double wrap. The deciding factor for whether one or two layers or sequential wrapping is required is the degree of barrier provided by the wrapper or preferred method.

67. Nonwoven wrappers eliminate the need for washing, inspecting, and patching. Quality is consistent because wrappers are used only once and then discarded.

68. Nonwoven, cellulose-based wrappers are compatible with steam and EtO, but are not compatible with hydrogen peroxide gas plasma sterilization. Polypropylene wrappers must be used. To determine appropriate wrappers for ozone and vapor-phase hydrogen peroxide sterilization, the sterilizer manufacturer should be consulted.

69. Nonwoven wrappers may display undesirable memory, as wrapper edges try to return to their original fold when packages are opened. This creates the potential for contamination of package contents when a wrapper edge that has been handled folds back into the package and contaminates the sterile contents.

70. Some nonwoven packaging materials may require a longer sterilization time than woven packaging materials. This information must be supplied by the manufacturer.

Pouches: Plastic/Paper, Plastic/Tyvek

71. A combination of plastic and paper—and, in the case of hydrogen peroxide gas plasma sterilization, a combination of plastic and Tyvek (material made from high-density polyethylene fibers)—pouches or "peel packs" may be used to wrap items in preparation for sterilization. The plastic/paper combination is appropriate for steam or EtO sterilization. Tyvek/plastic combinations are used with EtO and hydrogen peroxide gas plasma sterilization. With both types of pouches, the plastic film is fused to the paper or Tyvek so that one side is clear and the other opaque.

72. Advantages of combination plastic and paper or Tyvek wrappers are that they are inexpensive, permit visualization of the contents, are lint free, provide an effective barrier against airborne microorganisms, and are suitable for packaging a limited number of lightweight, small items.

73. Disadvantages are a tendency to display memory. In addition, the paper and plastic combination provides little resistance to punctures.

74. Items packaged in pouches are either single or double pouched depending on the manufacturer's guidelines and individual institutional

policies. Where double pouching is used, the inner pouch should fit into the outer pouch without being folded (AAMI, 2011 p. 60) (Figure 4-1).

75. Where double pouching is used, the pouches should be positioned so that plastic faces plastic, and paper faces paper (AAMI, 2011 p. 60). The sterilant penetrates the paper or Tyvek portion of the pouch, while the plastic portion allows the item to be viewed.

76. Pouch packages should be processed in a vertical position and should not be placed inside wrapped instrument trays.

Rigid Container Systems

77. Rigid container systems are packaging receptacles made from aluminum, stainless steel, heat-resistant plastic, or a combination of materials. The rigid container system contains perforations that are sealed with a bacterial filter or a valve system that allows entry and exit of the sterilant. The lid and base are held together by a latch mechanism with a tamper-evident seal (Figure 4-2).

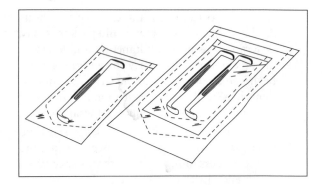

Figure 4-1 Examples of single/double packaging with paper/plastic pouches

78. Rigid containers are durable and protect instruments from damage. They are more resistant than other packaging materials to contamination during storage. Container packaging also eliminates the necessity for a wrapper.

79. Disadvantages of rigid containers include their weight. An empty container can weigh up to 10

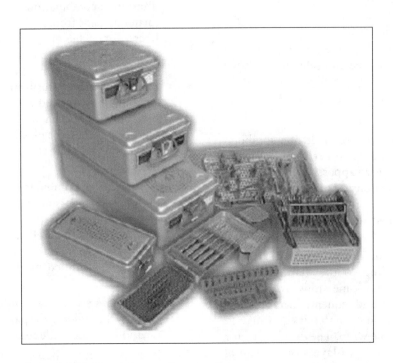

Figure 4-2 Rigid containers and accessories

pounds. If condensation occurs within the container, it is referred to as a "wet pack." When the scrub person opens a package in preparation for surgery and discovers a "wet pack," the instruments are not considered sterile and must not be used. The entire package should be returned to the SPD and sterile processing personnel informed of the problem.

80. Rigid container systems must be cleaned prior to filling. The gaskets, valves, and filters must be checked and changed according to the manufacturer's recommendation. The filters and valves must be inspected for integrity before and after sterilization.

81. Information on compatibility with sterilization technologies and cycles, arrangement of instruments within containers, sealing, labeling, temperature, exposure times, and cleaning instructions must be obtained from the manufacturer.

Section Questions   www

1. Discuss criteria for packaging materials appropriate for any process or device. [Ref 55]

2. Describe the characteristics of muslin that is used for packaging instruments. [Ref 57]

3. Differentiate between sequential and simultaneous double wrapping. [Ref 58]

4. Explain the concept of "memory" in relation to wrapping materials. [Ref 60]

5. Which sterilization method is incompatible with woven wrappers? [Ref 63]

6. What are the goals of a program to monitor woven fabrics? [Ref 64]

7. Describe nonwoven wrappers. [Ref 65]

8. Identify the benefits of nonwoven wrappers relative to woven wrappers. [Ref 67]

9. With which sterilization methods are nonwoven wrappers compatible and incompatible? [Ref 68]

10. What are the advantages of plastic/paper or Tyvek/paper pouches for instruments? [Ref 72]

11. What is the proper protocol for using two pouches to contain an instrument? [Refs 74–75]

12. How should pouches be arranged for processing? [Ref 76]

13. Describe a rigid container system. [Ref 77]

14. Explain the advantages and disadvantages of using container systems for instruments. [Refs 78–79]

15. Which criteria for use of container systems are determined by the manufacturer? [Ref 81]

Principles of Packaging: Steam

Instruments

82. Instruments and other items are arranged in sets and are placed in a tray with a perforated or mesh bottom or other specially designed container that permits steam to penetrate and also prevents air from being trapped (Figure 4-3). A non-linting absorbent towel or tray liner may be placed in the bottom of the tray to help absorb condensate that is formed during sterilization and to help speed the drying process (Figure 4-4).

83. A critical factor in arranging instruments and other items is to place them so that all surfaces of each item will be exposed to the sterilant (Figure 4-5).

84. Joints and hinges of instruments must be opened and detachable parts disassembled unless the manufacturer provides validated instructions for sterilization when the device is assembled (AORN, 2012, p. 516). Racks, pins, or stringers may be used to assist in arranging instruments and to secure them in an open position.

85. To prevent damage, heavy instruments are placed on the bottom of the tray, and delicate instruments are placed on top. Alternatively, multiple perforated trays/baskets may be used (Figure 4-6).

86. The combined weight of an instrument set, including the container, tray, and/or wrapper,

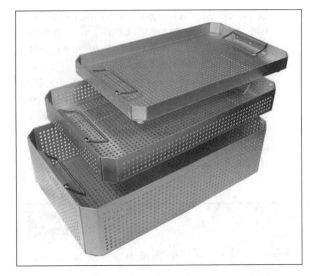

Figure 4-3 Instrument trays
Source: Courtesy of Case Medical, Inc., South Hackensack, NJ.

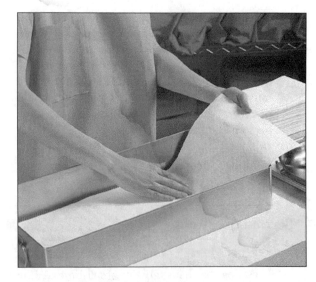

Figure 4-4 Tray liner in instrument tray
Source: © 2005 Kimberly-Clark Worldwide, Inc. Used with permission.

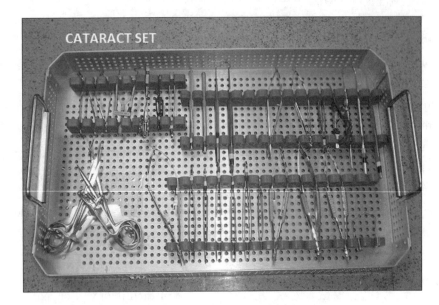

Figure 4-5 Instrument set arranged for sterilization
Source: Courtesy of Case Medical, Inc., South Hackensack, NJ.

should not exceed 25 pounds—an appropriate weight from an ergonomic standpoint (AAMI, 2011, p. 76). Sets heavier than 25 pounds should be repackaged or divided into two sets. In addition to employee safety concerns, instrument sets that are too heavy may concentrate too much metal mass and compromise drying.

87. Paper/plastic pouches should not be used within wrapped sets or containers because pouches cannot be positioned vertically—an orientation that is essential to ensure adequate air removal,

steam contact, and drying. When a pouch is necessary to hold an instrument within a tray or container, a paper-only bag may be used for this purpose if paper is compatible with the intended sterilization modality (AAMI, 2011, p. 73).

Other Items

Basins, Bowls, Cups

88. Basins, bowls, and cups can be nested one inside the other if they are separated by a porous

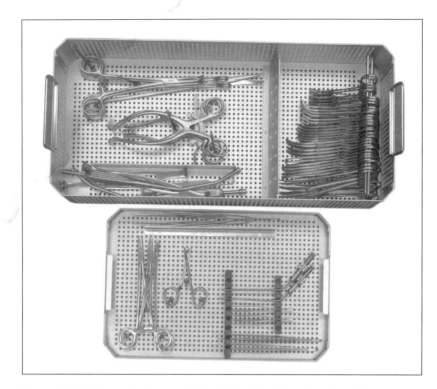

Figure 4-6 Instrument set arranged for sterilization. Note that ringed instruments are held open on a stringer, pins hold larger instruments in place, and more delicate instruments are arranged in a separate tray that fits on top.

Source: Courtesy of Case Medical, Inc., South Hackensack, NJ.

material such as gauze or an absorbent towel. The porous material permits sterilant entry, contact of the sterilant with all surfaces, and exit of the sterilant.

89. Basins, bowls, and cups should be positioned vertically in the steam sterilizer to prevent water from pooling in them and to prevent wet packs.

90. Nested items should be placed facing in the same direction to prevent air pockets, allow circulation of the steam, and permit condensate to drain out.

Impervious Material, Tubing, Items with a Lumen, Wood Items

91. Rubber sheeting or other impervious material is not folded on itself. In preparation for steam sterilization, it is covered with a porous material (e.g., gauze) of the same size, loosely rolled, and then wrapped. This allows steam contact with the entire surface of the rubber or other impervious material.

92. Items with a lumen, such as ventricular and irrigation needles, must be cleaned and rinsed thoroughly.

93. Items made from wood are rarely used in surgery today; however, they deserve special mention because resin can be forced out of wood during steam sterilization, condense onto other items, and cause a tissue reaction when contacted by a mucous membrane. Therefore, unless specific validated processing instructions are available from the device manufacturer, items made with wood should not be sterilized.

Reusable Textiles: Linen Packs

94. Textile packs should be composed of materials that permit air removal, steam penetration, and drying. The size and density of textile packs should be determined in consultation with the textile manufacturer. Many materials are used in the manufacture of textiles, and no one guideline is appropriate for all textiles.

95. Prior to sterilization, linen must be hydrated by laundering and must be stored at a humidity level of 30% to 60% and room temperature of 68°F to 73°F (20°C to 23°C). Linen that is not laundered or stored under these conditions may be dehydrated and subject to superheating

during the steam-sterilization process. Super-heating occurs when the temperature of the fabric exceeds the temperature of the surrounding steam. Superheating destroys cloth fibers and causes linen to deteriorate.

96. Reusable textiles have a limited life, and after repeated use will lose their barrier qualities. For this reason, a wrapper should not be used beyond its intended life. An evaluation and tracking or marking system to indicate the number of uses should be in place where reusable textiles are used.

Packaging for Alternative Methods of Sterilization

97. For hydrogen peroxide gas plasma:
    - All items must be thoroughly dry.
    - Appropriate packaging includes polypropylene wrap or rigid container systems validated for this sterilization method.
    - Cellulose-based material—such as gauze, linen, or towels—absorbs hydrogen peroxide and should not be included within the load.
    - Paper and cloth may not be used.
    - Trays and containers compatible with this technology may be used. The sterilizer manufacturer's and device manufacturer's guidelines must be followed when selecting trays and containers.

98. Information regarding packaging for ozone and vapor-phase hydrogen peroxide sterilization must be obtained from the sterilizer manufacturer.

99. For ethylene oxide (EtO) sterilization:
    - Cleaning and packaging for EtO sterilization is the same as for steam sterilization, with few exceptions.
    - Ethylene oxide in contact with water forms ethylene glycol, a toxic residue. Therefore, items prepared for gas sterilization must be dry. To ensure drying, items with a lumen should be blown dry with compressed air.
    - Oil-based lubricants may not be used, as ethylene oxide cannot penetrate the film left by these lubricants.

Section Questions [www]

1. Which type of tray is used to contain instruments for steam sterilization? [Ref 82]
2. What is the purpose of putting a towel in the bottom of the tray holding instruments for steam sterilization? [Ref 82]
3. In arranging instruments for sterilization, what is one critical factor to consider? [Ref 83]
4. How are instruments with joints and/or detachable parts prepared for sterilization? [Ref 84]
5. What is the maximum total permissible weight of an instrument set? [Ref 86]
6. Why are paper/plastic pouches not placed in instrument sets? [Ref 87]
7. How are basins, bowls, and cups arranged for proper sterilization? [Refs 88–90]
8. How is impervious material prepared for sterilization? [Ref 91]
9. What is important about preparing instruments with lumens for sterilization? [Ref 92]
10. Why are items made with wood not sterilized with steam? [Ref 93]
11. Discuss the role of hydration and the concept of "superheating" related to linen. [Ref 95]
12. Why must an evaluation/tracking system be in place for linen wrappers? [Ref 96]
13. List five criteria for preparing items to be sterilized with hydrogen peroxide plasma. [Ref 97]
14. Explain the necessity of thoroughly drying items that will be sterilized with EtO. [Ref 99]
15. Why can oil-based lubricants not be used on instruments that will be sterilized with EtO? [Ref 99]

Package Information and Identification

Chemical Indicators and Integrators

100. Chemical indicators vary in their ability to detect sterilizing conditions (AAMI, 2011, pp. 102–103).

    - A Class 1 indicator (process indicator) indicates that the unit has been exposed to the sterilization process and distinguishes between processed and unprocessed units. Such indicators are also referred to as external chemical indicators. They include heat-sensitive tape, labels, or strips used on the outside of a package. A process indicator should be visible on the outside of all packages. Pouch packaging often includes an external indicator as part of the pouch.

    - Single-variable indicators (Class 3) measure one of the critical variables and are intended to indicate exposure to a sterilization process at a stated value of the chosen variable.

    - Multiple-variable indicators (Class 4) react to two or more of the critical variables.

    - Integrators (Class 5) react to all critical variables.

101. Parameters of the sterilization process:

    - Steam sterilization: time and temperature
    - EtO sterilization: time, temperature, gas concentration, and relative humidity
    - Hydrogen peroxide gas plasma: hydrogen peroxide concentration, pressure, time, and temperature

102. A chemical indicator or integrator specific to the sterilization process should also be placed inside and outside of each package to be sterilized (AORN, 2012, p. 562). The internal indicator should generally be placed in the center of the package, not on top of it. An indicator should be placed in each layer of multilevel wrapped sets.

103. Process indicators do not guarantee sterility. They demonstrate only that the items have been exposed to the physical conditions within the chamber that are monitored by the indicator.

104. The perioperative nurse must understand the nature of the process indicator used and be able to interpret the reading to determine whether an item has been subjected to the requirements for sterilization.

105. Where there is no visible indicator, the package must be considered contaminated.

Sealing

106. All items intended for sterilization must be securely sealed.

107. Pressure-sensitive tape is used for both woven and nonwoven wrappers. Plastic/paper and plastic/Tyvek pouches may be either heat sealed, self-sealed, or sealed with pressure-sensitive tape. Self-sealing often provides the most secure seal. When heat sealers are used, it is important that the temperature be appropriate for the type of pouch being sealed. Application at the incorrect temperature may result in a weak or incomplete seal.

108. To prevent damage or loss of package integrity, seals must not permit resealing once the pouch has been opened.

Labels

109. Items packaged for sterilization should be clearly labeled with the contents, initials of the package assembler, and lot control number. The lot control number indicates the sterilization date, sterilizer used, and cycle or load number. Lot control numbers, in conjunction with computerized instrument tracking systems, facilitate inventory control, stock rotation, and retrieval of items in the event of sterilization or sterilizer failure.

110. Indelible, nonbleeding, and nontoxic markers may be used to mark packages. Marking should be on the plastic side of the pouch (AORN, 2012, p. 541).

Shelf Life

Storage Considerations

111. Sterilized items should be stored in a well-ventilated, limited-access area with controlled temperature and humidity.

112. Sterile items should be stored in a designated area with a barrier from clean items. They should not be stored under or next to sinks or other areas where they might become wet. The area should be clean and dust free.

113. Wrapped packages should not be bent, crushed, crammed, or stacked.

114. To reduce dust accumulation, wire mesh shelving may be preferable to closed shelving.

115. Closed cabinets are best for items that are used infrequently. Cabinets and shelves should permit adequate cleaning and air circulation. Storage cabinets and shelves should be far enough away from floors, ceiling fixtures, vents, sprinklers, and lights to prevent contamination. Shelves should be at least 18 inches below the ceiling, 2 inches from outside walls, and 8 to 10 inches above the floor (AAMI, 2011, p. 87).

Determining Factors

116. Shelf life is the amount of time an item may be considered sterile.

117. Event-related sterility: Theoretically, if an item is not contaminated during storage, it will remain sterile indefinitely. Shelf life is related to the events that can occur that will cause an item to become contaminated. Actual shelf life is event related, not time related; in other words, events are what determine shelf life. A package is sterile until opened or an event happens to render that package unsterile.

118. Only proper packaging, handling, and storage can prevent contamination. The poorer the quality of the wrapper, the poorer the storage conditions, the more a package is handled, and the longer a package is stored, the greater the possibility for an event to occur that will cause contamination.

119. A small percentage of institutions have policies that require that an expiration date to be placed on stored items. Most institutions have eliminated the use of expiration dates and instead have identified the conditions that must be achieved to consider a package sterile. Before any package is opened for surgery, it must be visually inspected to determine whether sterility appears to have been maintained. A stain, a pinhole, or a tear are several obvious examples of contamination and would preclude using the item in surgery.

120. Shelf life is determined by many factors:
    - Type and configuration of packaging material: Items packaged in rigid container systems may have a longer shelf life than items packaged with woven and nonwoven materials.
    - Use of dust covers: Dust covers can extend shelf life.
    - Conditions of storage: Dust, temperature, humidity, and traffic can affect shelf life.
    - Number of times a package is handled before use: The more the package is handled, the greater the risk of contamination.

121. When commercially prepared items do not have an expiration date, they are considered sterile provided the package is intact. Expiration dates on commercially prepared items may indicate that the integrity of the device or material will be compromised (material degradation) after the indicated date, and the item should not be used once this date has been reached.

Reuse of Single-Use Devices

122. Under current Food and Drug Administration (FDA) regulations, any hospital that chooses to reprocess single-use Class III devices (devices that carry a significant risk in the event of failure) that have been opened and used will be held to the same standard as the original manufacturer of that item. The requirements for the original manufacturer are extremely stringent and virtually impossible for a hospital to replicate.

123. The perioperative nurse in the operating room should never attempt to reprocess a single-use device. When a question arises about whether a single-use device will be reprocessed, a group including infection preventionists and risk management should determine the facility policy.

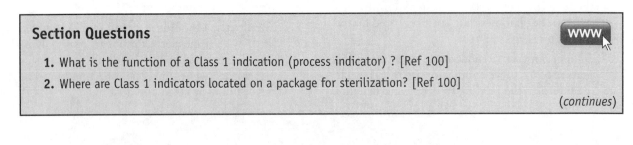

Section Questions   www

1. What is the function of a Class 1 indication (process indicator) ? [Ref 100]

2. Where are Class 1 indicators located on a package for sterilization? [Ref 100]

(continues)

Section Questions (continued)

3. How do Class 3 (single variable), Class 4 (multiple variable), and Class 5 indicators differ? [Ref 100]

4. Compare sterilization parameters among steam, EtO, and hydrogen peroxide plasma technologies. [Ref 101]

5. Where is the chemical indicator placed on the inside of a package to be sterilized? [Ref 102]

6. For which purpose is a process indicator used? [Ref 103]

7. What would a circulating nurse do with a package that has no visible indicator? [Ref 105]

8. What is used to seal packages wrapped in woven or nonwoven wrappers? [Ref 107]

9. Why is the temperature of a heat sealer for pouches important? [Ref 107]

10. Which information should be included on the label of a sterile package? [Ref 109]

11. On which portion of the paper/plastic or paper/Tyvek pouch should writing be permitted? [Ref 110]

12. List five characteristics of an appropriate place in which to store sterilized items. [Refs 111–112]

13. What is the value of wire mesh shelving as opposed to closed shelving? [Ref 114]

14. What is the minimum distance from floor, walls, and ceiling that sterile packages can be stored? [Ref 115]

15. What is the definition of "shelf life"? [Ref 116]

16. Define "event-related sterility." [Ref 117]

17. How does the circulating nurse determine the sterility of a package before opening it for surgery? [Ref 119]

18. Which factors affect the shelf life of a sterilized item? [Ref 120]

19. How does a circulating nurse assess a commercially prepared sterile item when the package has no expiration date? [Ref 121]

20. Under which circumstances can a hospital reprocess Class III devices that are identified as single-use items? [Ref 122]

• • • References

American National Standards Institute (ANSI)/Association for the Advancement of Medical Instrumentation (AAMI) (2001). Processing CJD: contaminated patient care equipment and environmental surfaces. ST79: 2010 & A1:2010 & A2:2011 Annex C. Washington, DC: ANSI/AAMI.

ANSI/AAMI (2001). Comprehensive guide to steam sterilization and sterility assurance in health care facilities. ST79: 2010 & A1:2010 & A2:2011. Washington, DC: ANSI/AAMI.

Association of periOperative Registered Nurses (AORN) (2012). *Perioperative Standards and Recommended Practices.* Denver, CO: AORN.

Center for Biofilm Engineering at Montana University. (2011). BIOFILMS: The HyperTextbook. V4.3. Available at www.hypertextbookshop.com/biofilmbook/v004/r003/. Accessed September 2012.

Occupational Safety and Health Administration (OSHA) (2012). Occupational Safety and Health Standards (29 CFR Subpart Z): toxic and hazardous substances. 1910.1030 bloodborne pathogens. Available at: www.osha.gov/pls/oshaweb/owadisp.show_document?p_table=STANDARDS&p_id=10051. Accessed September 2012.

Rutala W, Weber D (2010). Guideline for disinfection and sterilization of prion-contaminated medical instruments. *Infect Control Hosp Epidemiol*;31(2):107–117.

Society of Gastroenterology Nurses and Associates (SGNA) (2009). *Standards of Infection Control in Reprocessing of Flexible Gastrointestinal Endoscopes.* Chicago, IL: SGNA; 2009. Available at:http://infectioncontrol.sgna.org/Portals/0/SGNA%20Resources/Guidelines&PositionStatements/InfectionControlStandard.pdf. Accessed September 2012.

World Health Organization (WHO). (2003). WHO manual for surveillance of human transmissible spongiform encephalopathies including variant Creutzfeldt-Jakob disease. http://www.who.int/bloodproducts/TSE-manual2003.pdf

Post-Test

www

Read each question carefully. Each question may have more than one correct answer.

1. A biofilm
   a. consists of microorganisms living within a polysaccharide matrix that adheres to a surface.
   b. prevents sterilants from contacting all surfaces of an instrument during the sterilization process.
   c. prevents antibiotics from reaching cells.
   d. is readily dissolved by disinfectants.

2. Which statement (s) is (are) true?
   a. In the operating room, any item that is not sterile is considered contaminated.
   b. Following surgery, items on the sterile field that have not come in contact with the patient are not considered contaminated.
   c. Decontamination is a process that renders a contaminated item safe for handling.
   d. Decontamination is an automated process.

3. Which statement (s) is (are) true about nursing responsibilities?
   a. Cleaning, packaging, and storing of sterile supplies requires judgment and a comprehensive knowledge of scientific principles.
   b. The SPD processes instruments and supplies and makes the final determination of what is sterile and what is not.
   c. The perioperative nurse assumes primary responsibility for high-level disinfection and IUSS.
   d. Assuming responsibility for ensuring that all instruments and supplies delivered to the sterile field are, in fact, sterile is part of the perioperative nurse's commitment to advocating for patient safety.

4. Sterilization is required for
   a. all semicritical items.
   b. all instruments that contact mucous membranes.
   c. all instruments that penetrate mucous membranes.
   d. anything used for an operative or invasive procedure.

5. The first and most important step in instrument decontamination is
   a. disinfecting with an enzyme soak.
   b. cleaning.
   c. decontamination.
   d. sterilization.

6. How should instruments be managed after a surgical procedure?
   a. Separate the used from the unused instruments.
   b. Close all clamps and scissors to protect the tips and blades.
   c. Use a damp towel, enzymatic soak, or spray to prevent debris from drying.
   d. Store contaminated instruments in a safe place before returning them to the SPD at the end of the day.

7. What should be used to keep instruments clean on the sterile field?
   a. Soak them in a basin of normal saline.
   b. Wipe them with a sponge and sterile water.
   c. Spray them with an enzymatic detergent.
   d. Wipe or flush them with sterile water.

8. Which statement (s) is (are) true about instrument cleaning?

    a. An instrument can be clean, but not sterile.

    b. An instrument can be sterile, but not clean.

    c. Instruments opened for a procedure should be washed immediately following the procedure, whether they were used or not.

    d. Instruments should be kept as clean as possible on the sterile field.

9. Which statement (s) is (are) true about postoperative cleaning?

    a. Used instruments from a set should be returned to the set before returning them to the SPD.

    b. Blood and debris allowed to dry on instruments can cause rusting and pitting.

    c. Instruments for IUSS can be washed in the scrub sink.

    d. Instruments can remain in water safely for an unlimited period of time.

10. Before instruments are sent to the SPD,

    a. instruments with blades should have disposable blades removed and be separated from less dangerous instruments.

    b. drill bits should be wiped clean.

    c. heavy instruments should be placed on the bottom of the tray, with lighter instruments on the top.

    d. scissors and clamps should be closed to protect blades and tips.

11. Which statement (s) is (are) true about manual cleaning?

    a. It can be done in the operating room or in the SPD.

    b. All instruments should be soaked in water or an enzymatic detergent.

    c. Brushes, syringes, and compressed air should be available.

    d. Instruments should first be washed in hot water.

12. Immersible items should be cleaned below the surface of the water

    a. to be sure that all surfaces are wet.

    b. to minimize splashing.

    c. to prevent aerosolization of debris.

    d. to avoid wasting water.

13. Which statement (s) is (are) true about TASS?

    a. TASS is caused by foreign matter that is not removed from instruments during cleaning and sterilization

    b. TASS is a noninfectious inflammation of the anterior segment of the eye.

    c. TASS can result in blindness.

    d. Endotoxins from bacteria in ultrasonic cleaners have been associated with TASS.

14. Which statement (s) is (are) true about prions?

    a. A prion is an infectious protein particle.

    b. Creutzfeldt-Jakob disease, a prion disease of the central nervous system, is always fatal.

    c. Prions can be managed by routine sterilization and disinfection routines.

    d. Brain, spinal cord, and dura mater are considered high-risk tissue for transmission of prion disease.

15. Instruments that exposed to tissue at high risk for prions should be

    a. kept dry until cleaned or contaminated.

    b. kept separate from instruments not exposed to high-risk tissue.

    c. stored separately to be cleaned after all other instruments have been processed.

    d. soaked overnight in a phenolic solution.

16. Which statement (s) is (are) true about ultrasonic cleaning?
    a. Ultrasonic cleaning is used to flush all ports and articulations of robotic instruments.
    b. Ultrasonic cleaning removes tenacious debris through cavitation.
    c. Cavitation is the implosion of bubbles generated by sound waves.
    d. Ultrasonic cleaning is especially well suited to removing debris from box locks, serrations, lumens, crevices, and lensed and powered instruments.

17. Which statement (s) is (are) true about ultrasonic cleaning?
    a. Ultrasonic cleaning is a method of decontamination.
    b. It is especially useful for difficult-to-clean instruments.
    c. Instruments do not need to be free of gross soil before immersion in the ultrasonic cleaner.
    d. Instruments that rest on the bottom of the ultrasonic cleaner are subject to the strongest cavitation.

18. Which statement (s) is (are) true about lubrication and inspection?
    a. Oil-based lubricants are most protective and extend instrument life.
    b. Water-soluble lubricants permit penetration of sterilant.
    c. Items that are defective should be tagged before being placed in sets.
    d. Defective instruments can result in injury to the patient.

19. Which statement (s) is (are) true about packaging materials?
    a. Packaging materials must be compatible with the method of sterilization.
    b. Packaging materials must permit visibility or labeling of the contents.
    c. Packaging materials must be able to maintain an adequate seal.
    d. Packaging materials must allow for aseptic delivery to the field.

20. Which statement (s) is (are) true about woven fabrics?
    a. They are lint free.
    b. They can become superheated if not laundered between uses.
    c. They are compatible with all methods of sterilization.
    d. All woven materials require double wrapping to provide a tortuous path that provides a barrier to the migration of microorganisms.

21. Which statement (s) is (are) true about nonwoven wrappers
    a. They are virtually lint free, are tear resistant, and provide excellent barrier protection.
    b. They are disposable.
    c. They can display memory, creating a potential for contamination when packages are opened.
    d. They require double wrapping and longer sterilization times.

22. Which statement (s) is (are) true about pouches?
    a. Different pouches are used for steam and low-temperature sterilization.
    b. Pouches are inexpensive and permit visualization of the contents.
    c. One side of a pouch is clear and the other side is opaque.
    d. Plastic/paper and plastic/Tyvek pouches display memory and provide little resistance to puncture.

23. Which statement (s) is (are) true about pouches?
    a. They can hold multiple small items in a sealed inner pouch contained within an outer pouch.
    b. The inner pouch should be positioned within the outer pouch so that the contents of the inner pouch are visible.

    c. Pouches should be stacked loosely on top of one another in the autoclave to provide maximum penetration of the sterilant.

    d. Pouches can be used to contain small items within instrument trays.

24. Which statement (s) is (are) true about rigid containers?

    a. There may be a valve system to permit entry and exit of sterilant.

    b. Rigid containers are durable and protect instruments from damage.

    c. They are lightweight; an empty container weighs no more than 5 pounds.

    d. Cleaning before placing instruments inside a rigid container involves checking gaskets, valves, or filters.

25. Which statement (s) is (are) true about packaging for steam sterilization?

    a. Placing a towel in the instrument set creates condensate and delays drying.

    b. The surfaces of all instruments must be exposed to the sterilant.

    c. Scissors and clamps must be closed to protect tips and blades.

    d. Instruments with multiple parts may be assembled to prevent loss or misplacement of the individual pieces.

26. Which statement (s) is (are) true about packaging for steam sterilization?

    a. The combined weight of the tray and instrument cannot exceed 15 pounds.

    b. Pouches are used to contain small items within instrument sets.

    c. Pouches used within instrument sets should not be sealed.

    d. Basins and bowls should be positioned vertically to prevent pooling of water.

27. Which statement (s) is (are) true about reusable textiles?

    a. Textiles must be hydrated by laundering them before sterilization.

    b. Superheating is the result of the fabric temperature exceeding the temperature of the steam in the autoclave.

    c. Superheating enhances the barrier properties of textiles.

    d. Well-maintained textiles will maintain their barrier qualities indefinitely.

28. Which statement (s) is/are true about packaging for low-temperature sterilization?

    a. Items must be thoroughly dried before being placed in the sterilizer.

    b. Cellulose wrappers cannot be used with H_2O_2 sterilizers.

    c. Paper and cloth cannot be used with H_2O_2 or EtO sterilizers.

    d. EtO in combination with water forms a toxic residue.

29. Which statement (s) is (are) true about process indicators?

    a. A process indicator shows that a package has been exposed to the sterilization process.

    b. A process indicator is placed at the very center of the package or instrument set.

    c. Pouches sometimes have a process indicator as part of the pouch.

    d. Pouches with a built-in process indicator do not need a second indicator.

30. What are the parameters of steam sterilization?

    a. steam concentration, time, pressure

    b. relative humidity, time, temperature

    c. steam concentration, relative humidity, time

    d. time, temperature

31. What are the parameters for H_2O_2 sterilization?
    a. relative humidity, H_2O_2 concentration, time
    b. H_2O_2 concentration, time, pressure
    c. time, pressure, temperature
    d. H_2O_2 concentration, pressure, time, temperature

32. Which statement (s) is (are) true about indicators?
    a. A chemical indicator should be placed in the center of each sterile package.
    b. There should be an indicator on each layer of a sterile multilevel set.
    c. An indicator that functions properly will ensure that the set is sterile.
    d. If the indicator is questionable or the internal indicator is missing, the set can be used if the process indicator on the outside of the pack demonstrates that the set has been exposed to the parameters of sterilization.

33. Which statement (s) is (are) true?
    a. A pouch that has been opened but not used can be resealed if the type of seal permits it.
    b. Packages must be clearly labeled with the contents, initials of the assembler, and lot control number.
    c. Lot control numbers can be used to track packaged items from a "failed load."
    d. Packages should be marked on the paper side of the pouch.

34. Which statement (s) is (are) true about shelf life?
    a. Solid steel shelving is preferable to mesh shelving because it is durable and supports heavy sets.
    b. Shelves should be 8 to 10 inches above the floor and at least 18 inches from the ceiling.
    c. Event-related sterility is based on the theory that an item remains sterile until something contaminates it.
    d. Expiration dates on commercial packages indicate that the contents' integrity may degrade and should not be used after expiration date has been reached.

35. Which statement (s) is (are) true about reuse of single-use devices?
    a. The FDA holds facilities that choose to reprocess single-use devices to the same standards as the original manufacturer of the item.
    b. Perioperative nurses should choose single-use items carefully for resterilization, inspecting them carefully for contamination.
    c. Items opened but not delivered to the field are not considered contaminated and can be resterilized.
    d. The facility's infection preventionist can determine which single-use items can be resterilized.

Competency Checklist: Cleaning, Packaging, and Storage

WWW

Under "Observer's Initials," enter initials upon successful achievement of the competency. Enter N/A if the competency is not appropriate for the institution.

Name _____

	Observer's Initials	Date
1. Items are rinsed/wiped/irrigated during the procedure.	_____	_____
2. Contaminated instruments are contained during transportation to the decontamination area.	_____	_____
3. Enzymatic soak solution, spray, or gel is applied before transport to the decontamination area.	_____	_____
4. Personal protective equipment is worn during washing procedures.	_____	_____
5. Manual washing is accomplished below the surface of the water.	_____	_____
6. Decontamination equipment is operated according to the manufacturer's instructions.	_____	_____
7. The ultrasonic cleaner is operated according to the manufacturer's instructions.	_____	_____
8. Instruments are lubricated with water-soluble lubricant.	_____	_____
9. Instruments are inspected for:		
a. Cleanliness	_____	_____
b. Function—including ensuring all components are present	_____	_____
10. Instruments are packaged appropriately:		
a. Appropriate tray/container	_____	_____
b. Disassembled	_____	_____
c. Opened	_____	_____
d. Delicate on top of heavy	_____	_____
e. Nested items separated with porous material and placed facing the same direction	_____	_____
f. Instruments dried	_____	_____
g. Lumens rinsed for steam sterilization in the gravity-displacement cycle	_____	_____
h. Lumens dried for ethylene oxide and hydrogen peroxide gas plasma	_____	_____
i. Chemical indicator/integrator placed within the package	_____	_____
j. Appropriate wrapping material selected	_____	_____
k. No pouches within the tray/container	_____	_____
l. Process indicator visible on the outside of the package	_____	_____
m. Seal is secure	_____	_____
n. Labeled with contents, lot number, and initials	_____	_____
11. Rigid containers are used appropriately:		
a. Container washed between uses	_____	_____
b. Gaskets, valves, and filters checked prior to placement of instruments for sterilization	_____	_____
c. Items packaged in the container system according to the manufacturer's guidelines	_____	_____

Observer's Signature   Initials   Date

_____

Orientee's Signature

_____

5

Prevention of Infection
Aseptic Practices: Attire, Scrubbing, Gowning, Gloving, Draping, Prepping, Creating and Maintaining a Sterile Field Operating Room Environment, and Sanitation

LEARNER OBJECTIVES

1. Describe categories of surgical site infection.
2. Explain the relationship of aseptic practice to the prevention of infection.
3. Identify the perioperative nurse's responsibility for aseptic practice.
4. Identify four sources of infection.
5. Describe the precautions for contact, airborne, and droplet-transmitted infections.
6. Describe the purpose and technique of a surgical prep.
7. List the desired characteristics of topical antimicrobial agents.
8. Describe two processes for surgical hand antisepsis.
9. Describe open-gloving and closed-gloving techniques.
10. Identify restricted, semi-restricted, and unrestricted areas of the operating room.
11. Describe appropriate attire within the restricted, semi-restricted, and unrestricted areas of the operating room.
12. Discuss the term *surgical conscience*.
13. Discuss six guidelines for draping.
14. List the desired characteristics of surgical gowns and drapes.
15. Discuss four techniques to help maintain a sterile field.
16. Identify the recommended number of air exchanges per hour, temperature, and humidity in the operating room.
17. Describe the process for cleanup of small and large spills.
18. Discuss protocols for cleaning in the operating room.
19. Describe appropriate traffic patterns relative to movement around a sterile field.
20. Identify one nursing diagnosis related to a surgical incision.

www

Nursing Diagnosis: Desired Patient Outcomes

1. The chain of infection consists of those components that must be present for infection to occur: (a) presence of an infectious agent in a sufficient amount and virulence; (b) a susceptible host; (c) a portal of entry for the microorganisms; and (d) a mode of transmission.

2. Pathogenic microorganisms are ubiquitous, and a surgical incision creates the perfect portal of entry. As a result, a common nursing diagnosis for the patient undergoing surgical intervention is high risk for surgical site infection.

3. Activities in the operating room focus on breaking the chain of infection by reducing the presence of microorganisms and preventing a mode of transmission.

4. Infection may be evidenced by fever, erythema, tenderness, induration, cellulitis, purulent drainage, abscess, or dehiscence. The desired patient outcome is for the patient to exhibit none of the signs or symptoms of infection.

5. Although the exact incidence of surgical -site infection (SSI) is unknown, it is one of the most frequently reported healthcare-acquired infections. When patients develop an infection after discharge, the infection may not be reported. This is especially true for ambulatory surgery patients who leave the hospital before there is time to develop signs and symptoms of infection.

6. Surgical site infections are defined as superficial incisional, deep incisional, or organ/space.

   - Superficial incisional infection involves only the skin or subcutaneous tissue. It is the most common SSI, and is usually diagnosed after patient discharge. Removal of sutures or staples and drainage of the area are the usual treatment.

   - Deep incisional infection involves deep soft tissue (e.g., fascia and/or muscle). Deep incisional SSIs occur less frequently than superficial incisional SSIs, usually follow more extensive surgeries, and are usually diagnosed prior to discharge. Prolonged hospitalization or rehospitalization is common for deep incisional infections.

   - Organ/space infection involves the visceral cavity or anatomic structures not opened during the procedure. These infections are the most severe and require prolonged hospitalization, often with multiple reoperations. Organ/space SSI is associated with long-term morbidity and death.

7. Among surgical patients, SSIs are the most common hospital-acquired infections, developing in 2% to 5% of the more than 30 million patients undergoing surgical procedures each year, meaning one out of every 24 surgical patients develops a postoperative SSI. SSIs increase length of stay by 7 to 10 days and increase costs between $2000 and $4500 per patient (Anderson and Sexton, 2012). Patients with an SSI often require an extended stay or a readmission.

8. The National Nosocomial Infections Surveillance report lists rates of infection for various surgical procedures according to the number of risk factors a patient has for contracting an infection. For example, the SSI rate for low-risk patients having hip surgery is less than 1%, while the rate for high-risk patients is 2.4%. For low-risk colon surgery patients, the SSI rate is less than 4%, while the high-risk patient SSI rate is 9.47% (Edwards et al., 2009).

9. Many states have recently enacted legislation that requires hospitals to publish their infection rates. It is anticipated that mandatory reporting of risk-adjusted infection rates will permit better

gathering of statistics, create an increased awareness of the problem of infection, and champion efforts to reduce the incidence of healthcare-associated infections (HAIs).

10. Many variables contribute to the incidence of SSI; however, an in-depth discussion of these factors is beyond the scope of this chapter. Prevention of SSI in the operating room involves multiple interventions focused on adherence to aseptic practices related to attire, scrubbing, gowning, gloving, prepping, draping, creating and maintaining a sterile field, and sanitation of the suite. If these practices are not performed in accordance with accepted standards, the patient's risk of developing an SSI may increase.

Nursing Responsibilities

11. Asepsis refers to the absence of pathogenic organisms. Aseptic technique in the operating room refers to the practices by which contamination with microorganisms is prevented. Although it is impossible to eliminate all microorganisms in the surgical environment, strict adherence to aseptic technique is essential in preventing the patient and staff from acquiring an infection.

12. The perioperative nurse is responsible for creating and maintaining a sterile field and for monitoring the aseptic practice of all members of the surgical team. This role requires an understanding of infection sources, transmission modes, and the methods of reducing or eliminating microorganisms in the surgical setting. The perioperative nurse must have in-depth knowledge of principles and practices associated with attire, scrubbing, gowning, gloving, prepping, draping, maintaining a sterile field, and operating room sanitation.

13. Everyone working in the perioperative environment shares the responsibility for reducing the number of microorganisms in the operating room to the lowest level possible. However, the perioperative nurse assumes major responsibility for ensuring that each patient is provided with as aseptic an environment as possible and that risk for SSI is reduced to its lowest potential. The perioperative nurse continuously monitors all aspects of the operating room environment to ensure adherence to aseptic principles and compliance with aseptic practice.

Section Questions   www

1. What are the four links in the chain of infection? [Ref 1]
2. Why is a surgical site considered a high risk for infection? [Ref 2]
3. Identify some of the symptoms of an infection. [Ref 4]
4. Differentiate among the three types of surgical site infection: superficial incisional, deep incisional, organ/space. [Ref 6]
5. How frequently do surgical site infections occur? [Ref 7]
6. What are some of the ramifications of a surgical site infection? [Ref 7]
7. What are some perioperative practices focused on preventing infection? [Ref 10]
8. How would you define asepsis? [Ref 11]
9. Who is responsible for minimizing the number of microorganisms in the operating room? [Ref 13]
10. What does the perioperative nurse do to ensure that the risk for surgical site infection is as low as possible? [Ref 13]

Pathogenic Microorganisms

14. Pathogenic microorganisms are microorganisms that cause disease. The pathogens most commonly associated with SSI are *Staphylococcus aureus*, *Staphylococcus epidermidis*, coagulase-negative staphylococci, and *Enterococcus* spp. An increasing proportion of SSIs are caused by microorganisms resistant to antibiotics. These infections are difficult—and sometimes impossible—to resolve.

15. The more virulent the microorganism, the greater the potential for infection. More virulent strains of bacteria or bacteria with an

endotoxin in their outer cell membrane require a smaller inoculum to cause an infection than less virulent strains. An endotoxin is part of the outer wall of gram-negative bacteria such as *Escherichia coli* and *Pseudomonas*. Endotoxins are released when the bacteria cell is destroyed.

16. In 2010, encouraging results from a study conducted by the Centers for Disease Control and Prevention (CDC) showed that invasive, life-threatening healthcare-associated methicillin-resistant *S. aureus* (MRSA) infections declined 28% from 2005 through 2008. Decreases in infection rates were even more dramatic for patients with bloodstream infections. In addition, the study showed a 17% drop in invasive MRSA infections that were diagnosed before hospital admissions (community onset) in people with recent exposures to healthcare settings (CDC, 2012).

Sources of Infection (Endogenous)

17. Endogenous sources of infection are those present within the body. The patient is the source of endogenous infection due to the large number of microorganisms normally found on the skin, in mucous membranes, and in hollow viscera. In fact, the majority of SSIs are caused by the patient's own flora. However, if these microorganisms remain in their normal environment and if their numbers are not altered by external factors, they will not cause infection.

18. The skin serves as the first line of defense against the entry of microorganisms into the body. Incising the skin creates a portal of entry for pathogenic microorganisms and exposes the patient to the risk of infection. In addition, certain factors or conditions, if present, may significantly influence a patient's risk for developing an SSI. Among these are extremes of age, poor nutritional status, obesity, compromised immune system, preexisting disease (especially diabetes), preexisting infection, burns, and use of nicotine.

19. Length of surgery, type of procedure, surgical technique, and an extended preoperative hospital stay can also increase the risk of SSI. Colonization of the patient with healthcare-associated microbes is especially likely when the patient has extensive preoperative or postoperative hospitalization.

20. Geriatric and neonate patients have an increased risk of postoperative surgical site infection. Impaired healing in older adults is often related to inadequate circulation due to atherosclerosis or the presence of coexisting disease. Delayed healing increases the potential for surgical site infection. The premature infant has increased susceptibility to infection due to immature globulin synthesis, antibody formation, and cellular defense. The smaller the neonate, the less resistance to infection the child has. Invasive procedures increase the risk of infection.

21. The poor nutritional status that frequently accompanies drug or alcohol addiction or is attributable to disease entities or treatment can delay wound healing and increase risk for infection. Obesity is a risk factor because fatty tissue is not well vascularized, and avascular tissue is susceptible to infection.

22. Defense mechanisms are impaired in immunocompromised patients—for example, patients receiving radiation therapy, chemotherapy, or corticosteroids; those on immune-suppressive drugs; and those who have AIDS. Additional stress is placed on the immune system of patients with chronic conditions such as diabetes, cancer, and cardiac and respiratory diseases.

23. The presence of infection anywhere in the body significantly increases the risk of an SSI and is always a contraindication for elective surgery. Whenever possible, surgery should be postponed until any preexisting infection is resolved.

24. When skin integrity is destroyed, such as with a burn, the patient becomes susceptible to infection.

25. Smoking decreases the delivery of oxygen to the tissues, which delays wound healing and increases the risk for an SSI.

26. The risk of infection increases with the length of exposure of internal tissues to the environment (surgical time), the presence of implants, and the amount of ischemic tissue present.

27. Although necessary, catheters and drains can increase the risk of infection because they provide a pathway for pathogenic microorganism migration. The longer catheters and drains are left in place, the greater the risk for infection.

Sources of Infection (Exogenous)

28. Exogenous sources of infection come from outside the body—from the environment and personnel.

Personnel

29. Personnel are a major source of microorganisms in the operating room. The greater the number of personnel in the operating room, the greater the number of microorganisms present. A person who is colonized carries the organism but is not infected and can be a source of transmission of the microorganism, which can subsequently cause an infection. Many perioperative nurses and other personnel present in the operating-room suite are colonized with MRSA and could be sources of patient infection with MRSA.

30. The skin of all persons in the area of the patient is a potential source of infection. Cells and surface organisms are constantly being shed from skin surfaces. Certain body areas, such as the head, neck, axilla, hands, groin, legs, and feet, harbor an especially large number of microorganisms. Hair is a major source of *Staphylococcus*. The number of microorganisms present in hair is related to its length and cleanliness.

31. Talking, coughing, and breathing release numerous organisms into the environment.

32. Chipped fingernails can harbor pathogens in large numbers and should be removed prior to entry into the operating room environment (Association of periOperative Registered Nurses [AORN], 2012, p. 74). Due to the inability to continually monitor the state of fingernail polish, it should not be worn in the perioperative environment.

33. Other studies have found higher bacterial counts on the hands of nurses with long fingernails (more than ¼ inch) whether natural or artificial (World Health Organization [WHO], 2009, p. 141).

34. A growing body of evidence suggests that artificial nails may contribute to the transmission of healthcare-associated infection. Artificial nails are more likely to harbor gram-negative pathogens both before and after hand washing, and the longer the artificial fingernails are worn, the greater the number of microorganisms isolated (WHO, 2009, p. 141). Healthcare personnel who wear artificial nails may also limit hand hygiene and surgical hand scrub practices to protect their manicures (AORN, 2012, p. 74).

35. The Joint Commission's 2007 National Patient Safety Goals, the Association of periOperative Registered Nurses (AORN, 2012, p. 74), the Centers for Disease Control and Prevention (CDC, 2002, p. 78), and the World Health Organization (WHO, 2009, p. 66) all recommend against artificial nails for members of the surgical team.

Environment

36. The operating room is not sterile. Organisms are present in the air, on dust particles, and on dirt in the environment.

37. The walls, floors, overhead lights, light tracks, cabinets, door handles, and other stationary fixtures in the operating room may harbor microorganisms and, therefore, are potential sources of infection.

38. All instruments, supplies, and equipment that come in contact with personnel become potential sources for infection because personnel may transfer organisms to and from whatever instruments, supplies, or equipment they touch.

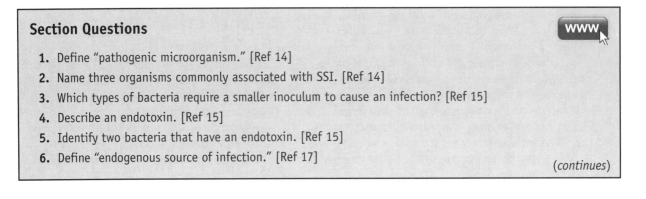

Section Questions   www

1. Define "pathogenic microorganism." [Ref 14]
2. Name three organisms commonly associated with SSI. [Ref 14]
3. Which types of bacteria require a smaller inoculum to cause an infection? [Ref 15]
4. Describe an endotoxin. [Ref 15]
5. Identify two bacteria that have an endotoxin. [Ref 15]
6. Define "endogenous source of infection." [Ref 17]

(continues)

Section Questions (continued)

7. How can endogenous microorganisms be prevented from causing an infection? [Ref 17]

8. List at least 10 factors or conditions that increase a patient's risk for developing SSI. [Refs 18–20]

9. Describe the increased risk for SSI in the geriatric and neonate populations. [Ref 20]

10. How does nutrition influence the risk for SSI? [Ref 21]

11. Describe one risk of obese patients for developing an SSI. [Ref 21]

12. Which conditions might impair a patient's immune system? [Ref 22]

13. Why might surgery be canceled if a patient is found to have an existing infection? [Ref 23]

14. How does smoking increase the risk for SSI? [Ref 25]

15. Why might catheters and drains increase the risk of developing an SSI? [Ref 27]

16. How do personnel affect the number of exogenous microorganisms present in the operating room? [Refs 29–30]

17. Which body areas harbor especially large numbers of microorganisms? [Ref 30]

18. Explain why AORN's recommended practices expect that the perioperative nurse will remove jewelry and avoid wearing nail polish and artificial nails? [Refs 32–34]

19. Which other organizations recommend against artificial nails for surgical team members? [Ref 35]

20. Besides personnel, which other sources of microorganisms are there in the operating room? [Refs 36–37]

39. Whenever dust particles in the air settle on instruments or supplies, the organisms on those dust particles are also deposited on those items.

Standard and Transmission-Based Precautions

40. Universal precautions were defined by the CDC in 1987. They are a set of precautions designed to prevent transmission of human immunodeficiency (HIV), hepatitis B (HBV), and other bloodborne pathogens. Blood and certain body fluids of all patients are considered potentially infected with bloodborne pathogens.

41. Universal precautions evolved into standard and transmission-based precautions in 1996. Standard precautions apply to blood and other body fluids containing visible blood, semen, and vaginal secretions. Standard precautions require that blood and body fluids of all humans (patients and personnel) be considered infectious and that the same safety precautions be taken whether or not the patient is known to have a bloodborne infectious disease. Because operating room personnel are often exposed to large amounts of blood, the term "standard precautions" is familiar in the perioperative environment.

42. The practice of standard precautions is a method of infection control that protects both the patient and operating room personnel. Standard precautions apply to blood, all body fluids, secretions, and excretions except sweat, regardless of whether they contain visible blood (Siegel et al., 2007, p. 66).

43. Standard and transmission-based precautions are methods of infection control that can be used to prevent the transmission of pathogens and protect both the patient and the healthcare worker from exposure to pathogenic microorganisms found in blood and body fluids and on nonintact skin and mucous membranes. Standard precautions should be used in the care of all patients.

44. Standard precautions include the use of personal protective equipment (PPE) and prompt and frequent hand washing. PPE includes use of gloves when touching blood, body fluids, secretions, excretions, and contaminated items can be anticipated, and use of masks, eye protection, and gowns during procedures with the potential to generate splashes of blood, body fluids, secretions, and excretions. Shoe and leg coverings may also be used as needed.

Hand washing should be done after touching blood, body fluids, secretions, excretions, and contaminated items, whether or not gloves are worn (Siegel et al., 2007, p. 66).

45. Transmission-based precautions are used in addition to standard precautions for patients who are known or suspected to be infected or colonized with infectious agents, including certain epidemiologically important pathogens that require additional control measures to effectively prevent their transmission (Siegel et al., 2007, p. 66).

46. There are three types of transmission-based precautions: airborne, droplet, and contact. Airborne precautions are appropriate against pathogens that spread by airborne transmission (particles 5 microns or smaller), such as rubeola, tuberculosis, and varicella. Airborne precautions include use of respiratory protection (e.g., a National Institute of Occupational Safety and Health [NIOSH]–approved N95 mask) and special air handling and ventilation. Persons susceptible to airborne pathogens should wear respiratory protection, and infected patients should wear a mask during transport.

47. Elective surgery should be postponed for patients who are on airborne precautions. If surgery cannot be postponed, if possible, it should be performed at a time during the day when fewer personnel are present. In addition, only personnel required for the surgery should be allowed to enter the room. Following surgery, the room should remain vacant and closed until the air in the room has been completely changed. The length of time required for this exchange will depend on the rate of air exchange in that operating room. Typically, it will require 28 minutes for 15 air exchanges with an efficiency removal effectiveness of 99.9% (Petersen, 2006, p. 648).

48. Droplet precautions are appropriate for protection against pathogens that are transmitted through droplets (particles 5 microns or larger), such as influenza and mumps. Droplet precautions include wearing a mask within 3 feet of an infected patient and positioning other patients at least 3 feet away from infected patients. Droplets are transmitted by sneezing, talking, and coughing. Infected patients should wear a mask during transport.

49. Contact precautions are used when caring for patients who are known or suspected to be infected or colonized with microorganisms transmitted by direct or indirect contact. Contact precautions include the use of gloves and gowns when contact with microorganisms is anticipated, wearing a mask if contact with aerosolized infectious organisms is possible, and cleaning and disinfecting patient equipment.

50. In 1992, the Occupational Safety and Health Administration (OSHA) established mandatory universal precautions practice standards. The three critical components of universal precaution standards are (1) use of personal protective barriers, (2) proper hand washing, and (3) precautions in handling sharps.

51. The standards include the following provisions:

- Employers must list job classifications, tasks, and procedures in which employees have occupational exposure to blood or other potentially infectious body fluids.

- Gloves must be worn when direct contact with blood or other potentially infectious body fluids is expected to occur.

- Masks with face shields or protective eyewear with side shields must be worn when splashes, splattering, or aerosolization of blood and body fluids is anticipated.

- Gowns, appropriate to the procedure being performed, must be worn when aerosolization or splattering of blood or other body fluids is anticipated. Gowns must not permit passage of blood or body fluids.

- Personal protective equipment (e.g., gloves, masks, face shields, gowns) must be provided by the employer at no cost to the employee.

- Hands and other skin surfaces must be washed as soon as feasible if contaminated with blood or body fluids.

- Contaminated needles are not recapped or removed unless required by a specific procedure. If recapping or removal is required, it must be accomplished with a mechanical device.

- Sharps are deposited in rigid, leak-proof, puncture-resistant containers that must be readily accessible.

- A written schedule of cleaning and appropriate disinfection of equipment and the environment must be implemented and maintained.

- Contaminated laundry is placed in labeled or color-coded laundry bags that prevent leakage.
- Infectious waste containers must be closable, prevent leakage, and be labeled or color coded as potentially infectious.
- The employer must provide a hepatitis B vaccination and a postexposure follow-up program. A preexposure vaccine must be offered free of charge.
- Training and education programs must be made available to all employees who may be exposed to blood or other body fluids that are potentially contaminated with hepatitis B virus (HBV) or HIV.

52. In addition, OSHA revised the Bloodborne Pathogens Standard (CFR 29 1910.1030) to include the requirement that employers identify, evaluate, and implement safer medical devices. The revision also requires that nonmanagerial healthcare workers must be involved in evaluating and choosing safer needle devices. A sharps injury log must be maintained as well (OSHA, 2011).

Section Questions   www

1. What is the purpose of standard precautions? [Ref 40]
2. What are the two major components of standard precautions? [Ref 41]
3. Which body fluids do standard precautions include? [Ref 42]
4. Describe personal protective equipment (PPE). [Ref 44]
5. Which patients require transmission-based precautions? [Ref 45]
6. Describe the three types of transmission-based precautions. [Ref 46]
7. A microorganism of what size particle determines the need for airborne precautions? [Ref 46]
8. Which type of mask is required for airborne precautions? [Ref 46]
9. If surgery must be performed on a patient on airborne precautions, which special interventions should be considered? [Ref 47]
10. How many air exchanges in which period of time result in a 99.9% air removal effectiveness? [Ref 47]
11. What are some diseases spread by droplet transmission? [Ref 48]
12. A mask is required within how many feet of a patient on droplet precautions? [Ref 48]
13. Which precaution should be taken when transporting a patient on droplet precautions? [Ref 48]
14. Describe the PPE required when managing patients on contact isolation. [Ref 49]
15. What are the three critical components of the universal precautions established by OSHA? [Ref 50]
16. What does OSHA say about the wearing of eye protection? [Ref 51]
17. How does OSHA say contaminated needles/sharps should be handled? [Ref 51]
18. According to OSHA, what are the requirements for containers of infectious waste? [Ref 51]
19. What does OSHA require of the employer in reference to hepatitis B vaccination? [Ref 51]
20. How does OSHA include the perioperative nurse in managing sharps safety? [Ref 52]

Control of Sources of Infection

53. Infection prevention in the operating room includes adherence to aseptic practices in relation to surgical attire, sterilization of instruments and equipment, staff and patient skin preparation, creation and maintenance of a sterile field, and control of the environment. A major responsibility of the perioperative nurse is to implement and ensure practices that are designed to prevent infection. Aseptic practice is what distinguishes the operating room from other clinical areas.

54. Some aseptic practices are mandated by regulatory bodies such as OSHA. Others are derived from standards-setting bodies such as the AORN and the Association for Advancement of Medical Instrumentation (AAMI).

55. Regardless of the source of the aseptic practices, they are only as good as the surgical conscience of the individual practitioner. A surgical conscience is a personal commitment to adhere strictly to aseptic practice, to report any break in aseptic practice, and to correct any violation, whether or not anyone else is present or observes the violation. A surgical conscience mandates a commitment to aseptic practice at all times.

56. Aseptic practice is the method used to prevent contamination from microorganisms. AORN has developed recommended practices to provide guidelines for establishing and maintaining a sterile field. The purpose of these practices is to decrease SSIs by preventing contamination of the open wound by creating a sterile field that is isolated from the surrounding unsterile areas. The AORN recommended practices are critical components of infection control and are addressed throughout this chapter.

Control of Patient Sources of Infection: Skin Prep

57. Efforts to reduce patient sources of infection are aimed at lowering the number of bacteria on the skin prior to surgery and reducing potential bacterial contamination from within the patient during surgery. Although the skin cannot be sterilized, the incision site and the area immediately surrounding it should be as free of microorganisms as possible prior to surgery.

58. Cruise and Foord (1980, pp. 27–40) performed the landmark study that demonstrated hair removal has been associated with increased risk of surgical site infection. Hair at the incision site should be removed only when its presence interferes with the intended procedure. If hair will interfere with the surgical procedure, hair removal should be done on the day of surgery, in a location outside the operating room (AORN, 2012. p. 451).

59. Before hair is removed from the surgical site, the patient's skin should be assessed for the presence of rashes, moles, warts, or other conditions. Trauma to these lesions can provide an opportunity for the colonization of pathogenic microorganisms.

60. Hair should be removed with single-use clippers or clippers with a reusable head that can be disinfected between patients—never a razor (AORN, 2012, p. 451). Clippers decrease the potential for nicks in the skin that can provide a portal of entry for microorganisms. The clipper should have a removable head and a new head should be used for each patient.

61. Hair removal may also be done with a depilatory cream.

62. Depilatory creams are infrequently used because of potential irritation to the skin. They also tend to be messy and time consuming.

63. To prevent airborne dispersal of hair and possible contamination of the sterile field, hair removal should be performed outside the room where surgery will be performed.

64. The operative site and the immediate surrounding area are cleaned and an antiseptic is used to prep the patient's skin prior to surgery. The objective of skin cleansing is to remove dirt and skin oils, to reduce the number of microorganisms on the skin to a minimum, and to prevent further microbial growth throughout the procedure.

65. The patient should be instructed to shower or bathe with an antimicrobial soap the night before surgery and/or just prior to surgery. Use of 2% chlorhexidine gluconate (CHG)–coated cloth or 4% CHG soap is recommended for reduction of the baseline microbial count on the patient's skin (Edmiston et al., 2010).

66. Skin antisepsis immediately before surgery needs to start with the patient's skin being clean. It may be necessary to remove adhesive residue, oils from skin, or other debris prior to the skin prep. The choice of antiseptic agent for the preoperative skin prep depends on the condition of the patient's skin, patient allergies, the intended incision site, and surgeon and hospital preference.

67. Acceptable antiseptic products should have the following properties:
    - Clean effectively
    - Reduce microbial count rapidly
    - Have a broad spectrum of activity
    - Easily applied
    - Nonirritating and nontoxic
    - Provide residual protection

68. The most commonly used antimicrobial agents include iodophors, chlorhexidine gluconate,

and alcohol preparations in concentrations of 60–90%.

69. The duration of the prep and technique used should be based on the manufacturer's recommendation and studies on the effectiveness of the antimicrobial agents.

70. Prior to the skin prep, the patient should be assessed for allergies or sensitivities to prep solutions. An alternate antimicrobial solution should be chosen if allergies or sensitivities are noted.

71. The area prepped should include the incision site and a substantial area surrounding it. Anticipated additional incision sites and potential drain sites must also be prepped (Figures 5-1, 5-2, 5-3, 5-4, 5-5, 5-6, and 5-7).

72. The following guidelines should be adhered to when performing the skin prep:

    • If the patient is awake, provide an explanation regarding the prep.

    • Avoid unnecessary exposure of the patient. To maintain patient dignity and to prevent unnecessary heat loss, expose only the area to be prepped.

    • Many skin prep products are available, and the person performing the prep should follow the manufacturer's instructions for application. Certain basic principles should be followed no matter which product is used. Some commercially prepared prep sets include both a soap preparation for cleansing the area and an antiseptic solution to be applied after cleansing.

    • Controversy exists over whether sterile gloves and a sterile prep kit are more effective than clean gloves or a clean prep kit. Insufficient research data exist to determine the effect on patient outcomes.

    • Do not allow prep solutions to pool beneath the patient or flow under a tourniquet cuff or electrocautery dispersive electrode. Pooled prep solutions have the potential to cause chemical burn. Folded towels should be placed at the periphery of the area to be cleansed to absorb excess fluid, to prevent saturation of drapes or linens, and to prevent pooling.

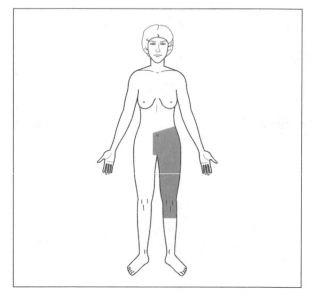

Figure 5-2 Hip prep
Source: Courtesy of Gina Beckman.

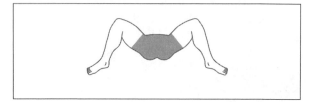

Figure 5-3 Perineum prep
Source: Courtesy of Gina Beckman.

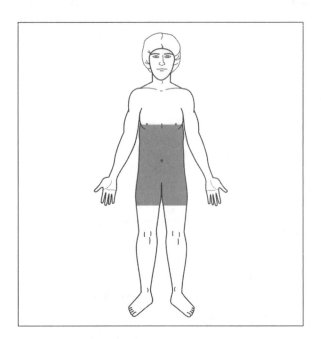

Figure 5-1 Abdominal prep
Source: Courtesy of Gina Beckman.

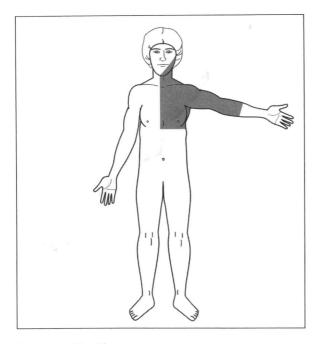

Figure 5-4 Shoulder prep
Source: Courtesy of Gina Beckman.

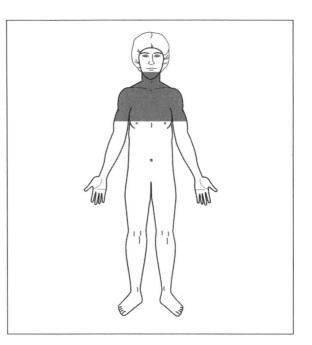

Figure 5-5 Head and neck prep
Source: Courtesy of Gina Beckman.

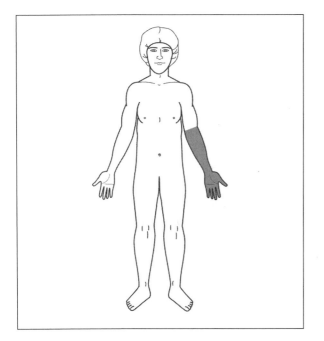

Figure 5-6 Hand prep
Source: Courtesy of Gina Beckman.

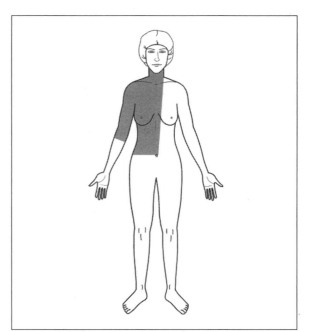

Figure 5-7 Breast prep
Source: Courtesy of Gina Beckman.

- The dirtiest areas are prepped last. In cases where skin is intact and open wounds and body orifices are not part of the area to be prepped, the prep begins at the proposed line of incision. In cases where potentially contaminated areas are included in the prep area, the prep begins at the surrounding skin area. The umbilicus is cleaned separately with cotton-tip applicators. A colostomy or stoma is covered until the surrounding area is prepped and then prepped with a separate sponge. In a perineal prep, the vagina and/or anus is prepped last with a separate sponge. In a shoulder prep, the axilla is prepped last.

- For unusual wounds or incision sites when it may be difficult to know where to begin, nursing judgment must be used to decide upon the prep process that will result in reducing the number of microorganisms at the incision site to the lowest level possible.

- Antiseptic contact time is an important consideration. Drapes should not be applied until the antiseptic contact time has been sufficient to reach maximum effectiveness. See the manufacturer's instructions to determine the required contact time.

73. In addition to the previous guidelines, the following considerations should be noted:

- Eyes are washed with cotton balls with a nonirritating solution. The prep is begun at the nose and continues toward the cheeks. Warm sterile water may be used to rinse off the solution. The solution should not be allowed to pool on the patient's eyes.

- Antiseptic solutions containing CHG should not be used near the eyes due to the danger of corneal ulcerations. CHG can cause deafness if it comes in contact with the inner ear. CHG is not recommended and should be used with caution on mucous membranes (AORN, 2012, pp. 448–449).

- For traumatic wounds, large amounts of irrigating solution may be used prior to and in addition to the prep to remove dirt and debris.

- Normal saline should be used to prep burned or denuded skin.

- When it is necessary to prep a limb, an additional person or an apparatus is needed to hold the limb securely so the entire circumference can be prepped adequately and safely.

- The brush part of the sponge or brush may be useful for areas such as hands and feet. Take care when using the brush to avoid irritating tender skin or creating scratches that could become a portal of entry for bacteria. Take care to prevent aerosolization of prep solutions and skin debris.

- Warm prep solutions are preferable. They may help maintain body temperature and are more comfortable for the awake patient. Take care not to overheat the prep solution, as the efficacy of the antiseptic may be compromised at elevated temperatures.

- Be gentle when prepping fragile skin sites and over pressure-sensitive areas such as the carotid body.

- If alcohol or alcohol-based prepping agents are used, the drapes should not be applied until the solution on the patient has dried. Evaporating fumes from prep solutions trapped by drapes are a potential fire hazard.

74. Documentation of the skin prep should include the following elements:

- Assessment of the skin at the operative site

- Hair removal, if performed, including site, method, time, location, and person who removed hair

- Patient skin allergies or sensitivities

- Prep agents or solution

- Area prepped

- Name of person performing the prep

- Skin condition postoperatively/patient response to prep, such as allergic reaction

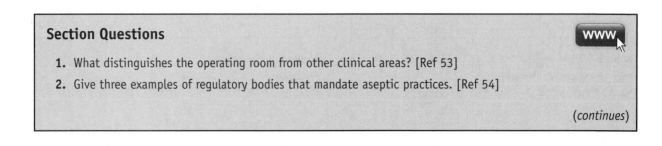

Section Questions   WWW

1. What distinguishes the operating room from other clinical areas? [Ref 53]
2. Give three examples of regulatory bodies that mandate aseptic practices. [Ref 54]

(continues)

Section Questions (continued)

3. Define the term "surgical conscience." [Ref 55]

4. Define "aseptic practice." [Ref 56]

5. What is the purpose of AORN's recommended practices? [Ref 56]

6. Discuss hair removal for a surgical procedure. [Refs 58–63]

7. What is the objective of skin cleansing prior to a surgical procedure? [Ref 64]

8. When should the patient shower before surgery? [Ref 65]

9. Which product is recommended for the preoperative shower? [Ref 65]

10. Which factors influence the choice of antiseptic agent for the skin prep prior to the procedure? [Ref 66]

11. Describe the ideal properties of an antiseptic agent for preoperative skin prep. [Ref 67]

12. What are the three most commonly used antimicrobial agents for skin prep? [Ref 68]

13. What determines the duration of the preoperative skin prep? [Ref 69]

14. Which assessment parameters are important prior to the skin prep? [Ref 70]

15. What determines how extensive the skin prep should be? [Ref 71]

16. Describe perioperative nursing responsibilities related to the preoperative skin prep. [Ref 72]

17. Which dangers are associated with allowing prep solutions to pool beneath the patient? [Ref 72]

18. Discuss the implications of the "dirtiest areas are prepped last" principle in relation to challenging preps. [Ref 72]

19. What is the perioperative nurse's responsibility related to the time required for the antiseptic solution to reach maximum effectiveness? [Ref 72]

20. Which special considerations apply when using CHG as a prep agent? [Ref 73]

21. Which additional considerations are involved in the prepping of a limb? [Ref 73]

22. What should the perioperative nurse take care to avoid when using a sponge or brush to prep hands or feet? [Ref 73]

23. What is the benefit of using warm prep solutions? [Ref 73]

24. Which special safety considerations apply to the use of alcohol-based prep solutions? [Ref 73]

25. Which information should be included when documenting the skin prep? [Ref 74]

Control of Personnel Sources of Infection

Attire

75. Personnel who work in restricted and semi-restricted areas of the surgical suite are required to change into special operating room or surgical attire designed to protect both patient and personnel. Scrub attire inhibits the passage of microorganisms from personnel to the patient and the environment and from patient to personnel. Attire for the restricted and semi-restricted areas is the same with one exception a mask must be worn in the restricted area when sterile supplies are open. For further discussion of restricted and semi-restricted differentiation, review references 194–199 in this chapter.

76. Appropriate surgical attire in the operating-room suite includes hats or hoods, scrub outfits (commonly referred to as "scrubs"), and shoe covers (optional).

77. Hats/caps or hoods are worn so that all head and facial hair is completely covered. Hair is a gross contaminant and major source of bacteria. It attracts and sheds bacteria in proportion to its length, oiliness, and curliness. A hat or hood should be worn in areas where supplies are processed and stored as well as in restricted areas where surgery is performed. Hats are frequently disposable (single use). Reusable hats should be covered with a disposable cap, or should be laundered between each wearing. Hats should be removed and single-use hats

or hoods deposited in a designated receptacle before leaving the operating-room suite (AORN, 2012, p. 62).

78. Scrubs are either a one-piece cover-up, such as a dress, or a two-piece shirt and pants set. To prevent shedding, the shirt should fit close to the body or be tucked into the pants. Scrubs may be made of a tightly woven reusable fabric that minimizes shedding, or they may be disposable. Reusable scrubs should be freshly laundered and changed daily.

79. Controversy exists over whether home laundering rather than hospital laundering is acceptable. Proponents of healthcare facility laundering cite controlled load mix, detergent, cycle time, and water temperature as reasons to mandate laundering in the healthcare facility. Recommendations against home laundering are extrapolated from laboratory data; however, no well-controlled studies have evaluated scrub-suit laundering as a risk for surgical site infection and no data are available to support improved patient outcomes as a result of mandatory healthcare facility laundering. Many healthcare facilities do permit home laundering of scrubs with the exception of grossly contaminated scrubs. AORN (2012, pp. 63–65) does not recommend home laundering of scrubs. OSHA (2001) mandates that garments penetrated by blood or other potentially infectious materials be removed immediately or as soon as feasible. In this event, the facility must supply a fresh scrub suit.

80. Scrub attire should completely cover any other garments that may be worn. In addition to scrubs, unscrubbed or nonsterile team members should wear a warm-up jacket with long sleeves to prevent shedding from bare arms. Operating rooms are cool, and warm-up jackets also serve to keep personnel warm. Warm-up jackets' sleeves should come down to the wrists and should be snapped or buttoned closed to prevent the edges from inadvertently contacting and contaminating sterile supplies (AORN, 2012, p. 62). Warm-up jackets may be reusable or disposable and made of the same type of fabric as scrubs. Fleece fabrics are not appropriate for warm-up jackets (AORN, 2012, p. 57).

81. Hospital policy dictates whether scrubs are to be removed when leaving the operating-room suite and fresh ones donned upon reentry, or if cover gowns or lab coats must be worn over scrubs outside the operating room. Changing

of scrubs or use of cover gowns has not been shown to influence the risk of surgical site infection (AORN, 2012, p. 60).

82. High-filtration masks are worn in the restricted area and in specifically designated areas according to hospital policy. They should be worn in the presence of open sterile supplies (AORN, 2012, p. 265). Masks contain droplets expelled from the mouth and nasopharynx during talking, sneezing, and coughing. Whether masks reduce risk of infection when worn by personnel who are not scrubbed and who are in forced ventilation systems is not clear and requires further research. For this reason, policies on wearing of masks may vary.

83. Masks should cover the nose and mouth completely and securely. Most masks contain a small malleable metal strip that should be pinched to conform to the nose to provide a secure, proper fit. The mask should be tied securely at the back of the head in a manner that prevents venting, which can allow unfiltered exhaled air to escape from the sides.

84. Masks with face shields or splash guards, or masks worn with protective eyewear such as goggles or glasses with side shields, are worn whenever splashes, sprays, or aerosols of potentially infectious agents, such as blood, are anticipated (AORN, 2012, p. 288).

85. Masks must be either on or off; they should never be left to dangle from the neck or be folded and placed in a pocket for future use. Masks should be removed and discarded when they become wet and after use. They should be removed and discarded by handling only the ties. Masks harbor bacteria, and handling of the material portion of the mask after use can transfer microorganisms from the mask to the hands; therefore, only the ties should be handled. Masks should be disposed of in a designated receptacle (AORN, 2012, p. 66). Hands should be washed after mask removal.

86. Shoe covers have not been shown to contribute to reducing surgical site infection rates. They are appropriate, however, when contact with copious or potentially infectious fluids is anticipated. Shoe covers are considered personal protective equipment and, as such, OSHA (2011) requires that they be worn in situations when gross contamination can be anticipated. Various-length high-top shoe covers that cover the shoe and lower leg are appropriate when

contact with copious or potentially infectious fluids is anticipated.

87. Shoe covers should be removed and deposited in a designated receptacle before leaving the operating-room suite. Removal of shoe covers can permit transfer of microorganisms from the shoe covers to the hands. Hands should be washed after shoe cover removal.

88. Jewelry increases bacterial counts on skin surfaces. Any jewelry that cannot be contained or confined within the surgical attire should not be worn. Removal of watches and bracelets allows for more thorough hand washing (AORN, 2012, p. 58).

89. Nails should be short and clean. Artificial nails should not be worn. Long nails may puncture protective gloves or scratch a patient during transfer.

90. Other attire worn to protect personnel from infectious agents includes gloves, liquid-resistant aprons, and gowns.

91. Personnel who scrub for surgery are referred to as "members of the sterile team" or "scrubbed personnel." In addition to wearing appropriate operating room attire, scrubbed personnel must perform surgical hand antisepsis, commonly referred to as "scrubbing," prior to donning a sterile gown and sterile gloves.

Section Questions   www

1. Attire for restricted and semi-restricted areas is the same with which exception? [Ref 75]
2. What is considered appropriate surgical attire in the operating-room suite? [Ref 76]
3. What are some considerations when choosing a hat, cap, or hood to wear? [Ref 77]
4. What is the current status of scientific evidence related to home laundering of scrub attire? [Ref 79]
5. Describe proper wearing of scrub attire. [Ref 80]
6. How is the warm-up jacket to be worn? [Ref 80]
7. What dictates the use of a cover gown or lab coat when leaving the operating room? [Ref 81]
8. What is venting and how does it influence the effectiveness of a surgical mask? [Ref 83]
9. When are face shields or other protective eyewear required? [Ref 84]
10. Why is it important to discard a mask as soon as it is removed? [Ref 85]
11. What is so important about the familiar phrase "masks are either on or off"? [Ref 85]
12. When are shoe covers mandated by OSHA? [Ref 86]
13. Which jewelry is permissible in the operating room? [Ref 88]
14. How do watches, bracelets, and rings affect hand hygiene? [Ref 88]
15. Describe appropriate care of fingernails for the perioperative nurse. [Ref 89]

Scrubbing, Gowning, and Gloving

Definitions

92. Definitions related to scrubbing, gowning, and gloving include the following:
    - *Alcohol-based hand rub*: A product containing alcohol intended for application to the hands for the purpose of reducing the number of microorganisms on the hands. Alcohol-based hand rub products are available as rinses, gels, and foams and are usually formulated to contain 60–95% alcohol.
    - *Alcohol-based surgical hand antiseptics*: A product containing alcohol and another antiseptic agent (such as CHG) that does not require the use of a scrub sponge/brush or sponge.
    - *Antimicrobial soap*: Soap containing an antiseptic agent.
    - *Antimicrobial surgical scrub agent*: A product intended for surgical hand antisepsis.
    - *Antiseptic agent*: An antimicrobial substance applied to the skin to reduce the number of resident and transient microbial flora.

- *Antiseptic hand wash*: A hand wash performed with a product formulated with an antiseptic agent.
- *Hand hygiene*: All measures related to hand condition and decontamination (AORN, 2012, p. 73).
- *Hand washing*: Washing hands with plain soap (soap without an antimicrobial) and water.
- *Resident microorganisms*: Microorganisms that are permanent residents of the skin.
- *Surgical hand antisepsis*: Antiseptic hand wash or antiseptic hand rub performed prior to surgery by surgical personnel to eliminate transient microorganisms and reduce resident hand flora. Products cleared for surgical hand antisepsis may be used in place of the traditional brush/sponge and antimicrobial surgical scrub agent.
- *Surgical hand antiseptic agent*: An antimicrobial product formulated to significantly reduce the number of microorganisms on skin. Surgical hand antiseptic agents are broad-spectrum agents and should exhibit both persistence and cumulative effect that prevents or inhibits proliferation or survival of microorganisms over time.
- *Transient microorganisms*: Microorganisms found on the skin that are easily removed with a soap and water hand wash or with an antimicrobial hand rub agent.

93. Hand hygiene is often considered the single most important step in preventing infection. Operating-room personnel, like all healthcare personnel, should perform hand hygiene before and after patient contact, before donning gloves, and after removing gloves.

94. Hand hygiene, other than in preparation for surgery, requires washing hands with either plain or antimicrobial soap and water or application of an alcohol-based skin rub. When hands are visibly soiled or contaminated with proteinaceous material, hand washing must precede application of an alcohol-based surgical hand preparation

95. Mechanical washing is the removal of dirt, oils, and microorganisms by means of friction. Antisepsis is the prevention of sepsis by the exclusion, destruction, or inhibition of growth or multiplication of microorganisms from body tissues and fluids.

96. Surgical hand antisepsis is an activity performed immediately prior to gowning and gloving in preparation for surgery. The purpose of surgical hand antisepsis is to remove dirt, skin oils, and transient microorganisms; to reduce the number of resident microorganisms on the nails, hands, and lower arms to as low a level as possible; and to prevent growth of microorganisms for as long as possible. This is accomplished through mechanical washing and chemical antisepsis. Personnel with respiratory infections should not function in the scrub role.

97. The objective of surgical hand antisepsis is to prevent the transfer of microorganisms from personnel to patients and from patients to personnel in the event of glove tears or gown penetration.

98. Prior to performing surgical hand antisepsis, all jewelry must be removed from hands and arms. All other jewelry should also be removed or be completely contained.

99. Hands and arms should be examined for cuts and other lesions that could ooze serum, which is a medium for microbial growth and serves as a potential means of transmission of microorganisms into the patient. Persons with cuts and abrasions should not function in the scrub role.

100. Protective eyewear should be worn when splash or splatter is anticipated. Goggles or face shields are considered appropriate eyewear protection. Regular eyeglasses do not always adequately protect against splashes or splatter that may occur. In the interest of safety, goggles or face shields should be worn for all invasive procedures.

101. Surgical hand antisepsis, traditionally referred to as "scrubbing," historically required that personnel scrub their hands and arms with a sponge/brush or sponge using an antimicrobial surgical scrub agent while adhering to either an anatomical timed scrub procedure or a counted stroke method procedure whereby each finger, hand, and forearm is visualized as having four sides and each side is scrubbed. This method has largely been supplemented by the use of alcohol-based surgical hand preparations that have been cleared by the FDA for use as surgical hand antiseptics.

102. Antimicrobial scrub agents are detergent-based products containing alcohol, iodine/iodophors, chlorhexidine gluconate, triclosan, or parachlorometaxylenol. Povidone-iodine and

chlorhexidine gluconate products are the most commonly used.

103. Alcohol-based products in combination with other products, such as chlorhexidine gluconate and emollients, add persistence and have been shown to be rapid, effective, and gentle to the hands.

104. Each institution should decide whether the traditional scrub procedure, the newer brushless, alcohol-based antiseptics, or a combination of these will be used by the sterile scrub team. Regardless of whether an alcohol-based antiseptic hand rub or a sponge/brush and surgical hand antiseptic hand agent is used, the hands should first be washed. Hands should also be washed after removing gloves (AORN, 2012, p. 75).

105. Surgical hand antiseptic agents should meet the following criteria:

   • Broad spectrum of activity (effective against gram-negative and gram-positive organisms)

   • Rapid acting

   • Nonirritating

   • Not dependent upon a cumulative effect (the first application is as effective as subsequent applications); however, they should demonstrate a cumulative effect

   • Significantly reduces microorganisms on the skin

   • Persistent activity—inhibits the rapid growth of microorganisms

106. Surgical hand antisepsis should be performed according to hospital policy, which should specify the agent and the method to be used. The manufacturer's recommendations and supporting literature regarding use of the agent should be incorporated into this policy.

Traditional Surgical Hand Antisepsis (Traditional Scrub Procedure)

107. Historically, scrub policies called for an anatomical scrub or a timed scrub. In either method, the scrub should include cleaning under nails and scrubbing of all surfaces of each finger, hand, and forearm.

108. Anatomical scrubs may indicate the number of strokes to be applied to each area to be scrubbed. The entire surface to be scrubbed is broken into specified areas with a specified number of strokes for each area. For example, each finger has four surfaces, each of which is scrubbed a specified number of times.

109. Timed scrubs specify the length of time a scrub should last and may specify how long the scrub should last on each specified surface. The number of strokes and time may both be incorporated into a scrub policy.

110. Basic steps in the traditional scrub procedure (scrub sponge/brush and antimicrobial surgical scrub agent) include the following:

   • Individually packaged commercially prepared product intended for traditional surgical hand antisepsis is selected. The product usually contains a sponge/brush combination impregnated with antimicrobial surgical scrub agent and a nail-cleaning tool.

   • The faucet is turned on with water set at a comfortable temperature.

   • Take care throughout the procedure not to splash water onto surgical attire. Wet surgical attire can cause the transfer of microorganisms from personnel to the sterile gown worn during surgery.

   • Hands and forearms are washed with soap and running water.

   • The packaged sponge/brush containing nail cleaner is opened.

   • The nail cleaner and sponge/brush are removed from the package.

   • The sponge/brush is held in one hand; under running water, the nail cleaner is used to clean nails and subungual spaces on the other hand.

   • The process is repeated with the opposite hand.

   • The nail cleaner is discarded.

   • The nails and hands are rinsed.

   • The sponge/brush, if it is impregnated with antimicrobial agent, is moistened. If it is not impregnated with antimicrobial surgical agent, an antimicrobial agent is added to the hands, usually from a foot-pump dispenser.

   • The arms are held in a flexed position with the fingertips pointing upward. Throughout the scrub, the hands are held up and away from the body/surgical attire. The elbows are flexed and the hands held higher than the elbows. Water and cleanser flow from the fingertips (the cleanest area) to the elbow and into the sink.

- Using circular motion and pressure adequate to remove microorganisms but not sufficient to abrade skin, the nails, fingers, hands, and arms are methodically scrubbed, beginning with the fingertips and continuing through the forearms. The scrub sponge/brush is discarded.

- The hands and arms are rinsed, keeping arms flexed with hands above elbows as the scrubbed person enters the operating room.

111. Three-minute surgical hand scrubs are as effective as five-minute scrubs (AORN, 2012, p. 78). The manufacturer's instructions for product use should be followed.

Use of Alcohol-Based Hand Preparations

112. Alcohol-based surgical hand products (either waterless or water aided) are more effective than traditional scrub products in killing microorganisms. They save time, require less time, and reduce costs compared to the traditional products, and added emollients make these products gentle to the hands (CDC, 2002, pp. 13, 19, 21; WHO, 2009, p. 41). Nevertheless, all three types—the traditional scrub sponge/brush and antimicrobial surgical scrub agent, the alcohol-based waterless surgical scrub, and the alcohol-based water-aided solution—are considered acceptable by the CDC.

113. Regarding surgical hand preparation, an alcohol-based waterless surgical scrub was shown to have the same efficacy and demonstrated greater acceptability and fewest adverse effects on skin compared with an alcohol-based water-aided solution and a brush-based iodine solution (WHO, 2009, p. 41).

114. Procedures for using an alcohol-based hand rub vary; however, it is critical that the manufacturer's instructions for use be followed. The scrub procedure should include the following measures:

- Hands and forearms are washed with soap and running water.

- The nails and subungual areas of both hands are cleaned with a disposable nail cleaner at a minimum at the start of the first scrub of the day.

- Hands and forearms are rinsed and thoroughly dried with a clean towel.

- Instead of scrubbing according to the traditional scrub, an alcohol-based hand rub product approved by the FDA for use as a surgical hand antiseptic is applied to the hands and forearms.

- The amount of product applied and the procedure for use must be strictly in accordance with the manufacturer's instructions.

- Hands and forearms are rubbed until dry (AORN, 2012, p. 77).

115. Product selection and policies and procedures for surgical hand scrub should be determined in conjunction with the end users, operating room managers, and the healthcare facility infection control practitioner/committee.

Section Questions

WWW

1. What is often considered the single most important step in the prevention of infection? [Ref 93]

2. Identify times when hand hygiene should be performed. [Ref 93]

3. When is hand washing with soap and water required? [Ref 94]

4. What is the purpose of mechanical hand washing? [Ref 95]

5. What are three outcomes of the surgical scrub prior to gowning and gloving? [Ref 96]

6. What is the objective of the surgical scrub? [Ref 97]

7. What should a scrubbed person do if he or she has a cut or lesion on the hands or arms? [Ref 99]

8. Why are regular eyeglasses not considered appropriate protective eyewear? [Ref 100]

9. Which antimicrobial scrub agents have demonstrated persistence as well as being rapid, effective, and gentle? [Ref 103]

(continues)

Section Questions (continued)

10. What determines whether a traditional sponge/brush product or a brushless alcohol-based antiseptic will be used for the surgical scrub? [Ref 104]

11. What are six criteria for an effective surgical and antiseptic? [Ref 105]

12. What dictates the method of surgical hand antisepsis and product used? [Ref 106]

13. Describe the areas that are included in the surgical scrub, whether it involves an alcohol-based product or a traditional sponge/brush product. [Ref 107]

14. Describe both the stroke method and the timed method appropriate to traditional surgical scrubs. [Refs 108–110]

15. What is the purpose of holding the arms in a flexed position during the surgical scrub? [Ref 110]

16. Which is more effective: a three-minute surgical scrub or a five-minute surgical scrub? [Ref 111]

17. Which is more effective in killing microorganisms: an alcohol-based antiseptic hand product or a traditional antiseptic hand product? [Ref 112]

18. How does the alcohol-based waterless scrub product compare to the alcohol-based water-aided and the brush-based povidone-iodine scrub? [Ref 113]

19. The manufacturer's instructions for using an alcohol-based hand rub should include which criteria? [Ref 114]

20. Who should participate in the selection of surgical hand scrub products? [Ref 115]

Gowning and Gloving Procedure

116. A gown package containing a sterile towel and sterile gown is opened on a small table, separate from the instrument or back table, within the operating room. The gown and towel are arranged so that when the package is opened, the towel is on top of the gown. The gown is folded inside out and from bottom to top in such a manner that the top inside portion of the gown is directly beneath the towel. The towel and gown may be reusable or single use/disposable.

117. If the traditional scrub procedure was performed, the hands and arms must be thoroughly dried before the gown is donned. If the hands and arms are not thoroughly dried, contamination of the gown may occur by strikethrough from organisms contained in moisture on the skin (Figure 5-8).

118. The scrubbed person grasps the sterile towel and lifts it straight up and away from the gown without dripping water on the gown or the sterile field. The scrubbed person steps away from the sterile gown and allows the towel to unfold without contacting the scrub attire. If the towel contacts an unsterile surface, the towel is considered contaminated and a new sterile one must be used.

119. Hold the top half of the towel in one hand and dry the opposite hand and forearm. Dry using a rotating blotting motion, beginning at the hand and working down toward the elbow. When the first hand and forearm are dry, grasp the unused lower half of the towel with the dry hand, and dry the opposite hand and forearm using the same rotating blotting motion from hand to elbow. Take care not to return to an area that has already been dried.

120. Sterile gowns may be reusable or disposable. The gown should be constructed of a material that provides a barrier to prevent the passage of microorganisms from the surgical team to the patient as well as from the patient to the surgical team. The gown manufacturer's data should verify that the materials used in the gown provide a protective barrier against transfer of microorganisms and fluids.

121. Gowns should be fire resistant, as lint free as possible, free from tears or holes, and fluid resistant or fluid proof. Fluid-proof gowns are coated or laminated with an impervious film that does not permit penetration of fluids. Fluid-resistant gowns provide an effective barrier and do not readily permit penetration of liquids. The barrier quality of gowns varies. For procedures where little or no exposure to blood or body fluids is anticipated, a gown

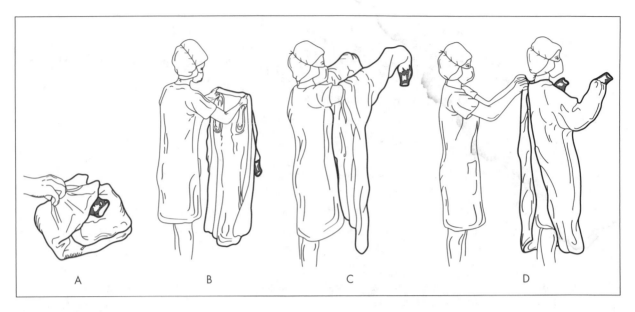

Figure 5-8 Gowning

Source: Reprinted with permission from S.S. Fairchild, *Perioperative Nursing: Principles and Practice*, 4th ed., p. 45, © 1996, Philadelphia: Lippincott Williams & Wilkins. Original illustration permission—J.R. Fuller, Surgical Technology: Principles and Practice, 2nd ed., © 1986, W.B. Saunders Company.

with minimal barrier protection is acceptable. Fluid-resistant gowns should be worn whenever splashes or spraying of blood or other infectious fluids is anticipated. Where large amounts of fluid are anticipated, fluid-proof gowns should be worn.

122. Surgical gowns should also have the following desirable characteristics (AORN, 2012, pp. 119–121):

    • Be resistant to penetration by blood and other body fluids.

    • Maintain their integrity and be durable—resistant to tears, punctures, and abrasions.

    • Be appropriate for the methods of sterilization available to the healthcare facility.

    • Resist combustion.

    • Be comfortable and contribute to maintaining the wearer's desired body temperature.

    • Have a favorable cost–benefit ratio.

123. Reusable gowns lose their barrier qualities with repeated laundering. Quality monitoring should be in place to ensure that only gowns of appropriate quality are used.

124. The cuffs are stockinette and fit tight to the wrist. Gowns may or may not be wraparound style and are held closed with cotton tapes, snaps, or Velcro fasteners.

125. The scrubbed person dons the sterile gown using the following procedure:

    • The scrubbed person grasps the sterile gown by the inside neckline and lifts it away from the gown wrapper.

    • Holding the gown by the neck edge, the scrubbed person moves away from areas of possible contamination and lets the gown unfold downward.

    • The scrubbed person locates the armholes, and both arms are simultaneously inserted into the sleeves. If a closed-gloving technique is to be used, the arms are inserted into the gown only until the hands reach the proximal edge of the cuff. If an open-gloving technique is used, the arms are inserted into the sleeves until the hands advance through the cuffs.

    • The gown is fastened in the back at the neckline and the waist by a nonsterile team member.

    • Gloves are donned.

    • After gloving is completed, the scrubbed person extends a paper tab attached to one of the gown ties to another team member (sterile or unsterile). The scrubbed person pivots away from the other team member, causing the gown to wrap around the scrubbed person. The scrubbed person grasps the tie and pulls it, releasing it from the paper tab, then ties the gown securely in front.

126. Sterile gloves are a barrier that is intended to prevent passage of microorganisms from the scrubbed person to the patient and from the patient to the scrubbed person.

127. Gloves should be selected according to desired strength, durability, and compatibility. Extra-strength specialty gloves are available and should be used for procedures such as bone and joint surgeries where there is high risk of percutaneous blood exposure. Policies and procedures within the facility should indicate when double gloving should be used (AORN, 2012, p. 88).

128. Latex-free gloves must be used when personnel or the patient have latex allergies. Hypoallergenic, powder-free gloves should be chosen to minimize sensitization to natural rubber latex and glove chemicals.

129. Sterile gloves without powder are preferred. The potential adverse effects from powdered gloves for patients include an inflammatory response, delayed healing, foreign body reaction, formation of granulomas, and peritoneal adhesion, especially with multiple surgeries. Powder/talc from latex gloves can serve as a carrier for airborne allergenic natural rubber latex proteins, potentially sensitizing patients and personnel. The use of low-protein, powder-free gloves significantly reduces occupational asthma and incidence of individuals developing allergies to natural rubber latex (FDA, 2011, p. 6). Powdered sterile gloves should be wiped with sterile water or saline prior to the surgical incision.

130. Closed gloving is one method of donning sterile gloves by yourself. Scrubbed hands remain inside the gown sleeve until the glove cuff is secured over the gown cuff (Figure 5-9).

131. Closed gloving begins with the hands inside the sleeves. Using the right hand that is still inside the right cuff, the scrubbed person grasps the everted cuff of the left glove.

132. The left forearm is extended with the palm facing up and the hand still inside the sleeve. The left glove is then placed palm-side down on the upturned left sleeve, palm to palm, thumb to thumb, with the fingers of the glove pointing toward the scrubbed person's body. Using the left thumb and index finger inside the stockinette, grasp the cuff of the glove to hold it in place. The fingers of the left hand must not extend beyond the stockinette cuff. Using the sleeve-covered right hand, stretch the cuff of the left glove over the open end of the left sleeve. The glove should totally encompass the stockinette portion of the sleeve. Using the sleevecovered right hand, pull gently but firmly on the left sleeve of the gown, causing the left hand to slide into the glove.

133. To glove the right hand, grasp the right glove with the already gloved left hand and placed on the right sleeve, palm to palm, thumb to thumb, with glove fingers pointing toward the scrubbed person's body. Grasp the right glove cuff through the stockinette cuff to hold it in place. The fingers of the right hand must not extend beyond the stockinette cuff. Stretch the right glove over the open end of the right sleeve. Using the left hand, pull lightly and evenly on the right sleeve, causing the right hand to slide into the right glove.

134. In the open-glove technique, the scrubbed person extends the hands through the stockinette cuff of the sleeves when donning the gown. During gloving, the surgically clean hand touches only the inside of the sterile glove and never contacts the exterior of the glove (Figure 5-10).

135. A nonscrubbed person opens the glove package on a clean, dry surface. Using the right hand, the scrubbed person grasps the everted cuff of the left glove and slides the fingers and thumb of the left hand into the glove, leaving the everted cuff of the glove over the hand and below the cuff of the gown sleeve. The scrubbed person then slips the fingers of the left gloved hand under the everted cuff of the right glove and slides the fingers and hand into the right glove. The everted glove cuff is brought up and over the cuff of the gown. Care is taken to prevent the sterile gloved hand from touching the skin of the wrist or hand. In the final step, using the gloved right hand, the everted cuff of the left glove is brought over the stockinette cuff of the left sleeve.

136. Although both the closed-glove and open-glove techniques are acceptable during initial gloving, the closed-glove technique is preferred because the open-glove technique affords a greater chance of the scrubbed person's bare hands contacting the outside of the sterile glove, thereby contaminating it.

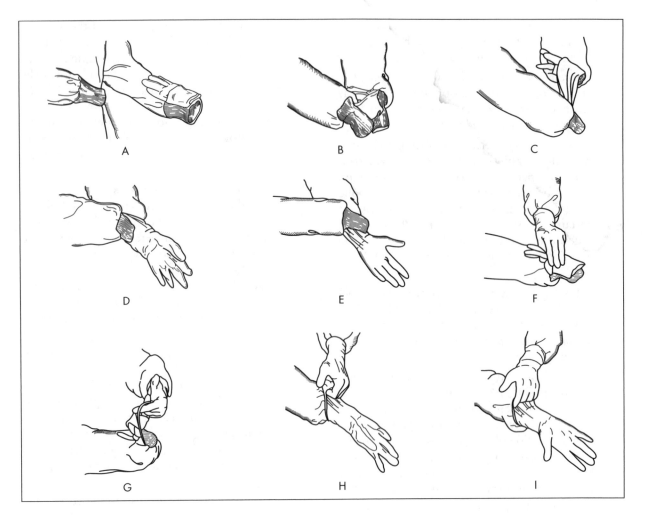

Figure 5-9 Closed gloving

Source: Reprinted with permission from J.R. Fuller, *Surgical Technology: Principles and Practice*, 2nd ed., p. 45, © 1986, Philadelphia: W.B. Saunders Company. Closed gloving. See text (refs 131 to 133) for precise instructions.

Assisting Others to Gown and Glove

137. After the scrubbed person has donned a gown and gloves, he or she assists other team members to gown and glove.

138. The scrubbed person extends a towel to a newly scrubbed person, being careful not to touch that person's hands. The towel should be presented by placing one end over the outstretched hand of the newly scrubbed person. A towel for drying hands is not necessary if an alcohol-based surgical hand product was used.

139. The scrubbed person then grasps the folded gown at the neck edge, lifts it away from the sterile field, and allows it to unfold. Keeping the hands on the outside of the gown and using the neck and shoulder area of the gown to form a protective cuff over the gloves, the scrubbed person offers the inside of the gown to the newly scrubbed team member.

140. The newly scrubbed person will don the gown by inserting the arms into the sleeves and extending the hands through the stockinette cuff of the gown. A nonsterile team member standing behind will then secure the gown at the neck and waist area (Figure 5-11).

141. The scrubbed person will then glove the newly scrubbed team member. The sterile glove is grasped under the everted edge and held so the thumb of the glove is in opposition to the thumb of the person being gloved. The cuff is then stretched open wide. The newly gowned person advances a hand into the glove, being careful to touch nothing but the inside of the

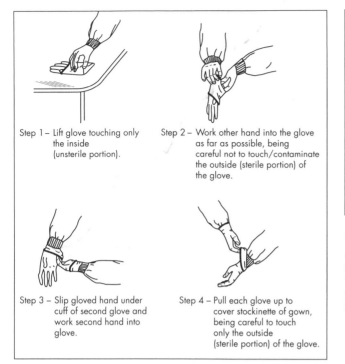

Step 1 – Lift glove touching only the inside (unsterile portion).

Step 2 – Work other hand into the glove as far as possible, being careful not to touch/contaminate the outside (sterile portion) of the glove.

Step 3 – Slip gloved hand under cuff of second glove and work second hand into glove.

Step 4 – Pull each glove up to cover stockinette of gown, being careful to touch only the outside (sterile portion) of the glove.

Figure 5-10 Open gloving

Source: Crooks, L. (1979). *Operating Room Technologies for the Surgical Team*, Boston: Little, Brown & Company. Used by permission of Lippincott Williams & Wilkins.

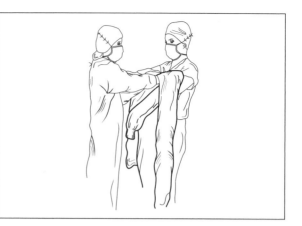

Figure 5-11 Gowning others

Source: Reprinted with permission from S.S. Fairchild, *Perioperative Nursing: Principles and Practice*, 2nd ed., p. 155, © 1993, Philadelphia: W.B. Saunders Company. Original illustration permission—J.R. Fuller, *Surgical Technology: Principles and Practice*, 2nd ed., p. 45, © 1986, Philadelphia: W.B. Saunders Company.

glove. The cuff of the glove must be stretched wide enough and high enough to cover the stockinette gown cuff entirely. This procedure is repeated to glove the other hand.

142. Wearing a second pair of gloves over the first is known as double gloving. Double gloving has been shown to reduce skin contact with the patient's blood and/or body fluids during surgery. This practice also greatly reduces the amount of blood on a needle if a puncture does occur. Double gloving is a widely practiced technique that decreases the risk of perforations of the inner glove. AORN (2012, p. 343) recommends double gloving for all invasive procedures.

143. If a team member's glove becomes contaminated, that person steps back from the sterile field and extends the contaminated hand to a nonsterile team member; the latter individual dons protective gloves and removes the sterile team member's contaminated glove by grasping the outside of the glove approximately 2 inches below the top of the glove and pulling the glove off inside out. The gown cuff must not be pulled down or slip down over the hand because the stockinette is considered

contaminated once the original gloves are donned. The scrubbed person may reglove the team member in the same manner as before, or the open-glove technique can be used to reglove without assistance.

144. If a team member's gown becomes contaminated, a nonsterile team member dons protective gloves and unfastens the gown at the neck and waist, grasps it in front at the shoulders, and pulls it forward and off over the scrubbed person's hands, which are still gloved. The gown should come off in an inside-out manner. The nonsterile team member then removes the sterile team member's gloves, and the scrubbed person regowns and regloves the sterile team member, or the sterile team member may regown and reglove without assistance. The contaminated gown should always be removed before the gloves are removed. This prevents microorganisms and debris that may be found on the gown from being dragged across unprotected, ungloved hands.

145. The closed-glove technique is not acceptable for changing a contaminated glove. During initial gowning and gloving, the scrubbed, but not sterile, ungloved hand passes through the gown cuff, contaminating the cuff. In the closed-glove technique, the cuff contacts the sterile glove; therefore, the new sterile glove would be contaminated by the contaminated cuff.

146. At the completion of surgery, gown and gloves are removed. The gown is removed first. It is grasped near the neck and sleeve and brought

forward over the gloved hands, inverting the gloves as it is removed. The gown is folded so the contaminated outside surface is on the inside. It is deposited in a designated linen or waste receptacle.

147. Gloves are removed in a manner that prevents the contaminated external glove from contacting skin. The gloved fingers of one hand are placed under the everted glove cuff of the opposite hand and pulled off. The fold on the remaining glove is grasped with the bare fingers of the opposite hand and the glove is pulled off. This technique must be performed carefully to prevent bare skin from contacting the contaminated glove surface. Gloves are deposited in a designated waste receptacle.

148. After gloves are removed, wash your hands. If desired, an antimicrobial product may be used. Hand hygiene lessens the chance of contamination of the hands that might have occurred from an invisible hole or tear in the glove.

149. Gown and gloves are not worn outside the operating room.

Creating a Sterile Field

Draping

150. Drapes serve as a barrier to prevent the passage of microorganisms between sterile and nonsterile areas. Sterile drapes are used to create a sterile area around the incision site that may be used for sterile supplies and equipment. This area is referred to as the sterile field.

151. The sterile field includes the patient, furniture, and other equipment that are covered with sterile drapes. The sterile field is isolated from unsterile surfaces and items. Only sterile items are placed on a sterile field (Figure 5-12).

152. Sterile drapes are positioned over the patient in such a way that only a minimum area of skin around the incision site is exposed.

153. Furniture draped to be part of the sterile field often includes instrument or "back" tables, Mayo stands, and ring stands that hold basins.

154. Drapes may be reusable or single use/disposable. Drapes should meet the following criteria:

- Resistant to blood, body fluids, and liquid penetration and provide an effective barrier to prevent passage of microorganisms from nonsterile to sterile areas

- Durable—resistant to tears

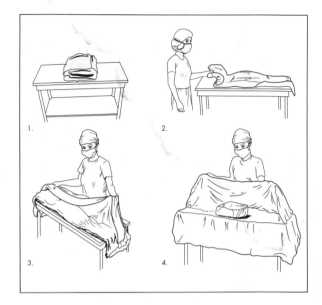

Figure 5-12 Draping a table

Source: Reprinted with permission from S.S. Fairchild, *Perioperative Nursing: Principles and Practice*, 2nd ed. pp. 235–236, © 1993, Philadelphia: W. B. Saunders Company.

- Lint free or low-linting to reduce airborne contamination or shedding into the operative site—microorganisms and dust particles may settle on airborne lint and shed into the operative site

- Flame resistant

- Memory free—easily conform to body and equipment contours or low memory

- Comfortable

155. As with gowns, drapes may be fluid resistant or fluid proof. Materials have varying degrees of resistance to liquids and should be selected based on the intended procedure and anticipated exposure to fluids.

156. Single-use/disposable drapes are more common than reusable drapes; however, both are appropriate for creating a sterile field. Reusable drapes are manufactured in a variety of fabrics with varying degrees of barrier effectiveness. All reusable drapes will lose their barrier qualities with repeated laundering and sterilizations. Laundering and steam sterilization swell fibers, and drying shrinks them. This reduces the tightness of the fibers and diminishes the barrier effectiveness. A quality monitoring program should be in place to ensure drape integrity

and barrier effectiveness. The program may include tracking the number of times a drape has been laundered. All reusable drapes must be routinely inspected for tears and punctures.

157. Single-use/disposable drapes are composed of nonwoven natural and synthetic materials and are manufactured with varying degrees of barrier effectiveness. These fabrics include a fluid-proof polyethylene film laminated between the fabric layers at strategic locations of the drape, usually around the drape fenestration. Nonwoven drapes are available in a variety of configurations and are commercially packaged and sterilized. They are designed for one-time use and are not resterilized.

158. Clear plastic drapes, with or without adhesive backings, are available in various sizes. They are available either plain or impregnated with an antimicrobial agent. These incise drapes are applied directly over the skin at the operative site. When applied securely to the skin around the incision site, incise drapes can aid in preventing migration of microorganisms into the wound. They may be partially applied over the drapes, in which case they assist in keeping the drapes in place without the use of towel clips. The incision is made through the plastic drape. Some plastic drapes include a fluid collection pouch to collect fluids. Pouches may prevent the accumulation of moisture under the drapes where bacteria can proliferate and contaminate the wound.

159. Plastic drapes are useful for draping irregular body areas such as joints, eyes, and ears. Plastic drapes may also be used to seal off a contaminated area such as a stoma.

160. Impervious plastic drapes are available for equipment, such as microscopes, portable C arm, and X-ray equipment, and for specialty needs such as to seal off the perineal area, to cover a tourniquet, or to contain body fluids and irrigation.

Draping Guidelines

161. The following guidelines should be followed during draping (Figure 5-13):
   - Only sterile drapes that are intact are used for draping. All defects in reusable materials must have been patched with a vulcanized heat seal patch.
   - Drapes should be handled as little as possible.
   - Drapes are placed gently; they must not be flipped or shaken. Shaking and flipping cause air currents that serve as vehicles for dust, lint, and other particles.
   - Drapes are carried folded to the operating table and held higher than the table (AORN, 2012, p. 88).
   - Draping begins at the operative site and progresses to the periphery.
   - Once a drape is placed, it is not moved or repositioned. Repositioning drapes can contaminate the incisional area that has been prepped. Drapes that are placed incorrectly are removed by an unscrubbed person.
   - When draping, a cuff is formed from the drape to protect the sterile gloved hands of the person draping (AORN, 2012, p. 88) (Figure 5-14).
   - The points of a towel clip that have penetrated a drape are contaminated and must not be removed until the procedure is complete. Use nonpenetrating towel clips when possible, as they do not interrupt the integrity of drapes and can be removed and repositioned.
   - Whenever the sterility of a drape is in doubt, it is considered contaminated and is discarded.

Standard Drapes

162. The number, type, and size of drapes selected for a procedure require careful planning. Selection factors include the type of procedure, the amount of area around the incision that needs to be included in the sterile field, and the furniture and equipment that will be draped. Cost considerations require that variety and number of drapes be kept to a minimum.

163. Standard drapes include the following options:
   - Flat sheets used to drape instrument tables and areas of the patient.
   - Mayo stand covers.
   - Towels used to drape the operative site.
   - Fenestrated drapes with openings of various sizes and configurations to drape for specific procedures or specialties (typical drapes include abdominal laparotomy, chest/breast, head and neck, total hip joint, and extremity). Fenestrations are generally reinforced with an impervious barrier. The

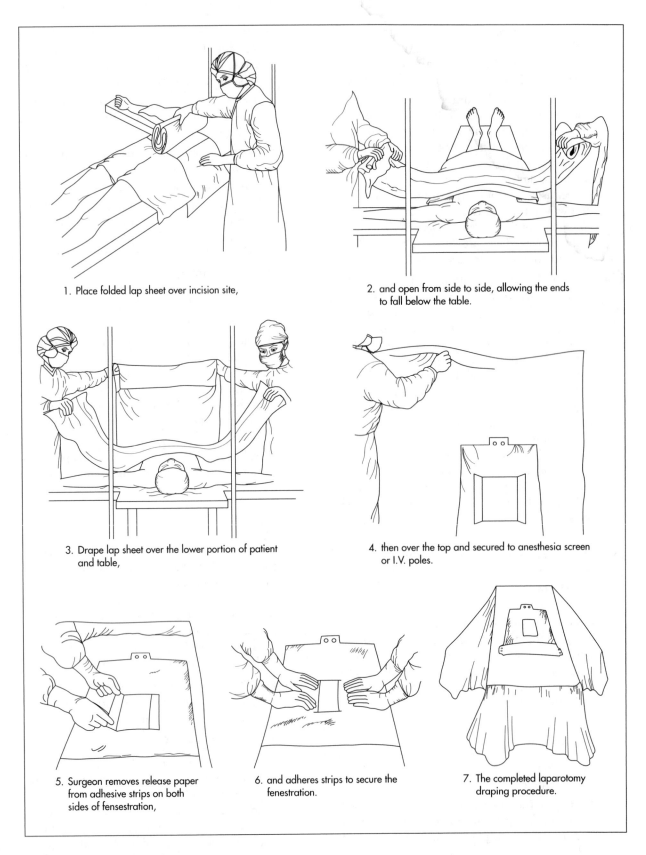

1. Place folded lap sheet over incision site,

2. and open from side to side, allowing the ends to fall below the table.

3. Drape lap sheet over the lower portion of patient and table,

4. then over the top and secured to anesthesia screen or I.V. poles.

5. Surgeon removes release paper from adhesive strips on both sides of fensestration,

6. and adheres strips to secure the fenestration.

7. The completed laparotomy draping procedure.

Figure 5-13 Draping the patient

Source: S.S. Fairchild, *Perioperative Nursing: Principles and Practice*, 4th ed., p. 248, © 1996, Philadelphia: Lippincott Williams & Wilkins.
Original illustration permission—J.R. Fuller, Surgical Technology: Principles and Practice, 2nd ed., © 1986, Philadelphia: W.B. Saunders Company.

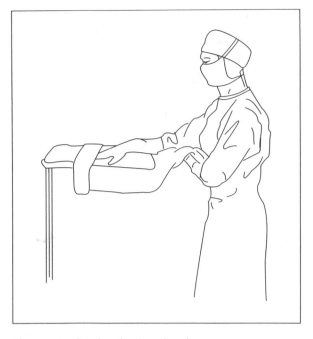

Figure 5-14 Draping the Mayo Stand
Source: Courtesy of Andrew Maillard.

fenestrated drape is large enough to cover the entire patient and the operating table with sufficient material to extend over the foot of the table, the ether screen at the head of the table, and the arm boards. If the drape does not cover sufficiently, flat sheets can be used to extend the sterile field.

- Aperture drape—a small clear fenestrated plastic drape frequently used in eye and ear procedures.
- Equipment drapes—clear plastic drapes that cover X-ray machines, microscopes, and other equipment.
- Stockinette used to drape feet and hands.
- Leggings—part of the drape set intended for surgery with the patient in the lithotomy position.
- Various specialty drapes (e.g., C/S, craniotomy, cardiac).

Section Questions

www

1. When gowning oneself, what are some precautions that prevent contaminating the sterile gown? [Refs 116–119]
2. List some essential qualities of gowns. [Refs 120–121]
3. What are some additional desirable gown characteristics? [Ref 122]
4. How does the scrubbed person wrap the gown around himself or herself and tie it? [Ref 125]
5. What is the value of hypoallergenic gloves? [Ref 128]
6. Which adverse outcomes have been associated with glove powder? [Ref 129]
7. Why is the closed method of gloving preferable to the open method? [Ref 136]
8. What is the value of wearing a second set of gloves (double gloving)? [Ref 142]
9. Why is the contaminated gown always removed before contaminated gloves? [Ref 144]
10. Why is the closed method of gloving not used to change a contaminated glove during a procedure? [Ref 145]
11. Why must hands be washed (or an antimicrobial product used) after gloves are removed? [Ref 148]
12. Why are the contaminated gown and gloves removed inside the operating room after a procedure and never worn outside the operating room? [Ref 149]
13. What is the purpose of sterile drapes? [Ref 150]
14. What does the sterile field encompass? [Ref 151]
15. What are some desirable characteristics of sterile drapes? [Ref 154]
16. What is the purpose of a quality monitoring program for laundering reusable drapes? [Ref 156]
17. Describe several reasons for using incise drapes. [Refs 158–159]

(continues)

Section Questions (continued)

18. How is the sterile field protected when items such as X-ray equipment and microscopes are used? [Ref 160]

19. In what ways are impervious plastic drapes used? [Ref 160]

20. How are defects in reusable drapes managed so that they can be used on the sterile field? [Ref 161]

21. Why is flipping or shaking drapes during the draping process prohibited? [Ref 161]

22. Which part of the patient is draped first? [Ref 161]

23. Why are drapes not moved once they have been positioned? [Ref 161]

24. Why are nonpenetrating towel clips preferable to towel clips with sharp points? [Ref 161]

25. List at least six types of standard drapes. [Ref 163]

Creating and Maintaining a Sterile Field

164. Only scrubbed persons can enter the sterile field. Personnel in the sterile field wear sterile gowns and gloves. Surgical gowns and gloves establish a barrier that minimizes the passage of microorganisms between nonsterile and sterile areas.

165. Scrubbed personnel should don sterile gowns and gloves from a sterile area separate from the sterile instrument table to avoid contamination of the sterile field. Once donned, the gown is considered sterile in front from the chest to the level of the sterile field. The sleeves are considered sterile from 2 inches above the elbow down to the top edge of the cuff. The neckline, shoulders, axilla, and cuffed portion of the sleeves may become contaminated by perspiration and, therefore, are not considered sterile. The back is considered nonsterile because it cannot observed by the scrubbed person to ensure that it has not been contaminated. The cuffs are considered contaminated once the hands have passed through them (AORN, 2012, p. 87).

166. Sterile drapes are used to create a sterile field (AORN, 2012, p. 88). Sterile drapes are placed on the patient and on all furniture and equipment that will be part of the sterile field. Sterile drapes serve as a barrier to the passage of microorganisms, isolate the sterile field from the surrounding environment, and minimize passage of microorganisms between sterile and nonsterile areas.

167. Items used within a sterile field must be sterile (AORN, 2012, p. 88). Items for use during surgery are wrapped and sterilized prior to surgery. On occasion, "just in time" sterilization will provide an unwrapped item that is taken directly from the autoclave to the sterile field.

168. Sterility of items must be ensured both by the person dispensing them and by the person accepting them. The circulating nurse should check the integrity of the wrapper, the expiration date (if there is one), and the color of the indicator tape. The chemical indicator or integrator inside the package is checked by the scrubbed person to ensure that items were exposed to the sterilant or, depend ing on the type of indicator used, that parameters of sterilization were attained during the sterilization process. If an item is taken directly from the autoclave, the circulating nurse must ensure that the proper technique is used to transfer items to the sterile field.

169. Whenever the integrity of a sterile barrier is broken, the contents must be considered unsterile. Wrappers, gowns, gloves, and drapes are all examples of sterile barriers. Examples of sterile barriers that have been permeated include a tear or hole in a wrapper or glove; a wet, scorched, or stained wrapper; and a barrier that looks questionable.

170. The contents of wet or stained wrappers may have been subject to strike-through, which occurs when liquids soak through a barrier from a sterile to an unsterile area, and vice versa. Strike-through allows for passage of microorganisms through the barrier, so the contents must be considered contaminated. When strike-through occurs, it might not be noticed initially and the item might dry. Therefore, items contained in wrappers that are stained should be considered contaminated.

171. If the sterility of any item is in doubt, it is considered contaminated and is discarded. Items that become contaminated must not be permitted on the sterile field. Items that remain on the drapes during the procedure, such as suction and cautery, are secured to prevent them from sliding below the level of the sterile field. An item that slides below the level of the sterile field is considered contaminated and must be discarded and replaced.

172. A sterile field should be prepared and maintained for every surgical patient. Items introduced to a sterile field should be opened, dispensed, and transferred by methods that maintain sterility and integrity (AORN, 2012, p. 89).

173. When dispensing an item to the sterile field, the unscrubbed person should open the wrapper flap that is farthest away first and the wrapper flap that is closest last. This prevents an unsterile body part from having to reach across a sterile field (Figure 5-15).

174. All wrapper edges should be secured to prevent accidental contamination of the scrubbed person or sterile field with a wrapper edge. If an item cannot be carefully placed or easily flipped onto the field, the item should be presented to the scrubbed person or opened on a separate surface.

175. Sterile gowns and drapes and other similar items may be placed onto the sterile field;

176. however, the portion of the unscrubbed person's hand that may extend over the sterile field is covered by an everted portion of the sterile wrapper.

176. Heavy, awkward, or sharp items should not be tossed onto the sterile field because they may roll off the edge, displace other items from the sterile field, or penetrate the sterile barrier. These items should be opened on a separate table or stand or received directly by the scrubbed person (Figure 5-16).

177. Solutions delivered to the sterile field should be first verified with the scrubbed person, then poured into a receptacle placed near the table's edge or held by the scrubbed person. The scrubbed person should label the container, verifying the label with the circulating nurse. The entire contents of the container should be poured slowly to avoid splashing. This eliminates the need to reach across the sterile field and decreases the risk of splashing the sterile field and creating the potential for strike-through.

178. Because the edge of a bottle is considered contaminated, once its cap is removed, the cap should not be replaced. Solutions remaining within a bottle or container should not be used. Drops may have contacted the unsterile outside of the bottle or container during initial pouring and could contaminate solutions if they are poured later. Therefore the entire contents of the bottle should be poured into the receptacle (Figure 5-17).

179. Transfer devices, such as a sterile vial spike, should be used to dispense medications to the

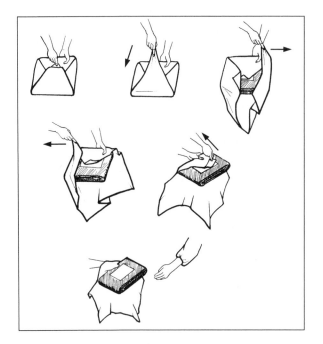

Figure 5-15 Opening a package

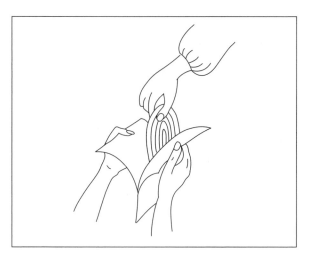

Figure 5-16 Retrieving an item

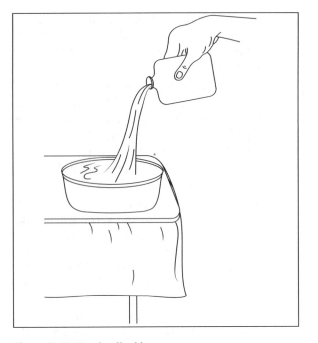

Figure 5-17 Pouring liquid

sterile field. The stopper of the medicine vial should not be removed, and the medication should not be poured into a medicine glass on the field (AORN, 2012, p. 272).

180. Rigid container systems should be opened on a separate surface. The external indicator should be verified for appropriate color change. Locks should be inspected for security to verify no breach of the container seal has occurred prior to its use. The lid should be lifted toward the person opening the container and away from the container. The filter should be checked and changed according to the manufacturer's written instructions.

181. Boundaries between sterile and unsterile are not always clearly defined. Good judgment and keen observation will ensure that only sterile items are introduced to the sterile field.

182. A sterile field should be maintained and monitored continuously (AORN, 2012, p. 90).

183. A sterile field should be set up as close to the time of surgery as possible. The longer sterile items are open to the environment, the greater opportunity there is for contamination to occur. There is no standard for how long a sterile field may remain open before it is considered contaminated. Institutional policy may dictate a time frame.

184. In the event that a sterile field is created in anticipation of surgery and the surgery is delayed, the sterile field should be under constant visual observation. In the absence of an institutional policy, the perioperative nurse must use good judgment to determine when a sterile field should no longer be considered suitable for use. The nature of the surgical procedure should be considered. For example, if the surgery is emergent and a delay caused by having to set up another sterile field would seriously compromise patient safety, the best decision may be to continue monitoring and preserve the sterile field.

185. Covering a sterile field to prevent contamination is a questionable practice and should be discontinued. It is difficult to remove a cover without contaminating the field because removing a cover requires that a portion of the cover that has been below the level of the sterile field be drawn up over the top of the sterile field. Some institutional policies may permit covering using two drapes. Each drape is positioned to cover half of the sterile field and to meet in the middle, where an everted cuff is formed from each drape. Using the cuffs, each drape is removed from the center outward, rather than up and over the field. This is not an AORN-recommended practice, however, and where it is practiced strict guidelines should be provided on application and technique.

186. Once a sterile field has been created, it should be monitored by all team members for possible contamination. For this reason, the sterile field should not be left unattended.

187. All personnel moving within or around a sterile field should do so in a manner that will maintain the sterility of the field (AORN, 2012, p. 91). Scrubbed personnel should remain close to and always face the sterile field (Figure 5-18).

188. Unscrubbed personnel should face sterile fields on approach, should not walk between two sterile fields, and should be aware of the need for distance from the sterile field. By establishing patterns of movement around the sterile field and keeping sterile areas in view, accidental contamination can be reduced.

189. Scrubbed personnel should keep their arms and hands above the level of their waists at all times. Hands should remain in front of the body above waist level so the hands remain

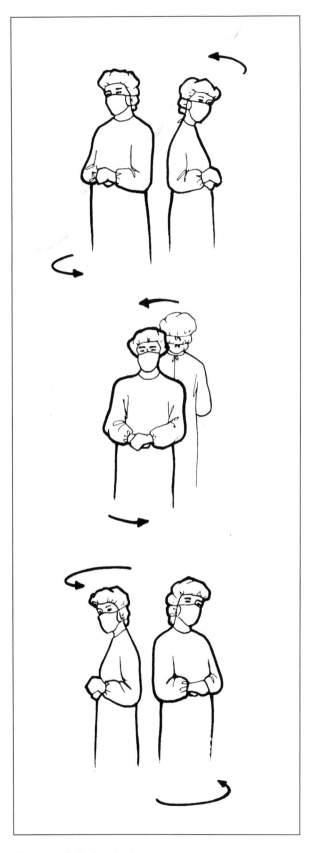

Figure 5-18 Back to back

visible. Contamination may occur when arms and hands are moved below waist level. Arms should not be folded with the hands in the axilla. This area has the potential to become contaminated by perspiration, allowing for strike-through of the gown and, ultimately, contamination of the gloved hands. Scrubbed personnel should avoid changing levels and should be seated only when the entire surgical procedure will be performed at that level. When changing levels, exposure of the nonsterile portion of the surgical gown is likely.

190. The number and movement of individuals involved in a surgical procedure should be kept to a minimum.

191. The patient is the center of the sterile field. All additional sterile equipment is grouped around the patient within view of the scrubbed person.

192. Unscrubbed persons contact only unsterile items. They should keep a safe distance from the sterile field to prevent accidental contamination. Determining a safe distance requires astute judgment. Unscrubbed persons who approach the sterile field do so by facing the sterile field; they do not walk between two sterile fields.

193. When a break in sterile technique occurs, corrective action should be taken immediately unless the patient's safety is at risk. If the patient's safety is at risk, correct the break in technique as soon as it is safe to do so. When a break in sterile technique occurs and cannot be corrected immediately, it should be reported and recorded, and the wound classification should be adjusted accordingly and documented on the operative record.

Control of Environmental Sources of Infection

Traffic Patterns

194. The operating room itself is divided into three areas that are defined by the activities that occur within each area. These areas are restricted, semi-restricted, and unrestricted (AORN, 2012, p. 95).

195. The restricted area is where surgical procedures are performed and sterile supplies are stored. This area includes the operating and procedure rooms, the substerile area where the autoclave may be located, and the clean core where sterile supplies are stored. Scrub attire

Section Questions

1. Who may enter the sterile field? [Ref 164]

2. Where does the scrubbed person don gown and gloves? [Ref 165]

3. Which parts of the gown, once donned, are considered sterile and which are considered unsterile? Give rationale for your response. [Ref 165]

4. Who is responsible for assuring the sterility of a sterile item—the person delivering the item or the person accepting it? [Ref 168]

5. How does the circulating nurse determine that an item is sterile and safe for delivery to the sterile field? [Ref 168]

6. How does the scrubbed person determine that an item is safe to accept onto the sterile field? [Ref 168]

7. What is done with an item of questionable sterility? [Refs 169, 171]

8. What is strike-through and why is it a reason to consider an item contaminated? [Ref 170]

9. When might suction tubing or an electrosurgical pencil that remains on the sterile field during the procedure be considered contaminated? [Ref 171]

10. How are items that remain on the sterile field during a procedure protected from becoming contaminated? [Ref 171]

11. When opening a sterile package, which flap is opened first and what is the rationale for doing this? [Ref 173]

12. How are items that are difficult to place or flip onto the sterile field delivered? [Ref 174]

13. How does an unscrubbed person protect the sterile field from his or her contaminated hand and arm when delivering a sterile item to the sterile field? [Ref 175]

14. What might happen if heavy, awkward, or sharp instruments are tossed onto the sterile field? [Ref 176]

15. How should heavy, awkward, or sharp instruments be delivered to the sterile field? [Ref 176]

16. How does the circulating nurse deliver liquids to the sterile field safely? [Refs 177–178]

17. Why do you think all containers into which liquids are poured should be labeled? [Ref 177]

18. Why must the entire contents of a bottle be delivered at once? [Ref 178]

19. How are medications in vials delivered to the sterile field? [Ref 179]

20. What is involved in opening instruments in a rigid container for the sterile field? [Ref 180]

21. When should a sterile field be set up and what determines the length of time a sterile field can remain set up before it is used? [Refs 183–184]

22. Why is covering a sterile field to protect it a questionable practice? [Ref 185]

23. Who is responsible for monitoring the sterile field? [Ref 186]

24. What is the protocol for unscrubbed personnel to navigate around a sterile field? [Ref 188, 192]

25. What should scrubbed persons do to ensure that they do not contaminate themselves? [Ref 189]

and hair covering are required in the restricted area. A long-sleeved cover-up jacket that is buttoned or snapped closed is recommended as well. A mask is required when sterile supplies are opened. The patient is not required to wear a mask except when transmission-based airborne or droplet precautions are necessary.

196. Persons entering the semi-restricted or restricted areas for a brief time for a specific purpose may wear a disposable coverall (jumpsuit) over street attire in place of scrub suit (AORN, 2012, pp. 58–59).

197. The semi-restricted area includes storage for clean and sterile supplies, instrument-processing

areas, scrub sinks, and corridors leading to restricted areas. Scrub attire and hair covering are required in the restricted area. A long-sleeved cover-up jacket that is buttoned or snapped closed is recommended as well. Depending on the design of the suite, lounges may be included in the semi-restricted area. Only authorized personnel and patients are permitted in this area.

198. The unrestricted area is where operating-room personnel interact with outside departmental personnel; it includes locker rooms, patient reception areas, and areas where supplies are received. Street clothes are permitted in the unrestricted area.

199. Movement from unrestricted to restricted areas should be through a transition zone such as a locker room, office, or holding area.

200. Operating-room suites should be secure to protect patient privacy; ensure the safety of patients, personnel, and visitors; and protect supplies and equipment from tampering and theft (AORN, 2012, p. 96).

201. Talking and numbers of personnel present during surgery should be kept to a minimum to reduce the number of microorganisms shed that settle on dust particles in the air.

202. Items that are considered contaminated, soiled, or dirty should not be transported through the same corridors as clean and sterile items. The flow of supplies should be from the clean core to the operating room and from the operating room to a peripheral corridor, and not back into the clean or sterile area. For example, supplies for a procedure should be taken from the clean core into the operating room, and after the procedure all instruments and other contaminated items should exit the operating room into a peripheral corridor where they are transported to an area for discard or transported to a decontamination area. In healthcare facilities where design does not permit this—for example, where only one door into the operating room exists—contaminated, soiled, or dirty items should be contained/covered and transported to the decontamination area at times other than when clean or sterile items are transported through the same area.

203. A common modern operating room design is one with a sterile core surrounded by operating rooms. This design eliminates having to move both sterile and contaminated supplies through the same space.

204. Items delivered to the operating room from sources outside the healthcare facility should be removed from external shipping cartons before being permitted into the operating room. Outside shipping cartons may harbor insects and dirt collected during transport (AORN, 2012, pp. 96–97).

205. Items and supplies prepared or selected for surgical cases that are delivered to the operating room from departments within the healthcare facility should be transported in closed or covered carts to reduce the potential for contamination.

Operating-Room Environment

206. The operating room is considered a clean environment. The design of the operating room, its location within the healthcare facility, limited access, traffic patterns, and policies and procedures for control and environmental cleaning help to maintain its cleanliness.

207. The operating room should have a separate ventilation and air filtration system. All air is filtered through a special filter system. Filters are designed to remove dust and aerosol particles from the air. All air flow is from ceiling to floor.

208. Air in the operating room is maintained under positive pressure. The air pressure is higher in each operating room than in the hallways so that the more contaminated hallway air is not pulled into the room. (The exception to positive-pressure air flow occurs in rooms specifically designed for procedures that should be performed in a negative-pressure environment, such as a bronchoscopy on a patient with tuberculosis.) Because of this pressure difference, doors to each operating room must be kept closed to prevent disruption of the air flow.

209. To maintain the cleanest air possible, a majority of operating rooms adhere to the standards identified by the American Institute of Architects (AIA), which require an air flow rapid enough to change the total volume of air in each operating room a minimum of 15 times per hour with at least 3 exchanges of outside air. A rate of 20 to 25 air exchanges per hour is recommended, and many newer facilities comply with this recommendation (AIA, 2006, p. 130; ASHRAE/ASHE/ANSI, 2010, p.

3). Ventilation systems must comply with local, state, and national regulations. When these regulations vary in the requirement for the number of air exchanges per hour and the number of fresh air exchanges required, the most stringent of requirements prevail.

210. Laminar air-flow systems may be found in some operating rooms. A laminar air-flow system is a unidirectional ventilation system in which filtered, bacteria-free, "ultraclean" air is circulated over the patient from a filtered outlet and returned through a receiving air inlet. Air is filtered through high-efficiency particulate air (HEPA) filters that remove all particles equal to or greater than 0.3 micron in size with an efficiency of 99.7%. Laminar air-flow systems can deliver more than 200 air exchanges per hour. Only sterile items are permitted within the area across which the filtered air flows. Laminar air-flow systems are used most often for procedures where the risk of infection is high, or when an infection can cause a disastrous patient outcome, such as total joint replacement.

211. Room temperature is maintained between 68°F and 75°F (20°C and 24°C). This is comfortable enough for the surgical team, yet will inhibit bacterial growth. Relative humidity is maintained at 20% to 60% (ASHRAE/ASHE/ANSI, 2010, p. 3). Higher humidity can provide an opportunity for mold growth, and lower humidity can result in excessive amount of dust that can carry bacteria.

Operating-Room Sanitation

212. To promote a clean environment, surface materials in the operating room should be nonporous, smooth, washable, and easy to clean. Wall, ceiling, and floor joints are completely sealed. Floor coverings are nonporous.

213. Operating-room sanitation practices play a significant role in creating a surgical environment for patients and personnel that contains a minimum of microorganisms. Microorganisms can survive on many environmental surfaces; in fact, the inanimate environment may serve as a reservoir for infectious organisms. Methicillin-resistant *Staphylococcus aureus* (MRSA) can remain for months, and *Clostridium difficile* can form spores that survive for years on inanimate surfaces. Rigorous cleaning practices are essential to control and minimize the numbers of pathogens present in the suite.

214. Although cleaning and housekeeping protocols may vary among healthcare institutions, cleaning procedures are generally carried out prior to the beginning of the day's schedule, during the procedure, between procedures, at the end of the daily schedule, and periodically, such as weekly or monthly. Only products registered with the Environmental Protection Agency (EPA) as hospital-grade disinfectants should be used for cleaning inanimate surfaces in the operating room.

215. Persons responsible for cleaning and who, in the course of their work, have the potential to contact contaminated items, blood, or body fluids must practice standard precautions by wearing personal protective attire that is appropriate to the task to be performed. Such attire includes gloves, masks, eyewear, and gowns.

216. Prior to the first procedure of the day, the perioperative nurse should visually assess the room for cleanliness and if necessary notify housekeeping or environmental services. Furniture, equipment, and surgical lights should be damp dusted with a lint-free cloth moistened with an EPA-registered hospital-grade disinfectant. Alcohol and high-level disinfectants used for instrument processing should not be used for operating-room sanitation.

217. Particular attention should be paid to horizontal surfaces because dust and lint that transport microorganisms settle on these surfaces. Equipment from other areas, such as X-ray machines and tourniquet devices that are necessary for the procedure, are damp dusted before they are brought into the room. Video and computer monitors and plasma screens may not be compatible with the germicide used on other surfaces. The manufacturers of this equipment should be consulted to determine the most appropriate cleaning products.

218. If possible, patients known to have a latex allergy should be the first scheduled cases of the day. Latex products used during the day may cause latex particles to remain airborne for a period of time, and damp dusting may not be sufficient to remove all traces of latex protein.

219. Throughout the procedure, contamination is confined and contained to as small an area around the patient and sterile field as possible. During the procedure, spills or splashes of blood and body fluids may occur in the immediate vicinity of the sterile field. These should be promptly cleaned using a soft disposable cloth

and an intermediate-level germicide intended for hospital use. The germicide should be EPA registered and should have a tuberculocidal claim. Amount and dilution should be determined by the manufacturer's instructions for use. Spills or splatters of other organic debris, such as patient tissue, should also be promptly cleaned.

220. Spills that contain blood or potentially infectious material should first be absorbed with a soft cloth and then cleaned with an EPA-registered disinfectant (AORN, 2012, p. 242). Spill kits should be available for large spills of body fluids and for chemicals such as glutaraldehyde.

221. Persons responsible for cleanup should wear personal protective equipment appropriate to the activity.

222. Disposable items that become contaminated should be discarded into leak-proof and tear-resistant containers to prevent contact with the environment and with personnel who are responsible for handling operating room waste. Sponges are deposited into a plastic-lined bucket or other prepared surface. They are counted as soon as possible and sealed in an impervious receptacle. They are not left to hang over the sides of the bucket, where they can drip onto the floor. Many institutions use a pocket count bag to contain discarded sponges. This allows for visualization of all sponges during closing counts. Blood, body secretions, and other fluids from the sterile field are collected in leak-proof containers.

223. Specimens should be placed in clean leak-proof containers. Upon receipt of the specimen from the sterile field, seal the container and, if necessary, wipe the container with an EPA-registered hospital-grade germicide. Take care to prevent contamination of specimen documentation and other records.

224. Contaminated reusable items that fall or are removed from the sterile field should be wiped with a germicide and placed in an impervious container. Persons handling contaminated items must wear gloves.

225. All items that come in contact with the patient or the sterile field are considered contaminated and, if single use/disposable, should be discarded according to local, state, and national waste regulations, which specify what constitutes infectious waste. Disposable items contaminated with infectious waste are deposited in leak-proof containers or bags that are color coded, tagged, or labeled so as to be immediately recognizable as hazardous waste (OSHA, 2011). Examples of such waste include gowns, gloves, sponges, and suture threads.

226. Infectious waste fluids may be poured down a drain connected to a sanitary sewer if regulations permit. Alternatively, the collection container may be sealed and placed in a leak-proof container or bag that is color coded and tagged or labeled so as to be immediately recognizable as hazardous waste. Many institutions used chemical agents to solidify liquid waste to reduce the possibility of spills. Local regulations must be followed to ensure the safety of the entire community.

227. Disposal and treatment of infectious waste is significantly more costly than disposal and treatment of noninfectious waste. It is important to know the definition of infectious waste in the area in which one practices, and to deposit only those items that meet the definition of infectious waste into the hazardous-waste bag or container. Noninfectious waste should not be placed into hazardous-waste bags/containers. Not all items contaminated with blood are defined as infectious waste. Some regulations define infectious waste as items contaminated with blood or other materials that, if compressed, would release blood or other infectious material.

228. Noninfectious disposable items are deposited into receptacles not designated for infectious waste; these containers are then sealed and removed from the room.

229. Sharp items, such as needles, staples, and scalpel blades, are considered infectious waste. They are deposited in a designated leak-proof, puncture-resistant sharps container identified with a biohazard label (OSHA, 2011). Sharps containers are sealed and replaced by designated personnel.

230. Reusable linen that is identified as infectious is placed in a closeable bag that is color coded, tagged, or labeled as infectious waste (OSHA, 2011). When contaminated linen is wet, it should be placed in a bag that prevents leak-through. Reusable noninfectious items are transported, cleaned, and disinfected or sterilized according to the healthcare facility's policy.

231. Following the procedure, all instruments opened for the procedure, whether or not they were actually used, are considered contaminated and must be appropriately cleaned and processed. Instruments from sets should be kept together. All contaminated instruments should be placed in designated closed carts, labeled as a biohazard, and transported to instrument cleaning areas. When designated carts are not available, the instruments should be covered and transported.

232. Furniture, including operating lights, linen hamper frames, the operating-room bed and mattress, suction canisters, and other equipment used during the procedure is wiped with an EPA-registered hospital-grade germicidal agent intended for housekeeping purposes. Kick buckets are cleaned and relined. Patient transport vehicles, including straps, railings, and other attachments, are also wiped with an EPA-registered hospital-grade germicidal agent. Items in contact with the patient, such as blood pressure cuffs, positioning devices, and tourniquets, should be cleaned as well.

233. Any equipment or furniture that is visibly soiled is cleaned with an EPA-registered hospital-grade germicide. Walls, doors, push plates, handles, cabinets, lights, and other areas that are visibly soiled are cleaned. Visibly soiled areas of the floor are cleaned with an EPA-registered hospital-grade germicidal agent. If visibly soiled, the floor around the operating-room table should be cleaned with an EPA-registered hospital-grade germicidal agent.

234. A clean mop head should be used for each cleanup, and the mop should not be dipped back into the solution once it has been used. If the used mop is not dipped into the solution, the solution may be used for subsequent cleanups, provided a clean mop head is also used. A clean mop head should be used for each room/patient procedure. Individual institutional policies for cleaning the floor may vary, and floor cleaning when there is no visible soil may not be necessary after each procedure.

235. A number of hospitals have switched from string mops to microfiber mops because they are lightweight, require less water for rinsing, attract and retain negatively charged dust and dirt particles (AORN, 2012, p. 238), and are cost-effective when labor costs are calculated (EPA, 2002).

236. At the conclusion of the day's schedule, operating and procedure rooms, scrub-utility areas, corridors, furnishings, and equipment should be terminally cleaned.

237. Other areas that should be cleaned daily include the following:
    - Surgical lights and tracks
    - Equipment towers
    - Computer keyboards
    - IV poles
    - Scrub sinks, including the faucet head and aerator
    - Horizontal surfaces such as tables and countertops
    - Furniture—particular attention should be given to castors and wheels
    - Drawer, door, and cabinet handles
    - Push plates
    - Ventilation grills
    - Cabinet and operating-room doors
    - Utility carts
    - Floors in the operating room, scrub sink area, and corridor (floors in the operating room should be wet-vacuumed)
    - Any food left out in the lounge area should be discarded or sealed and/or refrigerated as appropriate

238. Reusable cleaning equipment is disassembled, cleaned, and dried prior to storage.

239. Many items and areas within the operating room are cleaned periodically. Cleaning may occur weekly, monthly, or as otherwise indicated in the facility's policies. Each facility should have written policies that address cleaning schedules, techniques, and persons responsible for the following:
    - Lounges, locker areas, and offices
    - Holding areas
    - Cabinet shelves
    - Walls
    - Ceilings
    - Air-conditioning vents, grills, and filters
    - Ice machines and refrigerators
    - Sterilizers
    - Restrooms
    - Storage areas

240. The anesthesia department is generally responsible for cleaning and caring for its own equipment. The AORN-recommended practices for cleaning, handling, and processing of anesthesia equipment can serve as guidelines for developing institutional policies and procedures (AORN, 2012, pp. 473–482).

Additional Considerations: Cleaning and Scheduling

241. CDC's standard precautions consider all surgical patients to be infectious and the potential for cross-infection exists for all procedures; therefore, no special cleaning technique is required after procedures on patients known to be infected with HIV or other infectious microorganisms. Routine cleaning, however, must be adequate and thorough.

242. At one time it was believed that patients known to be infected with HIV, hepatitis, or other infectious diseases should be scheduled as the last patient of the day to prevent possible cross-contamination with other patients who would subsequently be brought into the room where surgery had been performed on the known infected patient. Because standard precautions are used consistently and all patients are considered infectious, cleaning practices should be consistent for all patients and procedures. There is no need to schedule known infected patients as the last procedure of the day.

243. Patients with airborne-transmitted infectious diseases are an exception to this rule. These patients should be scheduled when personnel and patient traffic is minimal so that exposure is reduced. Scheduling as the last case of the day may be appropriate for these patients.

Special Considerations

Clostridium difficile

244. Although standard and transmission-based precautions are adequate in regard to cleaning of equipment and surfaces contaminated or suspected to be contaminated with resistant microorganisms such as MRSA, there is a heightened awareness of the need for strict adherence to cleaning protocols when organisms are resistant to antibacterial agents and pose an infection risk.

245. When caring for a patient infected with *C. difficile*, alcohol hand rubs are *not* recommended. Hand hygiene should consist of washing hands with antimicrobial soap and water.

246. *C. difficile* is a spore-forming bacterium that can survive for months on environmental surfaces (McDonald et al., 2012).

247. For surface areas where epidemiology indicates transmission of *C. difficile*, the Society for Healthcare Epidemiology of America (SHEA, 2010, p. 3) recommends using chlorine-containing cleaning agents or other sporicidal agents to address environmental contamination.

Creutzfeldt-Jakob Disease

248. While prions (infectious proteins) have been shown to bind tightly to surfaces and to be difficult to remove by cleaning, specific formulations of alkaline and enzymatic detergents can effectively eliminate the infectivity of prions (Rutala and Weber, 2010, p. 108).

249. Environmental surfaces (noncritical) contaminated with high-risk tissue or suspected to be contaminated with high-risk tissue (brain, spinal cord, eye) from a patient with known or suspected Creutzfeldt-Jakob disease (CJD) should be cleaned with a detergent and then spot-decontaminated with 5000 ppm sodium hypochloride or 1 N NaOH. Noncritical equipment contaminated with high-risk tissue should be cleaned and then disinfected with 5000 ppm sodium hypochloride or 1 N NaOH, depending on material compatibility (AAMI, 2011, p. 166). Whenever possible, disposable supplies and instruments should be used.

Airborne- and Droplet-Transmitted Infections

250. If possible, surgery should be postponed on patients with airborne- or droplet-transmitted infections. If the patient's condition is such that the surgery cannot be postponed, ideally the procedure should be done in a room with negative pressure. When the pressure in the operating room is lower than the pressure in the surrounding area, microorganisms are contained within the operating room.

251. Some healthcare facilities have a room in which the air pressure can be converted from positive to negative pressure on demand. In these operating rooms, it is critical to check that the air flow has been changed back to positive pressure for patients not on airborne or droplet precautions.

Section Questions

www

1. Describe each of the three areas of the operating room. [Refs 194–198]

2. What is the required attire for the restricted area? [Ref 195]

3. Where must personnel wear a mask? [Ref 195]

4. Who is permitted in the semi-restricted area? [Ref 197]

5. Describe the appropriate flow of supplies in the operating room. [Ref 202]

6. What is the purpose for removing items from external shipping cartons before their delivery to the operating room? [Ref 204]

7. How are items for surgical procedures delivered from other areas within the facility managed to prevent contamination? [Ref 205]

8. Describe the air flow in an operating room. [Ref 207]

9. Describe the concept of positive pressure for operating rooms. [Ref 208]

10. What is the AIA recommendation for exchanging the total volume of air in each operating room? [Ref 209]

11. Describe a laminar air-flow system. [Ref 210]

12. Describe the parameters and explain the rationale for temperature and humidity in the operating room environment. [Ref 211]

13. What is an appropriate schedule for cleaning procedures in the operating room? [Ref 214]

14. Who determines the appropriateness of the products used for cleaning inanimate surfaces in the operating room? [Ref 214]

15. What is involved in the assessment of cleanliness prior to the first procedure of the day? [Refs 216–217]

16. What is the best time of day to schedule a procedure for a patient with a known latex allergy? [Ref 218]

17. How is cleanliness maintained during a surgical procedure? [Refs 219–220]

18. How is contaminated waste collected? [Refs 222, 224–226]

19. How are specimens collected? [Ref 223]

20. How is liquid infectious waste managed? [Ref 226]

21. What are some practices that help to manage the costs of disposing of infectious waste? [Refs 227–228]

22. How are sharps managed? [Ref 229]

23. Describe the proper management of instruments opened for a surgical procedure. [Ref 231]

24. Describe appropriate cleaning measures following a surgical procedure. [Refs 231–234]

25. List items in the operating room that should be cleaned daily. [Ref 237]

26. Based on CDC's standard precautions, how do we determine the level of cleaning required for each surgical patient? [Ref 241]

27. Which method of hand hygiene is appropriate when caring for a patient with *Clostridium difficile* infection? [Ref 245]

28. Which cleaning protocols are appropriate for managing *Clostridium difficile*? [Refs 246–247]

29. Which types of products are effective in eliminating the infectivity of prions? [Refs 248–249]

30. What is the value of using a negative-pressure room for procedures on patients with airborne- or droplet-transmitted infections? [Ref 250]

• • • References

American Institute of Architects (AIA), Committee on Architecture for Health (with assistance from the U.S. Department of Health and Human Services) (2006). *Guidelines for Design and Construction of Health Care Facilities.* Washington, DC: AIA Press.

American Society of Heating, Refrigerating, and Air Conditioning Engineers (ASHRAE), American Society of Healthcare Engineering (ASHE), American National Standards Institute (ANSI) (2010). *Ventilation of Health Care Facilities.* Addendum to ANSI/ASHRAE/ASHE Standard I 70-2008. Atlanta: ASHRAE; Chicago: ASHE; Washington, DC: ANSI.

Anderson D, Sexton, D (2012). *Epidemiology and pathogenesis of and risk factors for surgical site infection.* Waltham, MA: UpToDate. Available at: www.uptodate.com/contents/epidemiology-and-pathogenesis-of-and-risk-factors-for-surgical-site-infection. Accessed September 2012.

Association for the Advancement of Medical Instrumentation (AAMI) (2011). *Comprehensive Guide to Steam Sterilization and Sterility Assurance in Health Care Facilities* (ANSI/AAMI ST79:2011). Arlington, VA: AAMI.

Association of periOperative Registered Nurses (AORN) (2012). *Perioperative Standards and Recommended Practices.* Denver, CO: AORN.

Centers for Disease Control and Prevention (CDC) (2012). *MRSA statistics.* Atlanta: CDC. Available at: www.cdc.gov/mrsa/statistics/index.html. Accessed September 2012.

Centers for Disease Control and Prevention (CDC) (2002). Guideline for hand hygiene in healthcare settings: recommendations of the Healthcare Infection Control Practices Advisory Committee and the HICPAC/SHEA/APIC/IDSA Hand Hygiene Task Force. *MMWR*;51(RR-16):1–44. Available at: www.cdc.gov/mmwr/preview/mmwrhtml/rr5116a1.htm. Accessed September 2012.

Cruse PJ, Foord R (1980). The epidemiology of wound infection. A 10-year prospective study of 62,939 wounds. *Surg Clin North Am 1980*; 60(1):27–40.

Edmiston C, Okoli O, Graham M, et al. (2010). Evidence for using CHG preoperative cleansing to reduce the risk of SSI. *AORN J*;92(5):509–518.

Edwards J, Peterson K, Mu Y., et al. (2009). National Healthcare Safety Network (NHSN) report: data summary for 2006 through 2008: issued December 2009. *Assoc Professionals Infect Control Epidemiol*;37:783–805.

McDonald LC, Lessa S, Sievert D, et al. (2012). Preventing *Clostridium difficile* infections. *MMWR*;61(09):157–162. Available at: www.cdc.gov/mmwr/preview/mmwrhtml/mm6109a3.htm?s_cid=mm6109a3_w. Accessed September 2012.

Occupational Safety and Health Administration (OSHA) (2011). *Bloodborne Pathogens* Standard 1910.1030 (d)(4)(iii)(b). 56 Fed. Reg. 64004. Washington, DC: OSHA. Available at: www.oshaz.gov/pls/oshaweb/owadisp.show_document?p_table=STANDARDS&p_id=10051. Accessed September 2012.

Petersen P (2006). Clinical issues: Air exchanges in the OR. *AORN J*;84(4):647–648.

Rutala W, Weber D (2010). Guidelines for disinfection and sterilization of prion-contaminated medical instruments. *Infect Control Hosp Epidemiol*;21(2):107–117.

Siegel J, Rhinehart E, Jackson M, et al. (2007). Guidelines for isolation: preventing transmission of infectious agents in healthcare settings. Atlanta: CDC. Available at: www.cdc.gov/ncidod/dhqp/gl_isolation.html. Accessed September, 2012.

Society for Healthcare Epidemiology of America (SHEA) (2010). Clinical practice guidelines for *Clostridium difficile* infection in adults. *Infect Control Hosp Epidemiol*;31(5):431–455. Available at: www.jstor.org/stable/10.1086/651706. Accessed September 2012.

U.S. Environmental Protection Agency (EPA) (2002). *Using Microfiber Mops in Hospitals.* Washington, DC: EPA. Available at: www.epa.gov/region09/waste/p2/projects/hospital/mops.pdf. Accessed September 2012.

U.S. Food and Drug Administration (FDA) (2011). Draft guidance for industry and FDA staff: recommended warning for surgeon's gloves and patient examination gloves that use powder. Silver Spring, MD: FDA. Available at: www.fda.gov/MedicalDevices/DeviceRegulationandGuidance/GuidanceDocuments/ucm228557.htm. Accessed September 2012.

World Health Organization (WHO) (2009). *World Health Organization Guidelines on Hand Hygiene in Health Care.* Geneva, Switzerland: WHO. Available at: http://whqlibdoc.who.int/publications/2009/9789241597906_eng.pdf. Accessed September 2012.

• •

Post-Test

[WWW]

Read each question carefully. Each question may have more than one correct answer.

1. In which two ways do activities in the operating room focus on preventing infection?
   a. Hand washing
   b. Reducing the presence of microorganisms
   c. Creating a sterile field
   d. Preventing a mode of transmission of microorganisms

2. What is the most common type of surgical site infection?
   a. Organ/space
   b. Deep incisional
   c. Superficial incisional
   d. Muscle and fascia

3. Asepsis means
   a. the absence of organisms.
   b. creating a sterile field.
   c. scrubbing gowning and gloving.
   d. the prevention of infections.

4. The key to prevention of surgical site infections in the operating room is
   a. strict adherence to aseptic practices.
   b. preoperative patient showers with an antimicrobial soap.
   c. operating-room attire.
   d. traffic patterns in the operating suite.

5. Which of the following is (are) endogenous source(s) of infection?
   a. A break in sterile technique
   b. Microorganisms that live within the patient
   c. A very long surgical procedure
   d. Extremes of age of patients

6. Which of the following is (are) risk factor(s) that predispose patients to infection?
   a. Compromised immune system
   b. Smoking
   c. Obesity
   d. Poor nutritional status

7. Risk factor(s) for increasing microorganisms in the environment that personnel can control include
   a. laughing and talking unnecessarily.
   b. artificial nails.
   c. shedding from skin and hair.
   d. chipped fingernail polish.

8. In the operating room, where might there be infectious microorganisms?
   a. On supplies and equipment that come in contact with personnel
   b. On walls and floors

    c. Wherever dust particles settle

    d. On overhead lights, cabinets, and door handles

9. Universal precautions

    a. were defined by CDC in 1987.

    b. are the same as standard precautions.

    c. were designed to prevent the transmission of HIV and other bloodborne pathogens.

    d. were incorporated into the more comprehensive standard and transmission-based precautions.

10. Choose the single BEST response. The purpose of standard precautions is to

    a. protect patients and personnel from exposure to pathogenic microorganisms found in blood and body fluid.

    b. protect personnel from exposure to patients with AIDS.

    c. be sure that all patients get the same standard of care.

    d. protect patients from surgical site infections.

11. Transmission-based precautions

    a. is another term for standard precautions.

    b. address protection from specific infectious agents that a patient is known or suspected to have.

    c. are the same for all patients.

    d. include specific precautions for pathogens transmitted via the airborne, droplet, and contact routes.

12. Which practices related to surgery on patients who are on airbone precautions is (are) correct?

    a. Perform the procedure with only the required personnel.

    b. Do not use the room for 2 hours following the procedure.

    c. Postpone the surgery if possible.

    d. Following the procedure, leave the room vacant until a complete air exchange has occurred.

13. Wear a mask with a patient on droplet precautions if you are within

    a. 3 feet of the patient.

    b. 5 feet of the patient.

    c. 10 feet of the patient.

    d. 15 feet of the patient.

14. What are the three components of OSHA's mandatory practice standard?

    a. PPE

    b. Proper hand washing

    c. Preoperative patient prep

    d. Proper management of sharps

15. Which practice distinguishes the operating room from other clinical areas?

    a. Scrub attire

    b. Traffic patterns

    c. Invasive procedures

    d. Aseptic practices

16. What is the purpose of the preoperative patient skin prep?

    a. Sterilize the skin.

    b. Define the operative site.

    c. Reduce the number of microorganisms at the surgical site.

    d. Remove pathogens.

17. Which statement(s) about preoperative hair removal is (are) correct?
    a. Hair at the incision site should always be removed.
    b. Hair removal has been associated with increased risk of surgical site infection.
    c. Hair should be removed the night before surgery.
    d. Use clippers—never a razor—to remove necessary hair.

18. What determines the area to be included in the preoperative patient skin prep?
    a. The possibility of extending the intended incision
    b. The possibility of drains
    c. An additional incision site
    d. The type of dressing planned

19. Which of the following statement(s) is (are) true about preoperative patient skin prep?
    a. It is recommended to start at the periphery and work toward the incision site.
    b. Pooling of prep fluids can cause patient injury.
    c. Drapes can be applied immediately following the prep.
    d. There is evidence that a sterile prep kit and sterile gloves has better outcomes than a clean prep kit and clean gloves.

20. Which statement(s) is (are) true about scrub attire?
    a. Hair is a gross contaminant and a major source of bacteria.
    b. Scrub caps should be worn where sterile supplies are stored.
    c. Scrub tops should be worn over scrub pants, not tucked in.
    d. Scientific studies have shown that home laundering is just as effective as commercial laundering in preventing the transmission of infection.

21. Which statement(s) is (are) true about surgical masks?
    a. Masks should always be worn with goggles or a face shield.
    b. Masks should be on or off, never left dangling around the neck or saved in a pocket.
    c. Used masks should be removed and handled only by the ties.
    d. Masks must fit securely to prevent the escape of microorganisms.

22. What is the difference between hand washing and hand hygiene?
    a. Hand washing refers to practices outside of the operating room.
    b. Hand hygiene refers to practices within the operating room.
    c. Hand washing is done with soap and water.
    d. Hand hygiene refers to all measures related to hand condition and decontamination.

23. What is the single most important practice to prevent the transmission of microorganisms?
    a. Washing hands at the start of a shift before doing anything else
    b. Using an alcohol-based hand product
    c. Performing a surgical scrub
    d. Hand hygiene

24. Which statement(s) is (are) true about surgical hand antisepsis (surgical scrub)?
    a. It removes the amount of transient microorganisms on the hands before donning sterile gown and gloves.
    b. It can be performed without removing a watch and rings.
    c. It should be performed using the "timed" or "stroke" method.
    d. It can be done with the traditional sponge/brush or a brushless alcohol-based antiseptic.

25. Glove powder
    a. can cause an inflammatory response.
    b. can delay healing.
    c. can cause a foreign body reaction.
    d. should be removed with sterile water or saline prior to the incision.

26. Which statement(s) is (are) true about draping?
    a. Drapes, once placed, should never be repositioned.
    b. Draping begins at the patient's head and progresses to the feet.
    c. Sheets are flipped carefully so that they open completely but do not touch any contaminated object.
    d. Perforating towel clips and can be removed and reused.

27. Once the sterile members of the team have been gowned and gloved, which parts of the gown are considered unsterile?
    a. Neckline
    b. Chest
    c. Elbow
    d. Cuff

28. When there is doubt about the sterility of an item,
    a. double-check the external monitor.
    b. reexamine the package, and then open and check the internal monitor.
    c. ask someone else what they think.
    d. consider the item to be contaminated and send it back for reprocessing or discarding.

29. Which statement(s) is (are) true about delivering solutions to the sterile field?
    a. Deliver solutions into receptacles, then label them.
    b. Recap the unused portion carefully, as the outside of the cap is contaminated.
    c. Lean carefully over the back table so you can reach the receptacle without dripping water on the table.
    d. Use a sterile spike to deliver medication instead of removing the rubber stopper and pouring the medication.

30. How does the perioperative nurse manage a sterile field?
    a. The sterile field is set up as close to the time of use as possible.
    b. If the surgery is canceled, close the room door and save the field for the next case.
    c. Covering the sterile field is permitted, but for no more than 2 hours.
    d. The sterile field should be monitored at all times.

31. How do personnel navigate in the presence of a sterile field?
    a. Scrubbed personnel can sit on a stool until the procedure begins.
    b. Unscrubbed personnel should never walk between two sterile fields.
    c. Unscrubbed personnel should keep a safe distance from the sterile field.
    d. Scrubbed personnel should keep hands and arms in front of them and not allow them to drop below the waist.

32. The restricted area is
    a. where preoperative holding is located.
    b. where surgery is performed.
    c. where scrub sinks are.
    d. where masks are required.

33. In the semi-restricted area,
    a. scrub attire is worn.
    b. scrub caps are required.
    c. locker rooms are located.
    d. street clothes are permitted.

34. The operating room
    a. is a sterile environment.
    b. has a separate ventilation and air filtration system.
    c. should have 10 air exchanges per hour.
    d. is maintained under positive pressure.

35. Prior to the first case of the day, the perioperative nurse
    a. assesses the room for overall cleanliness.
    b. wipes horizontal surfaces with a cloth moistened with alcohol or an EPA registered hospital-grade disinfectant.
    c. ensures equipment from other areas is damp dusted before it is brought into the room.
    d. mops the floor where the sterile field will be located.

36. Following the procedure,
    a. items opened but not used on the patient can be used again without reprocessing.
    b. all items that came in contact with the patient or the sterile field are considered contaminated.
    c. disposable items opened but not used can be sent to SPD for reprocessing.
    d. infectious waste fluids can be poured down a drain connected to a sanitary sewer if regulations permit.

37. For a procedure where the patient is known to have HIV,
    a. the room is cleaned with hypochlorite solution.
    b. the case is scheduled for the end of the day.
    c. routine cleaning is sufficient as long as it is adequate and thorough.
    d. HIV patients are treated no differently from other patients, as all patients are considered infectious.

38. Which statement(s) is (are) true about C. *difficile*?
    a. Hands should be disinfected with an alcohol-based hand rub.
    b. *C. difficile* is spore-forming and can survive on surfaces for months.
    c. Hands should be washed with soap and water.
    d. Surfaces should be cleaned with chlorine-containing cleaning agents.

39. Which statement(s) is (are) true about prions?
    a. Disposable supplies and instruments should be used and discarded.
    b. Prions bind tightly to surfaces and are difficult to remove by cleaning.
    c. Special formulations of alkaline and enzymatic detergents are available to inactivate prions.
    d. High-risk tissue includes the brain, spinal cord, and eye.

40. Which statement(s) is (are) true about airborne- and droplet-transmitted infections?
    a. Procedures should be postponed for patients with airborne- or droplet-transmitted infections.
    b. If a procedure is done, it should be done in a room with positive pressure.
    c. Positive pressure maintains the contaminants inside the operating room.
    d. Special PPE is available for use with patients who have an airborne-transmitted infection.

Competency Checklist: Asepsis

Under "Observer's Initials," enter initials upon successful achievement of the competency. Enter N/A if the competency is not appropriate for the institution.

Name _____

	Observer's Initials	Date

Standard and Universal Precautions

1. Blood and body fluids of all patients are considered infectious. Standard precautions are practiced as follows:
   a. Gloves worn when direct contact with blood and body fluids is expected to occur _____ _____
   b. Masks and protective eyewear worn when aerosolization or splattering of blood and body fluids is anticipated _____ _____
   c. Gowns worn that provide a barrier appropriate to the procedure _____ _____
   d. Needles not recapped _____ _____
   e. Sharps deposited in sharps containers _____ _____
   f. Infectious waste correctly identified _____ _____
   g. Infectious waste deposited in designated container _____ _____
   h. Contaminated laundry deposited in designated laundry bags _____ _____
   i. Performs hand hygiene as appropriate _____ _____

Skin Prep

2. Skin condition and sensitivities are assessed and assessment is documented. _____ _____
3. Prep is implemented as follows:
   a. Awake patient is informed _____ _____
   b. Unnecessary exposure is avoided _____ _____
   c. Follows the manufacturer's instructions _____ _____
   d. Prep progresses from clean to dirty and not in reverse _____ _____
   e. Prep solutions are not permitted to pool _____ _____
   f. Dirtiest areas are prepped last _____ _____
4. Prep is documented for:
   a. Skin assessment _____ _____
   b. Solution used _____ _____
   c. Person performing prep _____ _____
   d. If hair removed—site, method, time, and person _____ _____
   e. Person who performed prep _____ _____
   f. Patient response to prep _____ _____

Attire

5. Hat/hood is worn so that all head and facial hair is covered. _____ _____
6. Surgical attire that becomes visibly soiled is removed and fresh attire donned. _____ _____

		Observer's Initials	Date

7. Mask:
   a. Covers nose and mouth and does not permit venting _____ _____
   b. Is not left to dangle around the neck _____ _____
   c. Changed between cases _____ _____
   d. Worn in presence of open supplies _____ _____
8. Appropriate attire is worn in restricted and semi-restricted areas. _____ _____

Surgical Scrub

9. Jewelry is removed. _____ _____
10. Scrub includes all surfaces of nails, subungual areas, hands, and arms to inches above the elbow. _____ _____
11. Timed anatomical, stroke count scrub, or alcohol rub procedure adheres to institutional policy. _____ _____

Gowning and Gloving

12. Hands are dried without contamination of towel. _____ _____
13. Gown is donned correctly and without contamination. _____ _____
14. Open gloving is performed correctly and without contamination. _____ _____
15. Closed gloving is performed correctly and without contamination. _____ _____
16. Assistance in gowning and gloving other team members is performed without contamination. _____ _____
17. At end of procedure, gown is removed before gloves. _____ _____
18. Gloves are removed in manner so that bare skin does not contact contaminated glove. _____ _____
19. Hand hygiene performed after gown and glove removal. _____ _____

Draping

20. Equipment is draped without contamination:
    a. Back table _____ _____
    b. Mayo stand _____ _____
    c. Ring stand _____ _____
21. Patient is draped without contamination:
    a. Abdomen _____ _____
    b. Perineum (lithotomy) _____ _____
    c. Extremity _____ _____
    d. (Other) _____ _____
22. Patient is draped from the operative site to the periphery. _____ _____
23. A cuff is formed from a drape to protect gloved hand. _____ _____
24. Drapes applied after sufficient prep solution contact. _____ _____
25. Drapes are not repositioned once placed. _____ _____

	Observer's Initials	Date

Aseptic Practices

26. Gloved hands are kept in sight at or above the level of the sterile field.

27. (Circulating role) Items are checked for sterility prior to being dispensed to the sterile field (package integrity, chemical indicator, evidence of strike-through, expiration date if applicable).

28. Sterile field monitored for contamination.

29. (Scrub role) Sterility of items is checked prior to accepting for delivery to sterile field (packaging, chemical indicator, expiration date).

30. Items of questionable sterility and unsterile items are not entered into the sterile field.

31. Items are dispensed to the sterile field without contamination.

32. Ungloved hands and arms are not extended over the sterile field.

33. Fluids:

    a. Are dispensed to a receptacle placed at the edge of the sterile field

    b. Are poured carefully to prevent splashing

34. Sterile field:

    a. Is set up as close to the time of surgery as possible

    b. Is not left unattended

    c. Is not covered

35. Scrubbed nurse touches only sterile items.

36. Scrubbed nurse remains close to the sterile field.

37. Movement around the sterile field is back to back and front (sterile) to front (sterile).

38. Circulating nurse maintains a safe distance from the sterile field.

39. Circulating nurse approaches the sterile field by facing the sterile field.

Sanitation

40. Spills or splashes of blood and body fluids that occur in the immediate vicinity of the sterile field are promptly absorbed and cleaned with an EPA-registered disinfectant.

41. Soiled sponges are deposited into a plastic-lined bucket, counted, and sealed in an impervious receptacle.

42. Specimen containers are wiped as needed with EPA-registered hospital germicide.

Observer's Signature   Initials   Date

_____

Orientee's Signature

_____

6

Prevention of Injury
Positioning the Patient for Surgery

LEARNER OBJECTIVES

1. List three factors that in combination create the potential for tissue damage.
2. Identify potential injuries related to improper and prolonged positioning.
3. List the desired patient outcomes relative to positioning.
4. Describe the impact of positioning on the respiratory, circulatory, neuromuscular, and integumentary systems.
5. Explain the importance of normal capillary interface pressure to positioning.
6. Discuss the impact of a pressure ulcer.
7. Discuss the responsibilities of the perioperative nurse in patient positioning.
8. Describe five common surgical positions.
9. Discuss body structures at risk in the supine, prone, lateral, lithotomy, Trendelenburg, and sitting positions.
10. Describe the appropriate use of five positioning devices.
11. Describe nursing interventions to prevent patient injury in the supine, prone, lateral, lithotomy, Trendelenburg, and sitting positions.
12. List special considerations for positioning the morbidly obese patient.

WWW

LESSON OUTLINE

I. Overview
II. Desired Patient Outcomes
III. Impact of Surgical Positioning
   A. Overview of Injuries
   B. Respiratory and Circulatory System Compromise
   C. Neuromuscular Injury
   D. Integumentary System Injury
IV. Responsibilities of the Perioperative Nurse

A. Patient Advocate
B. Nursing Considerations
V. Additional Considerations for Positioning
   A. Anesthesia
   B. Patient Dignity
VI. Positioning Devices
VII. Implementation of Patient Care
   A. Transportation and Transfer
   B. Initial Position Techniques
VIII. Basic Surgical Positions

Overview

1. The primary reasons for placing a patient in a surgical position are to give the surgeon access to the operative site and to stabilize the patient on the operative table.

2. When the patient is properly positioned, the surgeon will have optimal access to the surgical site, the patient will be stable on the operating room bed, and the patient will not suffer injury.

3. Many factors combine to create the potential for patient injury related to positioning. The degree of risk for injury is determined by the type of anesthesia; the type and length of the procedure; the position required for exposure of the operative site; the patient's age, height, weight, nutritional status, level of mobility, comorbidities, and overall condition at the time of surgery; and whether the patient is positioned correctly and safely.

4. Impaired skin integrity, compromised respiratory effort, altered tissue perfusion, and neuromuscular and musculoskeletal injury are all possible consequences related to positioning. Improper positioning can result in severe—sometimes permanent—injury to the patient.

5. Safe patient positioning in preparation for surgery is a critical component of perioperative nursing practice. Although patient positioning is a team responsibility, it is most often the perioperative nurse who coordinates the positioning process.

Desired Patient Outcomes

6. The desired patient outcome related to positioning: The patient is free from signs and symptoms of injury related to positioning (Association of periOperative Registered Nurses [AORN], 2011, p. 178):

    - Skin—intact, smooth, free of ecchymosis, cuts, abrasions, shear injury, rash, or blistering
    - Cardiovascular status—heart rate and blood pressure within expected ranges; peripheral pulses present and equal bilaterally; skin warm to touch, capillary fill less than 3 seconds
    - Neuromuscular status—flexes and extends extremities without assistance; denies numbness or tingling of extremities (AORN, 2011, p. 178)

7. To achieve these outcomes, the perioperative nurse must have knowledge of the following:

    - Principles of anatomy and physiology
    - Anatomical and physiological changes related to anesthesia, surgical position, prolonged immobility, and pressure
    - The surgical procedure to be performed
    - Proper positioning technique
    - Selection and proper use of positioning equipment

8. Maintenance of patient comfort and dignity is a perioperative nursing responsibility.

9. Proper positioning includes preventing unnecessary exposure, maintaining the patient's anatomical body alignment, ensuring optimal airway accessibility, and adequate exposure of the surgical site.

Impact of Surgical Positioning

Overview of Injuries

10. The basic positions used for surgery are supine, lithotomy, sitting, prone, and lateral. Injury can occur in any of these positions. Each position is described later in this chapter.

11. Complications that can result from improper positioning are postoperative musculoskeletal pain, joint dislocation, peripheral nerve damage, skin breakdown including

necrosis, and cardiovascular and respiratory compromise.

12. The anesthetized patient is at increased risk for positioning injury. General anesthetic and regional blocks prevent the patient from responding to pain, which is the body's normal warning of exaggerated stretching, twisting, and compression of body parts. Damage to nerves and vascular structures, as well as compromise of respiratory and circulatory function, may occur without the patient being aware.

Respiratory and Circulatory System Compromise

13. Extreme or unnatural positions such as the Trendelenburg position, where the head and upper body are lower than the feet and lower body, affect circulation and oxygen–carbon dioxide exchange. Pulmonary capillary blood volume, and therefore the amount of blood available for oxygenation, is altered by gravity.

14. Unnatural positions may decrease compliance or stretchability of the lung and the ability of the thoracic cage to expand. Lung capacity is reduced and the amount of oxygen available for gas exchange diminishes. With compromised respiratory mechanics, muscles become fatigued as the patient attempts to compensate, and hypoventilation may occur. Even where respiratory function is supported through mechanical assistance, hypoxia and hypercarbia can still occur.

15. Certain positions may result in decreased lung expansion by mechanical restriction of the ribs or sternum. Lung expansion may also be decreased by the diaphragm's reduced ability to push down against abdominal contents, as in the Trendelenburg position, or against retractors that are used during surgery.

16. General and regional anesthetics may disrupt normal vasodilation and constriction. Dilation of peripheral blood vessels may result in a drop in blood pressure. Dilated vessels allow venous blood to pool in dependent areas, thereby reducing the amount of blood returned to the heart and lungs for oxygenation and redistribution. In some operations, certain body parts may be placed in a dependent position for an extended period of time, causing a significant amount of pooling to occur.

17. Both positioning and anesthetic agents may interfere with the heart's ability to contract. The result is a relaxation of the skeletal muscles that normally support vein walls and help to propel blood, which may result in a decrease in cardiac output.

18. Any position that hinders the flow of blood in the legs has the potential to result in the formation of a blood clot, limiting blood flow particularly in the deep veins (deep vein thrombosis [DVT]). DVT occurs primarily in the lower extremities; it is a risk factor for the development of pulmonary embolism (PE).

19. Three factors may cause formation of a DVT (AORN, 2012, p. 355):
    - Venous stasis that results in blood pooling and clot formation.
    - Injury to a vessel wall from the surgical procedure, trauma, or interventions such as venous access. General anesthesia also causes dilation of peripheral vessels, which may result in endothelial damage and the formation of a thrombus.
    - Hypercoagulability.

20. Patients who are at high risk for DVT formation include those with the following characteristics:
    - Any patient with a history of previous DVT
    - Prolonged hospitalization
    - Malignancy or immobility
    - Heart failure
    - Varicose veins
    - Leg ulcers
    - Stroke
    - Age (older than 40 years)
    - Lengthy procedure
    - Total hip procedure or revision of total hip procedure

21. Sequential compression devices (SCDs) are encouraged to prevent venous stasis in the immobile patient. An SCD consists of a sleeve that encompasses the leg and is automatically sequentially inflated and deflated along the extremity. This device encourages blood flow and discourages pooling of blood. Sequential compression devices should be applied and activated before induction of general anesthesia.

22. Patients should be assessed for DVT risk and sequential compression devices applied accordingly (Figure 6-1).

Section Questions   www

1. What are the two primary objectives for positioning the patient for a surgical procedure? [Refs 1–2]
2. Identify factors that increase the patient's risk for injury related to positioning. [Ref 3]
3. What are some of the adverse outcomes related to positioning? [Ref 4]
4. Who most often coordinates positioning of the patient for surgery? [Ref 5]
5. What are three body systems assessed for injuries related to positioning? [Ref 6]
6. Who is responsible for maintaining the patient's comfort and dignity? [Ref 8]
7. Identify four components of proper positioning. [Ref 9]
8. Why is the anesthetized patient at greater risk for positioning injury? [Ref 12]
9. How does gravity affect respiration and circulation in positions where the head is lower than the feet? [Refs 13–14]
10. Which type of mechanical restriction can impact lung expansion? [Ref 15]
11. How can general anesthesia disrupt normal circulation? [Refs 16–17]
12. Why is it important to prevent DVT? [Ref 18]
13. Which three factors can be involved in the formation of a DVT? [Ref 19]
14. Identify patients at risk for the development of DVT. [Ref 20]
15. How does a sequential compression device aid in preventing DVT? [Ref 21]

Neuromuscular Injury

23. In the awake patient, normal pain and pressure receptors of muscle groups warn against unnatural stretching and twisting of tendons, ligaments, and muscles. Opposing muscle groups also prevent strain on muscle fibers. The anesthetized patient is unable to communicate when subjected to an exaggerated range of motion. Anesthetic agents and muscle relaxants further exacerbate the potential for injury by inducing loss of muscle tone and exaggerated muscle relaxation that interferes with the normal defense mechanisms that warn against unnatural or excessive range of motion.

24. Most nerve injuries are due to compression or hyperextension. Evidence of hyperextension injury can range from mild postoperative joint pain to dislocation.

25. Musculoskeletal injury is minimized with adequate support of the extremities during positioning as well as adequate stabilization and padding during the procedure. Extremities should not be allowed to hang unsupported over the edge of an armboard or the operating table. Lower extremities should be moved slowly and together to prevent sacroiliac joint

dislocation. If resistance is met in positioning, do not force the movement.

26. Crushing and pressure injuries to fingers, toes, ears, and nose are possible whenever the operating table, instrument table, or Mayo stands are adjusted. Team members are encouraged to visualize these body parts when positioning and repositioning the patient. Equipment must not be allowed to rest or exert pressure on the patient. Surgical team members must not lean on the patient.

Facial Nerves

27. Injury to the facial nerve (buccal branch), resulting in motor injury to the mouth, can occur if the nerve is compressed from an improperly fitting face mask.

28. Injury to the suborbital nerve, resulting in numbness of the forehead, can occur from pressure on the nerve by endotracheal tube connectors.

29. Prolonged stretching or compression of nerves may result in postoperative numbness, tingling, or pain. Severe injury can result in permanent loss of sensation and paralysis in the affected area.

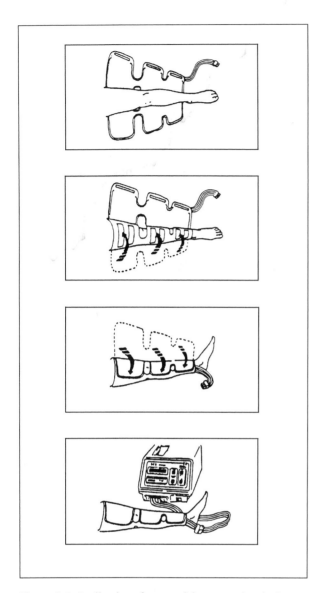

Figure 6-1 Application of sequential compression device
Source: Courtesy of Kendall Healthcare Products, Mansfield, MA.

Upper Extremity Nerves

30. Because of its superficial position and close proximity to bony structures, the brachial plexus nerve is vulnerable to injury as a potential complication of improper positioning.

31. Brachial plexus injury may result from improper positioning of the arm and/or armboard. The supine position, with one or both arms extended on armboards, is the most common surgical position. Brachial plexus nerve injury can occur in this position if the angle of the armboard causes hyperextension of the arm. Unintentional movement of

an armboard, causing the arm to be hyperabducted, might not be noticed because the arm is hidden by surgical drapes.

32. For supine patients, when an armboard is used, the armboard should be placed at an angle of less than 90 degrees. The palm should be facing up and the fingers extended. To minimize pressure on the brachial plexus, the patient's head may be turned toward the extended arm (AORN, 2012, p. 430).

33. Injury to the brachial plexus may occur when shoulder braces are improperly applied. In the Trendelenburg position, shoulder braces, which are used to prevent the patient from slipping from the table, can cause compression of the brachial plexus. If the brace is placed too far laterally and the arm is abducted, the head of the humerus can be pushed into the axilla, causing compression of the brachial plexus. If the brace is positioned too far medially and the arm is abducted, the plexus can be compressed between the clavicle and the first rib. Shoulder braces should not be used unless absolutely necessary and, if used, must be adequately padded.

34. Motor and sensory loss to the arm and shoulder may be evidenced postoperatively if damage has occurred to the brachial plexus.

35. The most common postoperative peripheral neuropathy is ulnar nerve compression caused by excessive flexion of the elbow or by external compression. Supination of arm is thought to be less damaging along with use of padded armboards. Do not allow the arm to slip off the mattress or edge of the operating room bed. Avoid compression in the area of the condylar groove (University of Pittsburgh, 2012) (Figure 6-2).

36. The radial or ulnar nerve may be injured if the elbow slips off the mattress onto the metal edge of the operating table and the nerve is compressed between the table and the medial epicondyle. Such an injury can occur when the surgical team leans against the table and is unaware that the patient's arm has slipped and is being compressed against the table.

37. The possibility of damage to the radial or ulnar nerve caused by compression against the table can be minimized by securing the arm with a draw sheet. The draw sheet begins from under the patient and is brought up over the arm and then tucked back under the patient, not under the mattress.

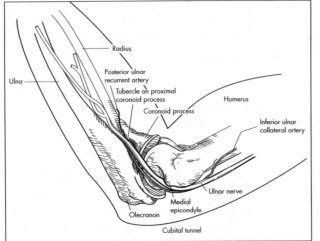

Figure 6-2 Ulnar nerve—most common postoperative peripheral neuropathy

38. The use of an automated blood pressure cuff on the arm may increase the risk of ulnar, radial, or median neuropathy (American Society of Anesthesiologists [ASA], 2011, p. 14).

39. Symptoms of ulnar nerve injury include tingling, pain, and numbness in the fourth and fifth fingers. Severe injury can result in a weak grip or contractures, leading to a "claw hand."

40. Radial nerve damage may be evidenced by wrist drop.

Lower Extremity Nerves

41. Improper placement in stirrups or improper movement of the legs can result in extension, flexion, compression, or stretching injuries to lower extremity nerves.

42. The peroneal, posterior tibial, femoral obturator, and sciatic nerves are at risk for injury in the lithotomy position (Figure 6-3).

43. Injury to the peroneal nerve on the lateral aspect of the knee can occur if the nerve is compressed between the fibula and a laterally positioned stirrup bar. This injury can result in foot drop.

44. Popliteal knee supports should be padded to prevent compression injury of the tibial and femoral obturator nerves that can cause foot drop.

45. Injury to the femoral obturator nerve, resulting in paralysis and numbness of the calf muscles, can occur if the nerve is compressed between a metal popliteal knee support stirrup and the medial tibial condyle.

46. Padding at these potential compression sites can prevent injury.

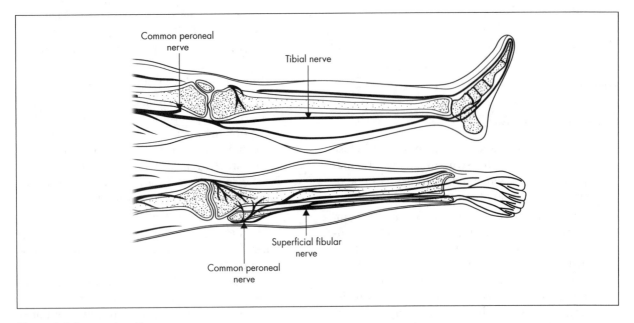

Figure 6-3 Lower extremity nerves

Adapted from: Photographic Atlas of Anatomical Models.

47. Foot drop from injury to the sciatic nerve can occur if the nerve is compressed or stretched by fully extending the legs in the high lithotomy position and flexing the thighs more than 90 degrees on the trunk.

Integumentary System Injury

48. Tissue damage, or pressure ulcers, result from a combination of immobility, pressure, and time—the longer the patient has been immobile, the higher the pressure; the longer the procedure, the greater the risk for tissue damage. The anesthetized patient is immobile and subjected to uninterrupted pressure during a surgical procedure. External pressure restricting blood flow can cause tissue ischemia that leads to tissue breakdown.

49. Friction, shearing, and pressure cause injury to tissues. Friction injuries occur when the skin moves across coarse surfaces such as bed linens or blankets. Such injuries can also be caused from excessive rubbing. Friction injuries are usually superficial and result in an abrasion or blister. These wounds, however, can contribute to the more serious injury of a pressure ulcer.

50. Shearing injuries occur when the skin remains stationary while the tissue beneath it moves. This can occur when the patient is pulled rather than lifted or when linen or blankets are pulled from underneath the patient. For example, when the anesthetized patient is repositioned incorrectly or slides down or up on the table when it is adjusted, shear injury occurs. Shearing injuries result in the stretching or tearing of subcutaneous capillaries and can lead to ischemia and contribute to the development of a pressure ulcer.

51. Use of warming devices and standard operating room table mattresses increase the risk of pressure ulcer development (Aronovich, 2008). Other extrinsic risk factors that contribute to pressure injuries include length of procedure, position, sedation, anesthetic agents, retractors, warming devices, and pooled prep solutions. It is important to ascertain the efficacy of the operating room bed mattress and positioning devices when considering products for purchase.

52. Tissue damage occurs most commonly over bony prominences when capillaries are compressed between bone and the table surface, causing ischemia, cell death, and tissue necrosis. Although it varies among individuals, pressure greater than 32 mm Hg is considered the force needed to occlude capillary blood flow. Prolonged, unrelieved pressure during surgery can occlude blood flow, causing ischemia in even the healthiest of patients.

53. Many mattress pads and positioning devices on the market are designed to reduce pressure. Viscoelastic and gel mattresses are commercially available to help prevent pressure injuries to the surgical patient. Properly engineered foam products have been found to be more effective than traditional foam overlays or the standard foam-covered-with-vinyl operating room mattress (AORN, 2012, pp. 421–422). Manufacturers should produce test results documenting the effectiveness of these products.

54. The average incidence of pressure ulcer formation in surgical patients is estimated at 8.5% (Aronovich, 2008). Immobility in the preoperative period increases this risk, and the duration of unrelieved pressure affects the extent of the injury. The incidence of pressure ulcers rises markedly in procedures lasting for more than 2 to 2.5 hours (Goodman, 2012, p. 21).

55. One of The Joint Commission's (TJC) 2012 patient safety goals is to prevent healthcare-associated decubitus ulcers. The Joint Commission estimates the cost for treatment of a pressure ulcer is $14,000 to $40,000 per ulcer. Every facility must have a plan for prediction, prevention, and early treatment of pressure ulcers that includes identifying patients at risk, maintaining and improving tissue tolerance, protecting against adverse effects of external mechanical forces, and staff education (TJC, 2012), all of which are relevant to the perioperative nurse.

56. In 2008, the Centers for Medicare and Medicaid (CMS) implemented the Present on Admission (POA) indicator. Under this CMS policy, a hospital will not receive additional funds to care for a patient who has acquired a pressure ulcer during hospitalization that was not present on admission. This groundbreaking policy provides a significant impetus for ulcer prevention (Armstrong et al., 2008).

57. Deep tissue injury (DTI), or tissue necrosis occurring at the bone–tissue interface, is not uncommon in surgical patients (Figure 6-4). Muscle closest to the bone is affected first, while the skin remains intact. Over time, as

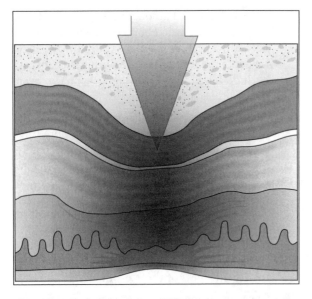

Figure 6-4 Deep tissue injury (DTI) from compression at the bone-tissue interface

Source: Reprinted with permission from T. Goodman (2012 p. 15). *Positioning: A Patient Safety Initiative: Study Guide for Nurses.* Dallas, TX: Terri Goodman & Associates.

the damage progresses to subcutaneous tissue and eventually skin rupture, the DTI appears as a bruise and rapidly progresses to an ulcer. Because a DTI that begins in surgery can go unnoticed for days, the connection between the injury and surgery is often missed. DTIs that appear within 72 hours postoperatively most likely can be attributed to the surgical procedure (Primiano et al., 2011, p. 556).

58. An area on the patient's skin that appears reddened after surgery may be an indication of the beginning of a superficial pressure ulcer, which can progress to involve deeper tissues. A reddened area may also be an indication of a self-healing transient reaction to pressure. In either case, the area should not be massaged. Massage may, in fact, compromise circulation to the affected area (Goodman, 2012, p. 23).

59. Areas most at risk for pressure ulcer formation are heels, elbows, scapula, sacrum, coccyx, occiput, iliac crest, ear, medial knee, malleolus, and toes, where there is little padding between skin and bone.

60. Intrinsic patient risk factors for pressure injury include age (older patients have less elastic, smaller blood vessels that hinder blood flow); weight (obesity causes additional weight and pressure on bony prominences); nutritional status (malnourished patients); and presence of diabetes or hypertension (both conditions are associated with diminished circulation).

61. Other intrinsic factors affecting the risk for pressure injury include immobility, infection, incontinence, impaired sensory perceptions, and comorbidities such as diabetes and peripheral vascular disease. Extrinsic factors that increase the risk of tissue damage are temperature, friction and shear, and moisture. Prevention of pressure ulcer formation is achieved through adequate padding and relief of pressure after 2 hours (Figures 6-5, 6-6, 6-7, and 6-8).

62. It is important to note that a patient can withstand a large amount of pressure for a shorter period of time better than the patient can withstand a small amount of pressure for a longer period of time.

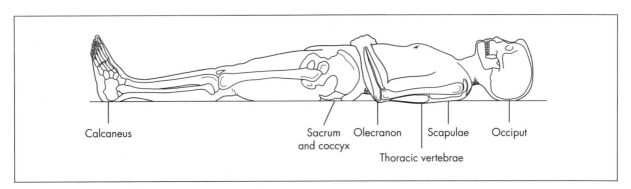

Figure 6-5 Potential pressure points in supine position

Source: Reprinted from L.K. Groah (1983) *Operating Room Nursing: The Perioperative Role*, p. 273. New York: Reston Publishing Company Inc. © 1983. Reprinted with permission of Appleton & Lange.

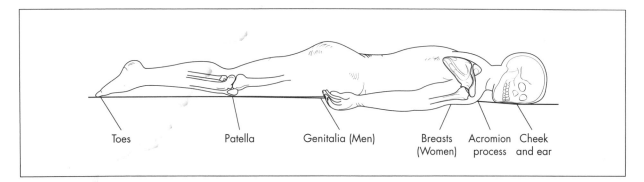

Figure 6-6 Potential pressure points in prone position

Source: Reprinted from L.K. Groah (1983) *Operating Room Nursing: The Perioperative Role*, p. 273. New York: Reston Publishing Company Inc. © 1983. Reprinted with permission of Appleton & Lange.

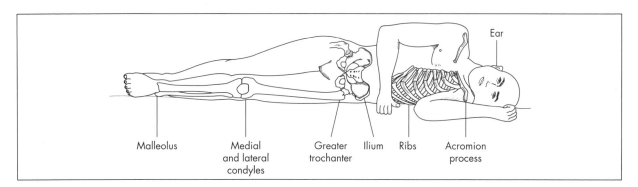

Figure 6-7 Potential pressure points in lateral position

Source: Reprinted from L.K. Groah (1983) *Operating Room Nursing: The Perioperative Role*, p. 273. New York: Reston Publishing Company Inc. © 1983. Reprinted with permission of Appleton & Lange.

Section Questions WWW

1. Explain why the anesthetized patient is at risk for neuromuscular injury. [Ref 23]
2. Which two conditions are responsible for most nerve injuries? [Ref 24]
3. How does the perioperative nurse provide adequate support, stabilization, and padding to prevent musculoskeletal injuries? [Ref 25]
4. How can crushing injuries occur during positioning and surgery? [Ref 26]
5. Which type of nerve injury can result from an ill-fitting face mask? [Ref 27]
6. What might be the outcome of prolonged stretching or compression of nerves? [Ref 29]
7. Why is the brachial plexus at particular risk for injury? [Ref 30]
8. Describe the most common cause of brachial plexus injury and explain how to prevent it. [Refs 31–32]
9. What causes ulnar nerve compression, and how can you prevent it? [Ref 35]
10. Which injury might be caused by leaning against the patient's arm during the procedure? [Refs 36–37]
11. Which precautions can prevent injuries when the patient's legs are in stirrups? [Refs 43–47]

(continues)

Section Questions (continued)

12. How do pressure, immobility, and time influence the development of pressure ulcers? [Ref 48]

13. What can be done to prevent friction injuries? [Ref 49]

14. Which steps can be taken to prevent shearing injuries? [Ref 50]

15. Which extrinsic factors related to surgery increase the risk of pressure ulcer development? [Ref 51]

16. Describe the pathophysiology of tissue damage that occurs when tissues over a bony prominence are compressed (deep tissue injury). [Refs 52, 57]

17. Why is it important not to massage a reddened area discovered on the patient's skin after surgery? [Ref 58]

18. Which parts of the body are at highest risk for tissue damage from pressure during positioning? [Ref 59]

19. Identify areas of the body at risk for pressure damage because there is little padding between skin and bone. [Ref 59]

20. Identify some intrinsic risk factors for tissue damage during surgery. [Ref 60]

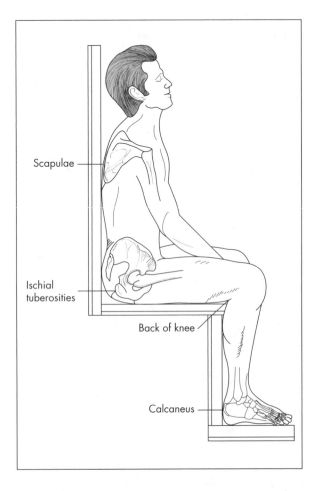

Scapulae

Ischial tuberosities

Back of knee

Calcaneus

Figure 6-8 Potential pressure points in sitting position

Source: Reprinted from L.K. Groah (1983) *Operating Room Nursing: The Perioperative Role*, p. 273. New York: Reston Publishing Company Inc. © 1983. Reprinted with permission of Appleton & Lange.

Responsibilities of the Perioperative Nurse

Patient Advocate

63. The patient undergoing surgery is vulnerable to positioning injury, particularly when the procedure is performed under general anesthesia and lasts longer than a few hours. Neuromuscular, musculoskeletal, integumentary, and physiologic systems can be severely compromised at a time when the patient is unable to indicate that there is a problem.

64. Although the surgeon, surgical assistants, anesthesia personnel, and other members of the nursing team may participate in patient positioning, it is most frequently the perioperative nurse who positions the patient.

65. The perioperative nurse is a crucial patient advocate, and at no time should the responsibility to ensure proper positioning be assumed to belong to another team member. The unconscious surgical patient is unable to respond to pain or discomfort, and responsibility for patient safety becomes a perioperative nursing responsibility.

Nursing Considerations
Patient Assessment

66. Planning for positioning begins with a nursing assessment of the patient, including the following considerations:

- Age

- Height, weight, and BMI
- Skin condition
- Presence of jewelry
- Nutritional status
- Allergies (including latex allergy, as tape is sometimes used as a positioning aid)
- Preexisting conditions (e.g., vascular, respiratory, circulatory, neurological, immune system, suppression)
- Physical or mobility limitations
- Prosthetic, corrective, or implanted devices
- Activity level (immobility places the patient at higher risk for pressure damage)
- Peripheral pulses
- Level of consciousness
- Perception of pain
- Psychosocial or cultural issues (AORN, 2012, p. 424)

Several risk assessment scales for pressure ulcer development are available (e.g., Braden [Exhibit 6-1], Gosnell, Abruzzese); however, no specific tool for the intraoperative patient population is available. Even patients with a low assessment tool–based risk score may develop a pressure ulcer within the operative period (Aronovich, 2008).

67. In a number of studies, increasing age, a diagnosis of either diabetes or vascular disease, and vascular procedures were found to be the most frequent predictors of perioperative pressure ulcers (Goodman, 2012, pp. 23–26). Reduction in blood perfusion may be responsible for increased incidence of pressure ulcers in patients undergoing vascular procedures lasting more than 2.5 hours.

68. Extrinsic risk factors include type and length of procedure, position, anesthetic agents, retractors, warming devices, and pooled prep solutions. The quality of the operating room bed mattress and positioning devices plays a significant role in preventing pressure damage (Goodman, 2012, pp. 40–48). In a number of studies, the most significant extrinsic risk factor was time on the operating room mattress.

69. The surgical procedure will determine the desired patient position. Lengthy procedures under anesthesia require extended periods of immobility and increase the risk for injury. Surgeries performed on areas where access is difficult may result in unnatural positions that increase the risk for injury.

70. Elderly patients have decreased muscle tone, poor skin turgor, and less subcutaneous fat and muscle to cushion bony prominences. These factors place elderly patients at increased risk for impaired skin integrity.

71. Height and weight are useful to determine appropriate positioning aids. Activity level and muscle tone provide information about how well the patient moves and the degree to which the patient may participate in transfer to and from the operating room bed.

72. Drugs and anesthetic agents can alter the patient's ability to move. Baseline data provide information that is useful for evaluating the impact of drugs and anesthesia on movement and muscle tone.

73. Patients with poor nutritional status are at increased risk for tissue injury. Malnourished patients lack the protein reserves necessary to maintain healthy skin cells and are at increased risk for skin impairment.

74. Obese patients may trap moisture and fluids from skin prep solutions in tissue folds, which may lead to skin breakdown. Adipose tissue is not well vascularized, and the pressure resulting from positioning can cause a decrease in circulation to peripheral body areas. Excess body weight increases the strain on joints and ligaments. Respiratory function is compromised in obese patients because of increased weight on the chest. Obesity also places an increased workload on the heart and circulatory system.

75. Anesthetic agents and positioning for surgery place additional strain on respiratory function.

76. Positioning that increases venous blood return to the heart can further compromise circulation.

77. Underweight patients experience greater than normal pressure on bony prominences and, therefore, are at greater risk for impaired skin integrity.

78. Patients with existing integumentary damage are at increased risk for further skin impairment. Diminished body fat provides little protection for peripheral nerves, and the underweight patient is at high risk for nerve damage.

79. Certain preexisting injuries or conditions and certain surgical procedures may require additional planning to prevent injury. Preexisting

Exhibit 6-1 Braden Scale for Predicting Risk for Pressure Damage

BRADEN SCALE FOR PREDICTING PRESSURE SORE RISK

Patient's Name _____   Evaluator's Name _____   Date of Assessment _____

	1	2	3	4
SENSORY PERCEPTION ability to respond meaningfully to pressure-related discomfort	**1. Completely Limited** Unresponsive (does not moan, flinch, or gasp) to painful stimuli, due to diminished level of consciousness or sedation. OR limited ability to feel pain over most of body	**2. Very Limited** Responds only to painful stimuli. Cannot communicate discomfort except by moaning or restlessness OR has a sensory impairment which limits the ability to feel pain or discomfort over ½ of body.	**3. Slightly Limited** Responds to verbal commands, but cannot always communicate discomfort or the need to be turned. OR has some sensory impairment which limits ability to feel pain or discomfort in 1 or 2 extremities.	**4. No Impairment** Responds to verbal commands. Has no sensory deficit which would limit ability to feel or voice pain or discomfort.
MOISTURE degree to which skin is exposed to moisture	**1. Constantly Moist** Skin is kept moist almost constantly by perspiration, urine, etc. Dampness is detected every time patient is moved or turned.	**2. Very Moist** Skin is often, but not always moist. Linen must be changed at least once a shift.	**3. Occasionally Moist:** Skin is occasionally moist, requiring an extra linen change approximately once a day.	**4. Rarely Moist** Skin is usually dry, linen only requires changing at routine intervals.
ACTIVITY degree of physical activity	**1. Bedfast** Confined to bed.	**2. Chairfast** Ability to walk severely limited or nonexistent. Cannot bear own weight and/or must be assisted into chair or wheelchair.	**3. Walks Occasionally** Walks occasionally during day, but for very short distances, with or without assistance. Spends majority of each shift in bed or chair	**4. Walks Frequently** Walks outside room at least twice a day and inside room at least once every two hours during waking hours
MOBILITY ability to change and control body position	**1. Completely Immobile** Does not make even slight changes in body or extremity position without assistance	**2. Very Limited** Makes occasional slight changes in body or extremity position but unable to make frequent or significant changes independently.	**3. Slightly Limited** Makes frequent though slight changes in body or extremity position independently.	**4. No Limitation** Makes major and frequent changes in position without assistance.
NUTRITION usual food intake pattern	**1. Very Poor** Never eats a complete meal. Rarely eats more than ⅓ of any food offered. Eats 2 servings or less of protein (meat or dairy products) per day. Takes fluids poorly. Does not take a liquid dietary supplement OR is NPO and/or maintained on clear liquids or IVs for more than 5 days.	**2. Probably Inadequate** Rarely eats a complete meal and generally eats only about ½ of any food offered. Protein intake includes only 3 servings of meat or dairy products per day. Occasionally will take a dietary supplement. OR receives less than optimum amount of liquid diet or tube feeding	**3. Adequate** Eats over half of most meals. Eats a total of 4 servings of protein (meat, dairy products) per day. Occasionally will refuse a meal, but will usually take a supplement when offered OR is on a tube feeding or TPN regimen which probably meets most of nutritional needs	**4. Excellent** Eats most of every meal. Never refuses a meal. Usually eats a total of 4 or more servings of meat and dairy products. Occasionally eats between meals. Does not require supplementation.
FRICTION & SHEAR	**1. Problem** Requires moderate to maximum assistance in moving. Complete lifting without sliding against sheets is impossible. Frequently slides down in bed or chair, requiring frequent repositioning with maximum assistance. Spasticity, contractures or agitation leads to almost constant friction	**2. Potential Problem** Moves feebly or requires minimum assistance. During a move skin probably slides to some extent against sheets, chair, restraints or other devices. Maintains relatively good position in chair or bed most of the time but occasionally slides down.	**3. No Apparent Problem** Moves in bed and in chair independently and has sufficient muscle strength to lift up completely during move. Maintains good position in bed or chair.	

Total Score _____

conditions requiring additional considerations include the following:

- Demineralized bone conditions such as osteoporosis and malignant metastasis—increased risk of fracture
- Diabetes, anemia, and paralysis—increased risk for skin breakdown
- Arthritis and joint prosthesis—limited joint movement
- Edema, infection, obstructive pulmonary disease, and other conditions that reduce respiratory and cardiac reserves
- Immunocompromise—increased risk of skin breakdown

80. Surgical procedures requiring additional considerations include:
- Surgeries lasting 2 hours or longer—increased risk for tissue damage
- Vascular surgery compromises blood perfusion to tissues—increased risk for skin breakdown
- Surgeries where prolonged traction or sustained pressure is required—increased risk for skin breakdown and nerve damage
- Warming devices placed under the patient may increase the potential for pressure ulcer (Seaman et al., 2012)

Planning Care

81. The perioperative nurse should communicate with surgical and anesthesia personnel to determine any specific needs related to patient positioning. This information, the procedure, assessment data, and nursing diagnoses serve as the basis for planning the care necessary to correctly position the patient. The perioperative nurse selects appropriate positioning equipment and makes decisions regarding the number of persons needed to assist with positioning and whether aspects of positioning can be assigned to ancillary personnel.

Additional Considerations for Positioning

Anesthesia

82. Patients who are awake or lightly sedated are able to communicate when they experience pain or discomfort. In contrast, patients under general anesthesia are totally dependent on the surgical team to protect them from injury. Patients who receive regional anesthesia will not feel or report pain and are at risk for injury to anesthetized regions that are improperly positioned.

83. The anesthesiologist or nurse anesthetist will perform a patient assessment prior to delivering anesthesia. The assessment data coupled with the specialized body of knowledge of anesthesia will determine the limitations to positioning with regard to anesthesia.

84. Anesthesia personnel (anesthesiologist or nurse anesthetist) are concerned with airway access, respiratory and circulatory functions, and monitoring lines. Anesthesia has a profound effect on cardiac and respiratory function.

Patient Dignity

85. Patient dignity should be a significant consideration during positioning. The patient should not be exposed unnecessarily, and once positioning is complete, a final check should be made to ensure that the patient is appropriately covered. Patients should be comfortable with the idea that, even when they are anesthetized, they will be appropriately covered. Traffic in the room should be limited, and the doors kept closed.

86. Provide privacy for the patient to speak openly to the perioperative staff while awake (AORN, 2012, p. 428).

87. For some patients, the response to entering the operating room is to relinquish control to their caregivers. Even an awake patient who feels a loss of dignity when exposed during positioning may not feel confident enough to cover an area inadvertently left exposed. The perioperative nurse, as patient advocate, must preserve the patient's dignity whether the patient is awake or asleep.

Positioning Devices

88. Even good positioning techniques can result in tissue damage when poorly designed positioning devices are used. When positioning equipment is purchased, manufacturers should provide evidence of the efficacy of products; evidence should demonstrate that a product

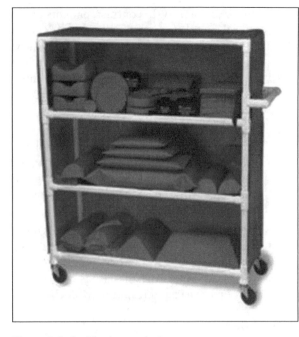

Figure 6-9 Positioning products
Source: Reprinted with permission from T. Goodman (2012 p. 50).
Positioning: A Patient Safety Initiative: Study Guide for Nurses.
Dallas, TX: Terri Goodman & Associates.

provides proper support and reduces pressure as expected (Figure 6-9).

89. Positioning equipment should be clean, in good repair, and used only by staff who are knowledgeable of the intended use of each piece of equipment.

90. Some type of operating bed or table is used for every surgical procedure. A table may be designed specifically for general, urologic, ophthalmic, dental, neurological, orthopedic, or minor surgery. Tables have multiple parts and specific functions. Table attachments are designed to hold a body part stationary and to facilitate access to the operative site. Personnel should have demonstrated competency to operate tables and utilize attachments appropriately.

91. Typical table attachments (Figure 6-10) may include the following items:
    - Head rest
    - Anesthesia screen
    - Padded armboards
    - Shoulder braces
    - Kidney brace
    - Table strap
    - Leg stirrups (Figure 6-11)

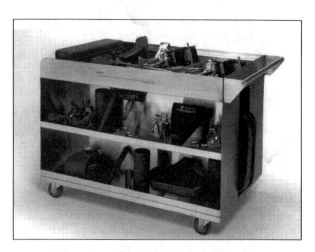

Figure 6-10 Table attachments
Source: Courtesy of Steris Corporation, Mentor, OH.

- Table extensions
- Table attachment holders

Specialized tables, such as those designed for major orthopedic procedures, have dedicated attachments necessary to achieve the desired patient position.

92. In addition to table attachments, positioning accessories are used to achieve certain positions and to provide patient safety and comfort:
    - Blankets and sheets are for patient warmth. They should not be used to form rolls and bolsters. A draw sheet under the patient's body can serve as a lift sheet. A draw sheet may be used to secure the patient's arms at the sides.
    - A pillow or contoured foam or gel headrest is used to position the patient's head and to protect the ears and nerves of the head and face. Donuts are not recommended as headrests or to support other high-pressure areas (Goodman, 2012, p. 41).
    - Pillows or contoured positioning devices may be used to support and elevate body parts.
    - Sandbags are used for immobilization.
    - A beanbag is a waterproof pillow filled with small plastic beads. A cloth cover to absorb moisture should be placed between

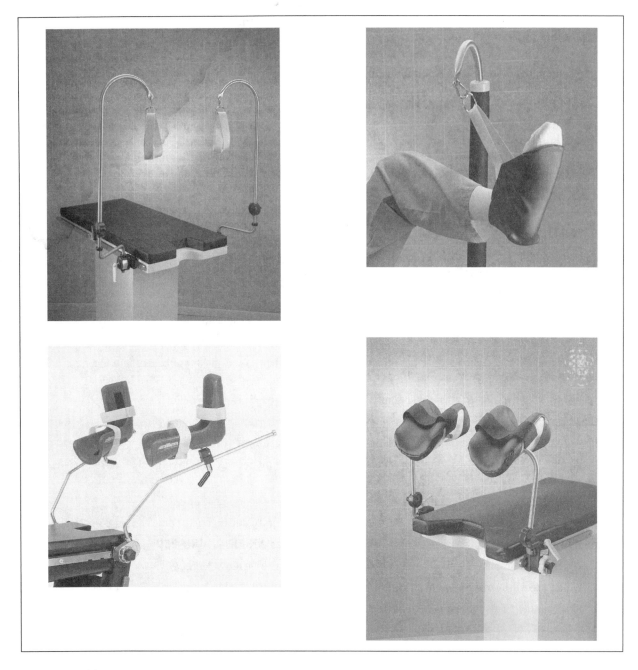

Figure 6-11 Stirrups

Source: Courtesy of Allen Medical Systems, Acton MA.

the patient and the beanbag (Dybec et al., 2011). Bony prominences that will be encased in the beanbag should be adequately padded. When the patient is positioned, the beanbag is molded to the patient. Air is then suctioned from the beanbag, leaving it rigid and holding the patient in position.

- Padding made of sheepskin, foam, felt, cotton, or contoured silicone gel can be used to protect bony prominences and pressure areas such as elbows, knees, and heels. Disposable foam and reusable contoured silicone gel pads are available in a variety of sizes and shapes.

- The firmness and density of foam padding determines its support capability. Soft foam "bottoms out" under pressure, providing little protection.

- Gel pads are made from oil-based chemical compounds or polymers sealed in a sturdy membrane-like, water-repellent covering.

- Tape is sometimes used to secure the patient or an extremity in position. Assessment for tape allergy should precede the use of tape as a positioning aid.

- A laminectomy frame (or chest rolls that extend from the acromioclavicular joint to the iliac crest) is used to support the body and allow for chest excursion while in a prone position.

- Eye pads may be used to protect the eyes and keep them closed.

- Pneumatic sequential compression devices (SCDs), elastic bandages, or antiembolectomy stockings reduce venous pooling and are frequently used to prevent deep vein thrombosis. In some facilities, one of these devices is used for every patient.

Section Questions www

1. How would you describe the perioperative nurse's responsibility for patient positioning? [Refs 64–65]

2. Which assessment parameters would you consider indicators of risk for pressure ulcer development? [Refs 66–67]

3. Name some extrinsic factors that are significant for pressure ulcer development. [Ref 68]

4. How do lengthy procedures affect risk for developing a pressure ulcer? [Ref 69]

5. Which characteristics of elderly patients place them at higher risk for developing pressure ulcers? [Ref 70]

6. How does nutritional status affect the risk development of pressure ulcers? [Ref 73]

7. Which characteristics of obese patients place them at higher risk for developing pressure ulcers? [Ref 74]

8. Which preexisting conditions increase the risk for skin breakdown? [Ref 79]

9. Which characteristics of surgical procedures might indicate higher risk for pressure ulcer development? [Ref 80]

10. Which two physiologic systems are most affected by anesthesia drugs? [Ref 84]

11. What are some interventions that preserve the patient's dignity during positioning? [Refs 85–87]

12. How can you know that a positioning device will perform as advertised? [Ref 88]

13. Which common positioning accessory should not be used as a headrest? [Ref 92]

14. Which precautions must be taken with a beanbag to protect the patient's tissues? [Ref 92]

15. What can be used to prevent deep vein thrombosis during a surgical procedure? [Ref 92]

Implementation of Patient Care

Transportation and Transfer

93. Verify the patient's identity. The surgical site should be marked and the procedure verified with the patient or a qualified patient representative, and the consent form signed, before the patient is transported to the operating room.

94. The patient's condition, the presence of invasive lines, the planned procedure, and institutional policy determine whether the patient may ambulate to the operating room or whether a wheelchair or stretcher is required.

95. Stretchers used for transportation should have side rails and a locking mechanism, and the head should elevate to alter the patient's position. Pediatric transport crib rails should be high enough to prevent a standing child from falling out (AORN, 2012, p. 426).

96. During transport, stretcher side rails are kept up and the safety strap, if present, is secured.

The patient is covered to maintain body temperature and to preserve dignity. The stretcher is pushed by the staff member at the head of the stretcher who is in close proximity to the patient's airway.

97. The nursing assessment will determine whether the patient's condition requires special equipment for transport, and whether additional personnel are required. (For example, patients on ventilators are transported to the operating room in a bed rather than on a stretcher, and additional personnel are required to wheel the bed and maintain the patient's respirations during transport.) Institutional policy may require the presence of nursing and/or medical personnel during transport of critically ill or ventilator-dependent patients.

98. Patient transfer from the stretcher to the operating table begins only when sufficient personnel are available. The stretcher is first brought adjacent to the operating table, and the side rail that is proximal to the table is lowered. Both the stretcher and the table are locked in place and raised or lowered to equal height. All patient intravenous lines and catheters need to be visible and free from entanglement. All team members must be ready for patient transfer.

99. During transfer to the operating table, one team member stands at the far side of the table to receive the patient. Another team member stands at the near side of the stretcher to assist the patient's move onto the operating room bed, and to ensure that the stretcher does not move away from the table should the lock fail. Operating room personnel must use good body mechanics to prevent injury to themselves.

100. If the patient is unable to move unaided, he or she is lifted from stretcher to bed; alternatively, the patient may be transferred with a roller or lateral transfer sheet/device. A patient lift may be more appropriate for obese patients. The patient is lifted—never pushed or pulled. Pushing and pulling create a shearing effect that compromises blood vessels and obstructs blood flow, creating the potential for a pressure ulcer.

101. Intravenous lines, monitoring devices, and endotracheal tubes are supported during transfer. The anesthesia provider typically supports the patient's head and indicates readiness for any move.

Initial Position Techniques

102. Prior to being anesthetized, the patient is positioned supine with careful attention to proper body alignment. Legs are secured with the table strap applied 2 inches above the knees. Venous thrombosis can result when superficial veins are occluded by pressure, straps, or other positioning devices. Safety straps should be tight enough to secure the patient but not so tight as to impair superficial venous return.

103. If necessary, the arms may be initially secured at the patient's side, with a draw sheet drawn over the arm and tucked under the patient (not under the mattress). The elbow should be padded and the arm should not be secured so tightly that it interferes with circulation or monitoring devices.

104. The patient is never left unattended while on the operating table.

105. If the patient is awake, all actions should be explained. The patient should be asked if he or she is comfortable; if the patient is not comfortable, make appropriate adjustments.

106. Because the temperature in the operating room is generally cool, a warm blanket should be available to the patient. Forced-air warming blankets are available in a variety of configurations and can cover the patient to help prevent hypothermia. Forced air devices are not used without the appropriate blanket. Maintaining normal body temperature can contribute to prevention of infection (Seaman et al., 2012).

107. Many patients are uncomfortable lying flat on their back. In such a case, pillows can be placed under the patient's knees and head.

108. To reduce the potential for compression injury and/or electrical burn, no part of the patient should contact a metal surface.

109. All body parts are supported and not allowed to hang free where they may be compressed or stretched.

110. To prevent compression and trauma to blood vessels, skin, and the tibial nerve, legs must not be crossed at the ankles.

www

Section Questions

1. When is the surgical site marked and consent form signed? [Ref 93]

2. Describe stretchers and cribs appropriate for transporting patients to the operating room. [Refs 95–96]

3. Which situations might require special equipment or personnel for transport? [Ref 97]

4. Describe the process for transferring the patient safely to the operating room bed. [Refs 98–101]

5. Where is the safety strap placed on the patient? [Refs 102, 118]

6. What is the proper way to secure the patient's arm at the side? [Ref 103]

7. What is an important caution about using forced-air devices with forced-air blankets? [Ref 106]

8. Other than comfort, what is an important reason for keeping the patient warm? [Ref 106]

9. What can we do to relieve pressure on the back in the supine position? [Refs 107, 117]

10. Why are we careful not to leave the patient's legs crossed at the ankles? [Ref 110]

Basic Surgical Positions

Supine (Dorsal Recumbent)

111. The supine position is the most common surgical position (Figure 6-12). Procedures in this position include abdominal surgeries and those that require an anterior approach. Head, neck, and most extremity surgeries, as well as most minimally invasive procedures, are done in the supine position.

112. In the supine position, the patient is positioned flat on the back with the head and spine in a horizontal line. Hips are parallel to each other, and the legs are positioned in a straight line, uncrossed, and not touching each other.

113. The head is supported by a headrest or pillow to prevent stretching of neck muscles.

114. Arms may rest on padded armboards or at the patient's side. Palms are either flat against the patient's side or palm down. When the arms are positioned at the patient's sides, the elbows should be padded and must not be flexed or

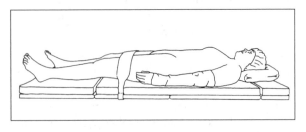

Figure 6-12 Supine position

Source: Courtesy of Reichart Consulting, Olmstead Falls, OH.

extend beyond the mattress. The arm is secured with a draw sheet that extends above the elbows and is secured under the patient (AORN, 2011, p. 345).

115. Take extra caution to be sure the sheet securing the arm is not so tight that it will interfere with the blood pressure cuff or IV line. The risk for infiltration of the intravenous line or compartment syndrome exists with the arms tucked.

116. When the arms are extended, armboards are positioned at less than a 90-degree angle from the body and palms are supinated (palms up) to prevent ulnar and radial nerve compression.

117. A small pillow may be placed under the lumbar curvature to prevent the back strain that occurs when paraspinal muscles are relaxed from anesthetic and muscle relaxant agents. An anesthetized patient lying on the back for hours will likely experience temporary lumbar pain without a lumbar support.

118. The table strap is applied loosely at least 2 inches above the knees to prevent hyperextension of the knees. The strap should be secure, but not constricting, and should never be placed over a bony prominence.

119. Appropriate protective padding is placed at pressure points. To prevent plantar flexion and crushing injuries to the toes, the table must extend beyond the toes. A table extension may be required for tall patients.

120. Pressure points at risk for skin injury in the supine position include skin over bony

prominences: occiput, spinous processes, scapulae, styloid process of the ulna and radius (elbow), olecranon process, sacrum, and calcaneus (heel). Skin breakdown from pressure is most common on the elbow, the sacrum, and the heel (Figure 6-5).

121. Nerves or nerve groups at risk include the brachial plexus, radial, ulnar, median, common peroneal, and tibial nerves.

122. Vital capacity can be reduced because of restriction of posterior chest expansion. If the patient is pregnant, a wedge may be placed under the patient's right side to prevent hypotension caused by pressure from the uterus on the aorta and vena cava.

Trendelenburg

123. Trendelenburg (Figure 6-13) is a supine position in which the table is tilted head down so that the patient's head is lower than the feet. This position is used for providing additional visualization of the lower abdomen and pelvis and is also indicated for patients who develop hypovolemic shock.

124. The patient is positioned supine with knees over the lower break in the table. All safety measures are initiated before the table is tilted. To help maintain this position, the lower part of the table may be adjusted so that the patient's legs are parallel with the floor.

125. Padded shoulder braces should not be used unless absolutely necessary because of the high risk of injury. Shoulder braces are positioned against the acromion and spinous process of the scapula. When placed incorrectly, they can cause brachial plexus injury.

126. Check the position of the patient's arm and hand to make certain that the elbow does not extend beyond the table and that the fingers are not too close to the lower break in the table where they might be crushed when the table is adjusted.

127. Before the table is tilted into Trendelenburg position, Mayo stands, tables, and other equipment are adjusted.

128. All movements are done slowly to allow the body enough time to adjust to the change in blood volume, respiratory exchange, and displacement of abdominal contents.

129. Before the procedure begins, ensure that the Mayo stand and other equipment are not touching the patient.

130. Respiratory and circulatory changes occur as a result of redistribution of body mass. Abdominal contents press against the diaphragm, limiting expansion and decreasing the ventilation–perfusion ratio.

131. Trendelenburg position increases intrathoracic and intracranial pressure. Because of these changes, the patient should remain in Trendelenburg position for as short a time as possible.

Reverse Trendelenburg

132. In reverse Trendelenburg (Figure 6-14), the table is tilted feet down. This position is used for head and neck procedures as well as to provide visualization in laparoscopic procedures in the upper abdomen.

133. The patient's feet may rest on a padded footboard, preventing the patient from sliding down on the table.

134. A pneumatic sequential compression device, elastic bandages, or antiembolectomy stockings prevent pooling of blood in the legs.

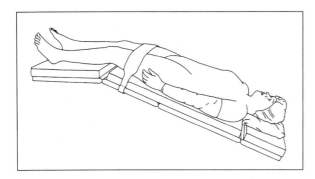

Figure 6-13 Trendelenburg position
Source: Courtesy of Reichart Consulting, Olmstead Falls, OH.

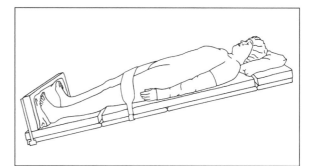

Figure 6-14 Reverse Trendelenburg position
Source: Courtesy of Reichart Consulting, Olmstead Falls, OH.

135. Movement in and out of reverse Trendelenburg is done slowly to allow sufficient time for the heart to adjust to change in blood volume.

Lithotomy

136. In lithotomy position (Figure 6-15), the patient is supine with the legs elevated, abducted, and supported in stirrups. This position is used for procedures involving the perineum region, pelvic organs, and genitalia.

137. The patient is positioned supine, with buttocks even with the lower break in the table.

138. For lengthy procedures, a sequential compression device or antiembolectomy stockings are applied to decrease pooling of blood in the lower legs.

139. Arms are secured on padded armboards to prevent crushing fingers and hands when the bottom section of the table is lowered or raised. Armboards should be positioned at an angle less than 90 degrees to the body.

140. Stirrups are attached securely to the table, positioned at equal height, and adjusted to the length of the patient's legs to prevent pressure at the knee and lumbar region of the spine.

141. Various types of stirrups are available, and their selection should be made carefully based on the type and length of the surgical procedure (Figure 6-11).

142. At-risk pressure points vary according to the type of stirrups used. Pay particular attention

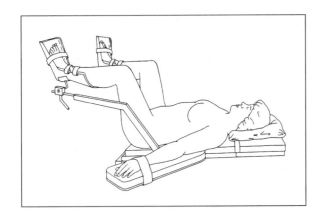

Figure 6-15 Lithotomy position
Source: Courtesy of Reichart Consulting, Olmstead Falls, OH.

to the femoral epicondyle, tibial condyles, and lateral and medial malleolus.

143. Padding on portions of the stirrups that contact the legs is appropriate to prevent external compression of nerves. Some stirrups come with a gel pad lining. To prevent injury from pressure on the peroneal nerve, the lower part of the leg should be free from pressure against the stirrup. To prevent injury to the femoral and obturator nerves, the inner thigh should be free of pressure from the stirrup.

144. Although rare, compartment syndrome—characterized by pain, muscle weakness, and loss of sensation—can result if calf muscles remain in prolonged contact with leg supports (AORN, 2012, p. 432).

145. To prevent hip dislocation or muscle strain from an exaggerated range of motion, the legs are raised and lowered simultaneously by two members of the surgical team. During leg elevation, the foot is held in one hand and the lower part of the leg in the other hand. The legs are flexed slowly, and the padded foot is secured in the stirrup.

146. After the legs are safely secured, the bottom section of the table is lowered or removed.

147. Padding may be placed under the sacrum to prevent lumbosacral strain.

148. Following the procedure, the lower section of the table is raised or replaced to align with the rest of the table. The patient's legs are removed from the stirrups simultaneously, extended fully to prevent abduction of the hips, and lowered slowly onto the table. The table strap is then applied.

149. When the legs are lowered, 500 to 800 mL of blood is diverted from the visceral area to the extremities, which can cause hypotension. Lowering the legs slowly will prevent severe sudden hypotension.

150. Lithotomy position reduces respiratory efficiency because pressure from the thighs on the abdomen and pressure from the abdominal viscera on the diaphragm restrict thoracic expansion. Lung tissue becomes engorged with blood, and vital capacity and tidal volume are decreased.

151. If nursing assessment suggests a limited range of hip motion because of contractures, arthritis, prosthesis, or another condition, the patient may be placed in lithotomy position while

awake so the patient can participate and ensure that the position is comfortable.

Sitting (Semi-Sitting, Semi-Fowler's, Lawnchair)

152. The sitting position (Figure 6-16) is used for certain cranial procedures.

153. The patient is initially positioned supine. The head is supported in a cranial headrest. The feet are supported on a padded footrest. The foot of the table is slowly lowered, flexing the knees and pelvis. The upper portion of the table is raised to become the backrest, and the torso is in either a semi-sitting or an upright position.

154. The torso and shoulders should be supported with a loose body strap. The arms may be flexed at the elbows and rest on a pillow on the patient's lap or on an adjustable padded platform in front of the patient. The arms should not fall into a dependent position.

155. Pressure points at increased risk for skin impairment include the scalp, scapulae, olecranon process, back of the knees, sacrum, ischial tuberosities, and calcaneus. Padding at these pressure points is essential.

156. The operating table should be well padded because most of the patient's body weight rests on the ischial tuberosities and the sacral nerve.

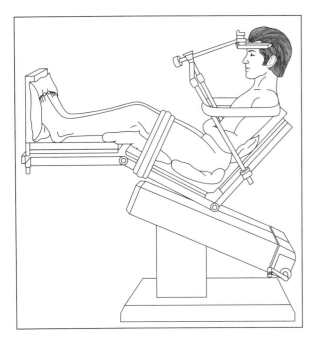

Figure 6-16 Sitting position
Source: Courtesy of Reichart Consulting, Olmstead Falls, OH.

157. Antiembolism stockings or a sequential compression device prevent postural hypotension and pooling of blood in lower extremities.

158. Because the sitting position causes negative venous pressure in the head and neck, the patient undergoing a craniotomy procedure in the sitting position is at risk for air embolism. A central venous catheter with a Doppler ultrasound flowmeter monitors the patient in this position. The Doppler device is used to detect an air embolism, and the central venous pressure line is used to extract the air.

159. In the semi-sitting (lawnchair) position, the patient's body is flexed at the pelvis and knees. The back of the table is not fully upright and the patient is in a reclining position. This position is used for nasopharyngeal, facial, breast reconstruction, and neck surgery. A roll may be placed under the patient's neck to hyperextend the neck and provide better access to the surgical site.

Prone

160. In the prone position (Figure 6-17), the patient is positioned on the abdomen. This exposure of the posterior body is used for procedures of the spine, back, rectum, and the posterior aspects of extremities.

161. The patient is initially positioned supine on the stretcher. The side rail closest to the operating table is lowered, and the stretcher is positioned adjacent to the operating table and locked. The other side rail is lowered, and anesthesia is administered while the patient is on the stretcher. Following induction, the anesthesiologist secures the endotracheal tube to prevent dislocation and applies ointment to the eyes and tapes them shut to prevent corneal abrasion. The anesthesiologist will indicate when the patient is ready to be moved onto the operating room table.

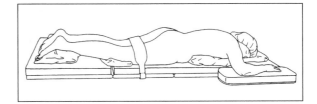

Figure 6-17 Prone position
Source: Courtesy of Reichart Consulting, Olmstead Falls, OH.

162. All necessary equipment—padded armboard, headrest, chest rolls or laminectomy frame, pillows, and padding materials—must be available prior to positioning. A minimum of four persons is necessary to safely turn the adult patient from a supine position on the stretcher to a prone position on the operating table: one person supports and manages the head, one supports and moves the torso, one supports and moves the lower body, and one person on the opposite side of the operating room table receives the patient as he or she is rolled onto the table.

163. All movement of the patient is done slowly and gently to allow the body time to adjust to the change in position. The anesthesiologist supports the head and neck and protects the patient's airway. A second person turns the patient from the stretcher onto the chest rolls or frame on the operating table and the waiting arms of the third person, who supports the patient's chest and lower abdomen. A fourth person supports and turns the patient's legs. During turning, the patient's arms and hands are placed at the sides. The body is maintained in anatomical alignment, and all team members work in concert to turn the patient in a single motion.

164. After the patient is supine, the arms are brought down and forward in a normal range of motion and then placed on armboards positioned next to the head. The arms are flexed at the elbows with the hands pronated (palms down) and elbows padded.

165. The anesthesiologist turns the patient's head to one side and supports it on a small pillow or headrest, secures the airway, and then checks that the patient's eyes are closed to prevent corneal abrasion and are free of pressure that can cause permanent eye injury. The ears must be not folded unnaturally. Neck and spine must be in good alignment.

166. The chest is supported by chest rolls or a laminectomy frame, such as the Wilson frame, which is positioned lengthwise from the acromioclavicular joint to the iliac crest. This positioning lifts the patient's chest off the operating table and facilitates respiratory expansion. Chest rolls that are too small or that are improperly positioned can result in restricted lung expansion. Female breasts and male genitalia must be free and not compressed.

167. A pillow under the ankles prevents stretching of the anterior tibial nerve and prevents pressure on the toes and feet that can cause plantar flexion and foot drop. A pillow also lifts the patient's toes, preventing pressure injury from resting on the table.

168. In the prone position, the table strap is placed over the mid-thighs, which are covered with a sheet, pad, and/or a blanket. The strap should be at least 2 inches above the knees to promote superficial venous return.

169. A small pillow or foam padding under the knees prevents pressure on the patellas.

170. If the patient has a stoma, take precautions to prevent ischemic compression of the stoma against the frame or chest rolls that can lead to tissue necrosis and sloughing.

171. If a Mayfield head positioned is used in the prone position, the patient must never be moved while the head is in the device.

172. Pedal pulses must be assessed to determine whether circulation to the lower extremities has been compromised by pressure at the iliac crest region from the positioning devices.

Jackknife (Kraske)

173. In the jackknife position (Figure 6-18), the patient is prone with the table flexed at the center break. This position is used for proctological procedures.

174. Venous pooling in the chest and feet can cause a decrease in mean arterial blood pressure. Restriction of diaphragm movement combined with increased blood volume in the lungs can cause a decrease in ventilation and cardiac

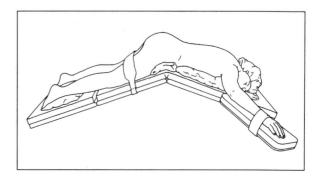

Figure 6-18 Kraske (jackknife) position
Source: Courtesy of Reichart Consulting, Olmstead Falls, OH.

output. Because of its adverse effect on the respiratory and circulatory systems, the jackknife position is considered one of the most precarious surgical positions.

175. For the jackknife position, the patient is first placed in the prone position on chest rolls with the hips over the center table joint. Arms are positioned on padded angled armboards placed next to the head. Elbows are flexed and padded, and palms are pronated. The head is turned to one side. (Chest rolls are not necessary if the patient is awake.) A pillow is placed under the ankles, knees are padded, and the table strap is applied to the thighs covered with a sheet or blanket. The table is then flexed to a 90-degree angle, causing the hips to be raised and the head and legs to be lowered.

176. All precautions appropriate for the prone position are applicable to the jackknife position.

Lateral

177. In the lateral (or lateral decubitus) position (Figure 6-19), the patient lies on one side. In the right lateral position, the patient lies on the right side for surgery on the left side of the body. The reverse is true for the left lateral position.

178. The lateral position is used to access the thorax, kidney, retroperitoneal space, and hip.

179. The patient initially lies supine on the operating table and anesthetized. A team of four persons then lifts and turns the patient onto the nonoperative side. The anesthesiologist initiates any movement, supports the head and neck, and guards the airway. A second person lifts and supports the chest and shoulders. The

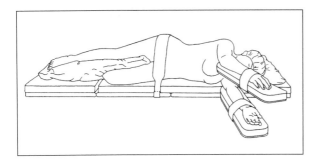

Figure 6-19 Lateral position

Source: Courtesy of Reichart Consulting, Olmstead Falls, OH.

third person lifts and supports the hips, while the fourth person supports and turns the legs.

180. The patient is lifted in supine position to the edge of the operative side of the table, then turned onto the side toward the center of the table. For kidney procedures, it is important that the patient's flank be positioned over the kidney rest with the iliac crest just below the table break. The patient's head is supported with a pillow or headrest, and the body is checked for proper alignment. The head must be placed in cervical alignment with the spine. The lower leg is flexed. The lateral aspect of the lower knee is well padded to prevent peroneal nerve damage that might result in foot drop caused by pressure from the fibula on the nerve. A pillow is placed between the legs, and the upper leg is extended out straight. Feet and ankles are padded and supported to prevent foot drop and pressure injuries of the malleolus. The patient is secured with the table strap or with wide tape applied across the upper hip and fastened to the table.

181. A small roll or padding is placed under the patient's lower axilla to relieve pressure on the chest and axilla, to allow sufficient chest expansion, and to prevent compression of the brachial plexus by the humeral head. The lower arm is slightly flexed and placed on a padded armboard. The upper arm may rest on a padded elevated armboard or other padded support. Take care not to abduct the arm more than 90 degrees, as a greater angle can cause brachial plexus injury.

182. For kidney procedures, the patient is supported on the operating table with well-padded braces, rolls, or sandbags. Extra padding is applied to ankles, knees, greater trochanter, iliac crest, shoulders, elbows, and wrists.

183. The table may be flexed at the center break. The kidney elevator (kidney rest) is raised to provide greater exposure of the area from the 12th rib to the iliac crest. Kidney braces that fit over the kidney elevator may be used to support and maintain the patient in this position. These devices must always be well padded.

184. Respiratory efficiency is affected by pressure from the weight of the body on the lower chest. The lower lung receives more blood from the right side of the heart in the lateral position, so

it has increased perfusion but less residual air because of mediastinal compression and weight from abdominal contents.

185. Circulation is compromised by pressure on abdominal vessels and pooling of blood in the lower extremities. In the right lateral position, compression on the vena cava impairs venous return. If the kidney elevator is raised, additional pressure on abdominal vessels can further compromise circulation.

186. Injury of the eye or ear is a special concern with the patient in the lateral position. The ear must be laid flat against the operating table and the eyelid must be closed.

Section Questions

1. Describe the proper positioning of the patient in supine position. [Refs 112–114]
2. What is one danger of securing the arms tightly at the patient's side? [Ref 115]
3. What is important about positioning the patient's arm on an armboard? [Ref 116]
4. What might happen if the patient's feet extend beyond the operating room table? [Ref 119]
5. Name the bony prominences at risk for pressure injury in the supine position. [Ref 120]
6. Which nerves are at risk for injury in the supine position? [Ref 121]
7. How do we relieve pressure on the vena cava when positioning a pregnant patient? [Ref 122]
8. How does the Trendelenburg position differ from the supine position? [Ref 123]
9. In which instances is the Trendelenburg position appropriate? [Ref 123]
10. What is the danger in using shoulder braces to keep the patient from sliding in Trendelenburg position? [Ref 125]
11. For which reason are changes in position done slowly? [Ref 128]
12. How are the patient's anatomy and physiology affected in Trendelenburg position? [Refs 130–131]
13. For which types of procedures is the reverse Trendelenburg position used? [Ref 132]
14. What can we use to keep the patient from sliding in the reverse Trendelenburg position? [Ref 133]
15. Describe the lithotomy position. [Refs 136–137]
16. What can be used to prevent blood from pooling in the lower legs? [Ref 138]
17. Which pressure points are at risk for injury when the patient's legs are in stirrups? [Ref 142]
18. Why are the patient's legs raised and lowered slowly and simultaneously? [Refs 145, 149]
19. How can a patient with an implant or limited range of leg motion be placed safely in the lithotomy position? [Ref 151]
20. Which pressure points are at risk in the supine position? [Refs 155–156]
21. Describe the danger of air embolism in the sitting position and explain how this risk is managed. [Ref 158]
22. Describe the process of moving the patient from the supine to the prone position. [Refs 161–169]
23. Why is it important to assess pedal pulses with a patient in the prone position? [Ref 172]
24. Why is the jackknife position considered precarious? [Ref 174]
25. The patient will be placed in the right lateral position for surgery on which kidney? [Ref 177]
26. Describe the precautions taken to prevent injury to the patient in the lateral position. [Refs 179–181]
27. What is the purpose of the kidney rest? [Ref 183]
28. Describe the impact on respiratory efficiency in the lateral position. [Ref 184]
29. Describe the impact on circulation in the lateral position. [Ref 185]
30. How are injuries to the eye and ear prevented in the lateral position? [Ref 186]

Positioning the Morbidly Obese Patient

187. The morbidly obese patient is an individual with a BMI of greater than 40.

188. Obesity places an increased workload on the heart and circulatory system, and respiratory function is compromised in obese patients because of increased weight on the chest.

189. Skim breakdown is a challenge with obese patients, as they may trap moisture and fluids from skin prep solutions in tissue folds. Adipose tissue is not well vascularized, and the pressure resulting from positioning can cause a decrease in circulation to peripheral body areas.

190. Bariatric and morbidly obese patients require special safety considerations:
    - The operating room bed must be capable of supporting the patient's weight and must be wide enough to contain the patient. Side extensions may be necessary. The manufacturer's recommendations must be followed for weight restrictions.
    - Lifting devices should be used to transfer the patient.
    - The safety strap must be long enough to secure the patient.
    - Two safety straps may be necessary—one for the upper portion of the legs and one for the lower portion.
    - The supine position may cause the patient to have difficulty breathing due to pressure of the viscera on the diaphragm. A wedge should be placed under the right flank to relieve pressure on the vena cava.
    - The lithotomy and Trendelenburg positions should be avoided, as they may also cause respiratory and circulatory compromise.
    - The prone position may cause pressure on the diaphragm.

Evaluating Implementation of Positioning

191. The anesthetized patient cannot report discomfort or pain related to positioning, and the effects of improper positioning will usually not be identified until the patient recovers from anesthesia and is able to report pain and injury. The patient relies on the surgical team to ensure that positioning injuries do not occur.

192. Once the patient is in position for the surgery, the perioperative nurse should do a thorough, once-over check to ensure that the patient's body is in alignment, extremities are not extended beyond their natural range of motion, bony prominences are appropriately padded, nerves where injury can occur are protected, respiratory and circulatory efforts are restricted as little as possible, and positioning devices are appropriately positioned and padded and holding the patient's body securely without excessive restriction on body structures. Intermittent reevaluation of the patient's position throughout the procedure is important. If the patient is repositioned during the procedure, a thorough reevaluation is critical, with adjustments made as necessary.

Postoperative Transfer

193. When surgery is completed and the anesthesiologist indicates that the patient is stable and can be moved, the postoperative bed or stretcher is brought adjacent to the operating table. It is raised or lowered to the level of the operating table and locked into place.

194. Ideally, four people should be available to transfer the anesthetized adult patient slowly and smoothly to the bed or stretcher with a roller or lateral transfer sheet/device, maintaining the airway and proper body alignment. Lines and catheters must be protected and kept free from entanglement.

195. The patient is lifted or rolled onto the bed or stretcher, avoiding pushing and pulling. Side rails are raised and locked for safe patient transfer.

Documentation of Nursing Actions

196. Nursing documentation related to positioning should include the following information:
    - Assessment and considerations for positioning—desired outcomes
    - Overall skin condition on arrival and discharge from the perioperative suite
    - Position
    - Placement of extremities

- Type and placement of positioning equipment and devices, such as stirrups, rolls, padding, and restraints
- Precautions to protect eyes
- Presence and placement of safety strap or equivalent

- Who positioned the patient
- Any changes made in positioning during the procedure
- Patient condition following surgery—whether desired outcomes were met
- Signature

Section Questions

www

1. What are some of the challenges the obese patient faces with positioning? [Refs 188–189]

2. Describe the safety considerations in planning for positioning of the obese patient. [Ref 190]

3. Once the patient is positioned, what is involved in the "once-over" check that is done by the circulating nurse? [Ref 192]

4. Which member of the surgical team determines when the patient can be moved following surgery? [Ref 193]

5. Which elements should be included in the nurse's documentation of positioning? [Ref 196]

• • • References

American Society of Anesthesiologists (ASA), Task Force on Prevention of Perioperative Peripheral Neuropathies (2011). Practice advisory for the prevention of perioperative peripheral neuropathies. *Anesthesiology*;114:1-1.

Armstrong D, Ayello E, Capitulo K, et al. (2008). New opportunities to improve pressure ulcer prevention and treatment. *J Wound Ostomy Continence Nurs*;35(5):485–492.

Aronovich S (2007). Intraoperatively acquired pressure ulcers: are there common risk factors? *Ostomy Wound Manage*;53(2):57–69.

Association of periOperative Registered Nurses (AORN) (2012). *Perioperative Standards and Recommended Practices*. Denver, CO: AORN.

Association of periOperative Registered Nurses (AORN) (2011). *Perioperative Nursing Data Set*, 3rd ed. Denver, CO: AORN.

Dybec R, Needler J, Pfister J (2011). *Basic Principles of Patient Positioning*. Aurora, CO: Pfiedler Enterprises.

Goodman, T (2012). *Positioning: A Patient Safety Initiative: Study Guide for Nurses*. Dallas, TX: Terri Goodman & Associates.

The Joint Commission (2012). National Patient Safety goals (Goal 14). Washington, DC: TJC. Available at: www.jointcommission.org/standards_information/npsgs.aspx. Accessed September, 2012.

Primiano M, Firend M, McClure C, et al. (2011). Pressure ulcer prevalence and risk factors during prolonged surgical procedures. *AORN J*;94(6):555–566.

Seaman M, Wobb J, Gaughan J, et al. (2012). The effects of intraoperative hypothermia on surgical site infection. *Ann Surg*;224(4):789–795.

University of Pittsburgh (2012). Nurse Anesthesia Program Surgical Positioning Website. *Complications and nerve injuries*. Pittsburgh, PA: University of Pittsburgh. Available at: www.pitt.edu/~position/complications.htm#Ulnar%20Nerve%20Injury. Accessed September, 2012.

Post-Test

Read each question carefully. Each question may have more than one correct answer.

1. Choose the two primary reasons for positioning a patient for a surgical procedure
   a. Preventing tissue damage
   b. Providing exposure to the operative site
   c. Keeping the patient comfortable
   d. Stabilizing the patient on the operating table

2. Which factors influence the potential for injury related to surgical positioning?
   a. Type of procedure
   b. Age of the patient
   c. Position required for the procedure
   d. Comorbidities

3. Which surgical team member most often coordinates the positioning of the patient?
   a. Surgeon
   b. Anesthesiologist
   c. Scrub nurse
   d. Circulating nurse

4. Which of the following positions is most likely to affect circulation and oxygen–carbon dioxide exchange?
   a. Supine
   b. Sitting
   c. Trendelenburg
   d. Reverse Trendelenburg

5. Which factors can lead to decreased lung expansion?
   a. Retractors
   b. Pressure of abdominal contents on the diaphragm
   c. Reverse Trendelenburg position
   d. Prone position on improperly placed chest rolls

6. Which of the following can result in brachial plexus injury?
   a. Tucking the arms too tightly at the patient's sides
   b. Hyperextension of the arm on an armboard
   c. An automatic blood pressure cuff cycling too often
   d. Pressure on the acromion process of the elbow

7. What is the correct way to position the patient's arm at the side?
   a. Padded elbow, palm up, sheet tucked under mattress
   b. Padded elbow, palm facing patient, sheet tucked under mattress
   c. Padded elbow, palm against the patient's side, sheet tucked under patient
   d. Padded elbow, palm against the mattress, sheet tucked under patient

8. Which of the following are symptoms of an ulnar nerve injury?
   a. Pain, tingling, or numbness in the ring finger and little finger
   b. Weakness of grip leading to a "claw hand"

   c. Pain, tingling, or numbness in the first and middle fingers

   d. Wrist drop

9. Which of the following are symptoms of a radial nerve injury?

   a. Pain, tingling, or numbness in the ring finger and little finger

   b. Weakness of grip leading to a "claw hand"

   c. Pain, tingling, or numbness in the first and middle fingers

   d. Wrist drop

10. Which injuries can result from improper placement of legs in stirrups and moving the legs improperly?

   a. Extension

   b. Flexion

   c. Compression

   d. Stretching

11. Which three factors contribute to pressure injuries to tissues?

   a. Immobility

   b. Pressure

   c. Time

   d. Surgical procedure

12. Skin moving across a course surface produces which type of injury?

   a. Shear

   b. Pressure

   c. Friction

   d. Deep tissue injury

13. Shearing injuries occur when

   a. there is pressure at the bone–tissue interface.

   b. skin is rubbed or pulled across a rough surface.

   c. the skin remains stationary while tissues beneath it move.

   d. the table strap is too tight across the thighs.

14. Extrinsic factors that contribute to pressure injuries include

   a. sedation.

   b. warming devices.

   c. length of surgery.

   d. obesity.

15. What is a deep tissue injury?

   a. A red area over a bony prominence that progresses from skin to deep tissues

   b. Stage IV ulcer

   c. Damage to the large muscles

   d. Necrosis at the bone–tissue interface that does not become evident until days after surgery

16. Which of the following are intrinsic factors that contribute to pressure injuries?

   a. Quality of the positioning equipment

   b. Age and weight

   c. Obesity and comorbidities

   d. Length of the surgical procedure

17. Which of the following place the elderly at great risk for tissue damage?
    a. Decreased muscle tone
    b. Less subcutaneous tissue to protect bony prominences
    c. Poor heat receptors
    d. Poor skin turgor

18. Why are obese patients at risk for tissue damage during surgery?
    a. Operating room beds cannot provide adequate support.
    b. Moisture and fluid can be trapped in skin folds.
    c. Adipose tissue is not well vascularized and pressure can decrease blood flow to peripheral areas.
    d. Excess weight increases strain on joints.

19. In which ways does the perioperative nurse advocate for the patient?
    a. Provides privacy
    b. Makes the patient comfortable
    c. Preserves the patient's dignity
    d. Takes responsibility to ensure proper positioning

20. How can blankets and sheets be used in positioning the patient?
    a. Draw sheet
    b. Provide warmth
    c. Provide privacy
    d. Rolled up to provide support

21. When can the patient be transferred from stretcher to operating room table?
    a. When the anesthesia provider says to make the transfer
    b. When the surgeon is available to assist
    c. When the perioperative nurse says to make the transfer
    d. When sufficient personnel are available to make the transfer

22. How can the patient be made comfortable prior to anesthesia?
    a. Place a pillow beneath the head and the knees.
    b. Provide a warm blanket.
    c. Leave the safety strap off until the patient is asleep.
    d. Explain all procedures.

23. What is the correct positioning when placing an arm at the patient's side?
    a. Palms up
    b. Palm against patient side
    c. Palm down
    d. Arm secured with draw sheet tucked under the patient

24. What is the correct positioning when placing an arm on an armboard?
    a. Extended more than 90 degrees
    b. Palms pronated
    c. Extended less than 90 degrees from the body
    d. Palms supinated

25. The table strap should be placed
    a. snugly across the patient's knees.
    b. loosely across the patient's knees.
    c. loosely 2 inches above the patient's knees.
    d. snugly 2 inches below the patient's knees.

26. The Trendelenburg (head down) position is used
    a. to provide good visualization of the abdomen.
    b. for obese patients, to keep them from sliding off the table.
    c. to manage hypovolemic shock.
    d. for foot surgery.

27. Some challenges in the Trendelenburg position include
    a. decreased intrathoracic pressure.
    b. decreased ventilation–perfusion ratio.
    c. increased intrathoracic pressure.
    d. Mayo stand can place pressure on the patient's legs and feet.

28. Why is movement out of the Trendelenburg position done slowly?
    a. To keep the patient from getting dizzy
    b. To prevent nausea and vomiting
    c. To prevent headache and increased intracranial pressure
    d. To allow the patient's heart to adjust to the change in blood volume

29. How are the legs protected from injury in lithotomy position?
    a. Stirrups are positioned at equal height adjusted to the patient.
    b. At-risk pressure points are properly padded.
    c. Legs are lifted and lowered simultaneously and slowly.
    d. The patient is positioned while still awake to confirm the comfortable position.

30. Craniotomy patients in sitting position are at risk for
    a. pressure damage at the ischial tuberosities.
    b. increased intracranial pressure.
    c. air embolism.
    d. sacral nerve damage.

31. How is cardiorespiratory expansion preserved in the prone position?
    a. Pillows are placed under the patient's chest.
    b. Shoulder braces hold the patient in place.
    c. The patient's chest is held off the table with chest rolls or a laminectomy frame.
    d. The patient's weight rests on knees and shoulders.

32. Which areas are at risk for injury in the lateral position?
    a. Eye
    b. Ear
    c. Peroneal nerve
    d. Brachial plexus

33. At the end of the procedure, which team member decides when the patient is ready for transfer from the operating room bed?

    a. Surgeon
    b. Anesthesia provider
    c. Perioperative nurse
    d. Scrub person

34. What is the ideal number of personnel to transfer the patient from the operating room bed while protecting lines and catheters?

    a. Two
    b. Three
    c. Four
    d. Five

35. Nursing documentation related to positioning should include

    a. the patient's skin condition before positioning.
    b. the patient's position and related equipment used.
    c. the presence and placement of a safety strap.
    d. who positioned the patient.

Prevention of Retained Surgical Items

LESSON OUTLINE

Description

1. Items opened and delivered to the sterile field that could be retained in the surgical wound are counted to prevent patient injury. Counted items include soft goods (radiopaque sponges and towels), sharps such as blades and needles, instruments, and miscellaneous items such as vessel loops and vein introducers.

2. The purpose of a count is to reconcile what was delivered to the sterile field before the initial incision and during the procedure with what remains at the end of surgery.

3. Each facility should have a documented system in place to prevent retained surgical items. A reliable system includes accurate counting, radiological confirmation, and the use of adjunct technology to promote operative perioperative patient outcomes (Association of periOperative Registered Nurses [AORN], 2012, p. 313).

Nursing Diagnosis: Desired Patient Outcome

4. Patients undergoing surgery are at risk for injury related to an unintentionally retained surgical item (RSI) (AORN, 2011, pp. 146–149; 2012, pp. 313–332).

5. A retained surgical item is considered a sentinel event or "never event"— an unexpected occurrence involving death or serious injury that is reasonably preventable by following

evidence-based guidelines. The Joint Commission (TJC) identified RSI as the most frequently reported sentinel event in 2010 (Norton and Martin, 2012, p. 110), and RSI is first on the Centers for Medicare & Medicaid Service's list of nonreimbursed hospital-acquired conditions (CMS, 2011, p. 9).

6. A retained surgical item causes unnecessary pain and suffering, extended stay or readmission to the hospital, additional surgery, delayed healing, and a significant increase in healthcare costs.

7. The abdomen and pelvis are the most common sites for retained items; however, there have been reports of items retained in the vagina, thorax, spinal canal, face, brain, and extremities (AORN, 2012, p. 313).

8. Gossypiboma (surgical complications related to the unintentional retention of soft goods) can be either acute or delayed. Acute presentations generally follow a septic course, with abscess or granuloma formation. Often these symptoms do not occur until after the patient has returned home. Delayed presentation may occur months or years after surgery with adhesion formation and encapsulation (AORN, 2012, p. 316).

9. A desired outcome following a surgical procedure is that the patient is free from signs and symptoms of injury caused by retained surgical items (AORN, 2011, p. 146).

Overview

10. In addition to causing harm to the patient, retained surgical items frequently result in malpractice litigation. Because a retained surgical item in a patient is almost always indefensible based on the doctrine of res ipsa loquitur ("the thing speaks for itself"), such cases usually do not come before a jury. Any or all members of the surgical team may be held liable.

11. Retained surgical items (e.g., sponges, needles, instruments) are sentinel events that occur in an estimated one in 5500 surgeries. Gauze sponges account for 48% to 69% of retained surgical items, and the abdomen is the cavity most often involved (Steelman and Cullen, 2011). In abdominal surgeries, the incidence is one in every 1000 to 1500 operations (American Hospital Association [AHA], 2011).

12. Counts are usually performed by the scrub person and the circulating nurse. The perioperative nurse is legally accountable for counts; however, the entire surgical team has a responsibility to participate in protecting the patient from injury.

13. AORN (2012, p. 314) asserts that a system that accounts for all items opened and used during a surgical procedure is a primary and proactive injury-prevention strategy.

14. Many healthcare facilities have established count policies that reflect the AORN's recommended practices for prevention of retained surgical items; however, there are also facilities whose count policies differ from the AORN-recommended practice. Count policies should specify when counts are to be taken, by whom, and what is counted.

15. Policies specifying what is counted are based on the nature of the procedure, the anticipated size of the incision, the probability of a retained item, and the supplies required for the procedure.

16. The perioperative nurse should be familiar with institutional count policies and procedures. Compliance with institutional policy and an understanding of the principles of and the techniques for surgical counts can provide a foundation for patient safety.

17. Determining when to count based on identifying procedures in which the possibility exists for a retained item requires critical thinking skills and a significant amount of experience. The perioperative nurse must be familiar with the intended surgical procedure and the risk associated with it to be able to assess the risk of a retained item. Facility policies provide clear direction even when the nurse does not have extensive experience in this area.

18. Some facilities use a count sheet to record count results. This count sheet may become part of the patient's operative record. Others use a wallboard where counts are recorded during the procedure and only the final results are documented as a permanent record.

Nursing Responsibilities

19. As patient advocates, perioperative nurses have a responsibility to ensure that count procedures are carried out according to facility policy.

20. Surgical counts are not a guarantee that items will not be retained in a patient. A retained surgical item lawsuit often includes documentation of a "correct count." The item was not retained intentionally, nor does the documentation intentionally misrepresent the count. The false "correct count" usually represents an error in the count process.

21. All counts must be performed carefully, and the scrub person and the circulating nurse must share the responsibility equally. Items being counted must be visible to both the scrub person and the circulating nurse. Counts must be done together and aloud. The scrub person and the circulating nurse must both view the sponges as they are counted. It is not acceptable for the scrub person to count the sponges and tell the circulating nurse how many are present.

22. Rowlands and Steeves (2010, p. 413) discovered three general themes that represented challenges to correct counts: individual behaviors, environmental factors, and communication difficulties. Challenges include the following issues (Figure 7-1):

- Unkempt, messy, or cluttered sterile field
- Disorganized documentation
- Distractions that interfere with concentration during the count (e.g., interruptions, conversations, loud music, telephones, pages)
- Multitasking
- Items may be delivered to the field by someone other than the circulating nurse and not documented or communicated
- Sponges saturated with blood may not be visible in the wound
- Sponges placed in cavities for packing can be overlooked
- Change in personnel when it is not possible to perform a total relief count; multiple changes of personnel during a procedure
- Emergency surgery
- An unplanned change in the procedure

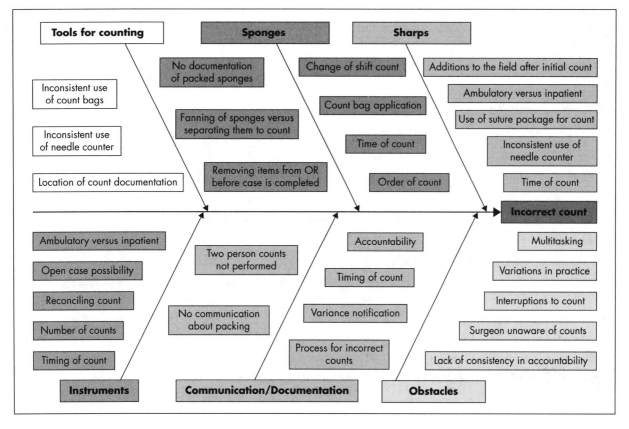

Figure 7-1 Ishikawa diagram showing factors affecting the accuracy of counts

Source: Reprinted from EM Edel (2012). Surgical count practice variability and the potential for retained surgical items. *AORN J;*95(2): 228–238. Copyright 2013 with permission from Elsevier.

- Patient obesity
- Signing for counts that were not performed (AORN, 2012, p. 314; Edel, 2012, p. 234; Rowlands and Steeves, 2010, pp. 413–414)

23. Counts should be performed as follows:
    - Before the procedure to establish a baseline and identify manufacturing and packaging errors (initial count)
    - When new items are added to the field
    - Before closure of a cavity within a cavity (e.g., the uterus)
    - When wound closure begins
    - At skin closure at the end of the procedure or at the end of the procedure when counted items are no longer in use (i.e., the final count)
    - At the time of permanent relief of either the scrub person or the RN circulator, although direct visualization of all items may not be possible (AORN, 2012, pp. 316–321)

24. When an incorrect count occurs, it is the responsibility of the nurse to inform the surgeon and for all team members to assist in locating the missing item before the wound is closed. The search should begin at the incision site and progress to the entire sterile field, and to the environment—sponge collection system, floor around and under the table, and the trash.

25. All surgical counted sponges should have a radiopaque marker. If the count remains unresolved, an X ray of the patient can verify that the sponge has not been retained in the wound.

26. In an extreme emergency situation, such as multiple trauma, it may not be possible to perform a count before the procedure. Omission of the count and the rationale should be documented, and institutional policy for this occurrence should be followed. Policy may mandate that an X ray be taken.

27. Counts should be verified when either the scrub person or the circulating nurse is relieved by a new team member.

28. Counted items should never be removed from the operating room until after the procedure when final counts have been completed. All counted items should be removed from the room at the end of surgery. Items left in the room may interfere with the count in a subsequent procedure in that room.

29. The nurse is responsible for documenting count information and for notifying the surgeon of the count results.

Section Questions   `WWW`

1. Which items have been identified as having potential for being retained in a surgical wound? [Ref 1]

2. What is the purpose of the surgical counts? [Ref 2]

3. What are some components of a facility policy for prevention of retained surgical items? [Ref 3]

4. Define a "sentinel event." [Ref 5]

5. What are some of the consequences to the patient of a retained surgical item? [Refs 6–8]

6. In litigation related to RSI, who is liable? [Refs 10, 12]

7. Who customarily performs surgical counts? [Ref 12]

8. How does the perioperative nurse determine what should be counted and who should participate? [Refs 14–17]

9. Explain how the surgical documentation can reflect a "correct count" during litigation relating to a retained item. [Ref 20]

10. Describe proper count procedure. [Ref 21]

11. Identify situations when correct counts might be a challenge. [Ref 22]

12. Explain the situations related to a surgical procedure when surgical counts should be done. [Ref 23]

13. When a count is incorrect, what are the responsibilities of the perioperative nurse? [Ref 24]

14. How is the situation managed when circumstances make required counts impossible? [Ref 26]

15. Why must all counted items remain in the room until after the final count? [Ref 28]

Count Procedures

Soft Goods Counts

30. "Soft goods" refers to sponges and towels—materials designed to absorb blood and fluids. All sponges placed on the sterile field should incorporate a radiopaque strip or thread that makes them X-ray detectable. Sponges should not be altered, and the radiopaque strip should never be removed. Sponges include the following items:

    - Lap pads (also referred to as lap sponges, tapes, and lap packs)—square or rectangular gauze pads with an X-ray-detectable tape sewn to the corner of the sponge. These sponges are used where moderate to large amounts of blood or fluid are encountered.

    - Gauze sponges (also referred to as raytec and swabs)—approximately 4¾-inch squares of gauze used where a small amount of blood or fluid is anticipated. They may also be folded and clamped to ring forceps (sponge stick) to be used for swabbing or deep dissection.

    - Peanuts—very small sponges approximately the size of a peanut. They are clamped to forceps and used for dissection or to absorb a small amount of fluid or blood on delicate tissue.

    - Kitner dissectors—a small roll of heavy cotton tape that is clamped to forceps and used for dissection or absorption.

    - Tonsil sponges—cotton-filled gauzes in the shape of a ball with a long tape attached that are used in tonsil surgery. They are inserted into the mouth to absorb blood and stop bleeding from the tonsil bed. The tape extends outside the mouth and is used for retrieval.

    - Cottonoid patties (also referred to as neuro sponges)—strips of compressed cotton in a variety of sizes that incorporate a long radiopaque thread. They are used for surgeries on delicate structures such as the brain and spinal cord. When patties become saturated with blood, they are difficult to see; the thread facilitates their location.

31. Before surgery begins, the scrub person and the circulating nurse count all sponges on the field aloud and together. Sponges must be handled so that both persons can visually verify the count. The circulator documents the count.

32. Sponges are generally supplied from the manufacturer in packs of five or ten and are held together with a paper strip. Never assume that the amount indicated on the package label is accurate. The paper strip must be removed and all sponges must be separated and counted individually.

33. If a commercially prepared package of sponges is found to be incorrect, it should be removed from the field, bagged, and labeled as such, and isolated from the rest of the sponges. These sponges may be removed from the room before the patient enters. If the patient is already in the room, the sponges must remain in the room, but are not included in the count (AORN, 2012, pp. 316–317).

34. If additional sponges are needed during the procedure, they are delivered to the sterile field and counted together and aloud; the addition is also recorded.

35. During surgery, the scrub person discards used sponges into a plastic-lined kick bucket or surface prepared for this purpose.

36. Pocketed sponge bags or a similar system should be used on all procedures where a soft goods count is performed (AORN, 2012, p. 318). When a unit of five or ten sponges accumulates, the circulating nurse counts them aloud with the scrub person and places them in the impervious pocketed bag to facilitate the ability to visualize the sponges for counting.

37. Soiled sponges are handled with an instrument and with gloved hands. Discarded sponges are never handled with bare hands.

38. After the final count, the bags containing sponges are discarded in a manner that reduces the risk of bloodborne pathogen disease transmission.

39. Individual healthcare facility policy and the U.S. Department of Labor, Occupational Safety and Health Administration (OSHA) Bloodborne Pathogen Standards 1910-1030 (2011) should be consulted for guidelines related to personal protective equipment and disposal of infectious waste. In some states, the state regulations for definition and disposal of regulated waste may be more stringent than the federal regulations. As a result, policies for managing soiled sponges will vary among facilities.

40. As wound closure begins, the scrub person and the circulating nurse count aloud and together all sponges on the sterile field and any that have been discarded from the field. The number of

sponges still in use plus the number of previously counted sponges should equal the total number supplied for the surgery.

41. The procedure for counting sponges should be consistent, following the same sequence each time. Typically the count starts at the surgical site, continues to the Mayo stand, moves to the back table, and finally goes to the discarded sponges. The count begins with the smallest type of sponge and progresses to the largest. Consistent practice promotes efficiency and continuity.

42. All sponges that were opened for the procedure should remain in the room until the procedure is completed and the patient has left the room. Trash and linen containers should also remain in the room. This practice will assist in locating a missing sponge in the event that the count cannot be immediately reconciled.

43. The surgical team is informed of the results of the initial closing count. If the count is accurate, closure will continue. As skin closure begins, a final count of sponges is conducted using the same procedure. The results are reported to the surgical team and are documented.

44. If the count is incorrect at the time of wound closure, the surgical team is notified and a thorough search is initiated, beginning within the wound and including the sterile field, the room, and the trash. If the sponge cannot be located, facility policy will determine if an intraoperative X ray is required.

45. According to The Joint Commission (and many states), a sentinel retained surgical item event is reportable if discovered after wound closure.

46. The following steps will minimize the possibility of an incorrect sponge count:

    • Keeping to a minimum the amount, size, and types of sponges opened for a procedure

    • Counting and bagging discarded sponges frequently

    • Containing all sponges in the room

    • Not removing any linen, trash, or supplies from the operating room until after the patient leaves the room

47. If the surgeon chooses to intentionally pack the surgical wound, X-ray-detectable sponges should be used, clearly documented with rationale, and communicated in the hand-off report. When the patient returns to surgery and the

sponge is removed, the count from the original surgery should be reconciled.

48. X-ray-detectable sponges should not be used for wound dressing. Should an X ray be required, an X-ray-detectable sponge used for dressing could appear to be a retained sponge.

49. Gauze sponges for dressings should not be delivered to the sterile field until the surgery and the counts are complete. Dressing sponges do not contain a radiopaque strip and are not counted. Keeping these sponges separate from sponges used during the procedure prevents them from accidentally being included in the count and potentially contributing to an incorrect count.

New Technologies

50. Several advanced adjunctive technologies are available to assist the perioperative team to eliminate RSI. Current technologies include computer-assisted bar code and radio-frequency identification (RFID) technology. With the emphasis in health care on patient safety, this is a highly competitive field and technologies are emerging rapidly.

Sharps and Miscellaneous Items Counts

51. Sharps include scalpel blades, suture needles, hypodermic needles, cautery blades, needles, and safety pins, among other items. Miscellaneous items include vessel loops, vein introducers, vessel clip bars, trocar sealing caps, electrosurgery tip scratch pads, and marking pens. Any item that could be inadvertently left inside the patient should be accounted for.

52. The procedure for counting sharps is the same as that for counting soft goods. Counting must be done concurrently, visibly, and aloud by the scrub person and the circulating nurse. The circulating nurse documents the sharps count.

53. Sharps pose a risk of inflicting injury and transmitting infectious disease to patients and personnel. The scrub person should account for and confine all sharps on the sterile field until the final count is reconciled. Used sharps should be kept in a puncture-resistant container (AORN, 2012, p. 320).

54. To prevent an excess of loose needles on the field, it is good practice to keep suture packets unopened until the suture is needed.

55. When delivering suture packages containing multiple sutures to the field, it is acceptable practice to count needles according to the number indicated on the packet label; however, once the scrub person opens a suture multipack, both the scrub person and the nurse must verify the number of needles inside.

56. Occasionally, a needle or blade will break during a surgical procedure. When this occurs, the sharp(s) in question must be accounted for in their entirety.

57. On occasion, the risk of injury to a patient may be greater if a needle or piece of a needle is retrieved than if it is left to encapsulate in tissue. The decision not to retrieve a needle rests with the surgeon. Individual institutional policy dictates documentation of such an occurrence.

58. If a sharp is removed from the sterile field for any reason during a procedure, the circulating nurse should isolate it and keep it in a designated place in the operating room until the final count is performed and the procedure is complete. Like the sponge count, the procedure for counting sharps should be consistent.

59. When a surgical procedure requires a large number of suture needles, frequent needle counts can help reduce the risk of an incorrect count.

60. Actual needles—not suture packets—should be used to verify counts. Empty suture packets should not be used to rectify a discrepancy in a closing needle count (AORN, 2012, p. 320).

61. Following the procedure, sharps must be disposed of in containers that are leak proof, puncture resistant, and color coded, or labeled as biohazardous waste (OSHA, 2011).

Instrument Counts

62. Instrument counts are a proactive injury-prevention strategy. Retention of surgical instruments accounts for approximately one-third of all retained item case reports (Greenberg et al., 2008). In procedures where risk of a retained instrument is either nonexistent or minimal, facility policy will determine whether an instrument count can be omitted.

63. Instrument counts should be completed before skin closure. In procedures where instrument count is not possible, facility policy will indicate if an intraoperative X ray is required.

64. In addition to being a means of providing safe patient care, instrument counts are a means of inventory control and cost containment. Instruments are less likely to be lost—inadvertently thrown out with drapes, taken from the room, and so on—if they must be accounted for.

65. The procedure for counting instruments is essentially the same as that for counting soft goods and sharps. However, instruments are generally counted only twice: once just prior to the procedure and once at wound closure.

66. Instruments should be accounted for in their entirety. Many instruments consist of multiple parts such as screws and retractor blades. Individual parts should be identified and accounted for separately.

67. Like all counts, instrument counts must be done concurrently, visibly, and aloud by the scrub person and the circulating nurse. The circulating nurse documents the instrument count.

68. Instruments removed from the sterile field should remain in the operating room until the final count is done and the patient leaves the room. Removal of an instrument from the room increases the potential for an incorrect count.

69. It is helpful when instrument sets are standardized and when the number of instruments in sets is kept to a minimum.

Documentation

70. Count sheets may be generic, specialty specific, or set specific (Exhibit 7-1 and Exhibit 7-2). When sets are standardized, count sheets can be preprinted so that the list of instruments on the count sheet is identical to the contents of the set. The count sheet may be delivered to the operating room along with the set or retrieved from a computerized database within the operating room (Exhibit 7-3).

71. Computerization of instrument set lists facilitates periodic review and modification of count sheets as appropriate. Preprinted count sheets may list only the names of instruments contained within the sets, or they may list both instrument names and the quantity included. Preprinted count sheets that list instruments and number are not a substitution for performing a count.

Exhibit 7-1 Instrument/Sponges/Needle Count Record Example

ST. VINCENT'S MEDICAL CENTER OF RICHMOND
INSTRUMENT/SPONGE/NEEDLE COUNT RECORD

OPERATION   DATE

SECTION A	COUNT BEFORE SURGERY	ADDED DURING SURGERY	COUNT BEFORE PERITONEUM	FINAL COUNT (BEFORE SKIN CLOSE)
Raytec Sponges (4x4)				
Laparotomy Sponges				
Cottonoid				
Peanuts				
Tonsil Sponges				
Umbilical Tapes				
Vessel Loops				
Scalpel Blades				
Reel Ties				
Retention Sutures				
Free Needles				
Atraumatic Needles				

SECTION B	BEFORE SURGERY	ADDED	BEFORE PERITONEUM	FINAL COUNT INSTS. AFTER PERITONEUM	SECTION B CONTINUED	BEFORE SURGERY	ADDED	BEFORE PERITONEUM	FINAL COUNT INSTS. AFTER PERITONEUM
Mosquitos (curv)					Richardson Retractors				
Criles					Deaver Retractors				
Kelly (med)					Ribbon Retractors				
Allis					Balfour, Blade, Screw				
Babcock					Self-Retaining				
Kelly (lg)					McBurney Retractors				
Allis (lg)					Vein Retractors				
Babcock (lg)					Allen (anastomosis)				
Kochers					Bowel (rt) Angle				
Adson					DeMartel Applier				
Mixters					DeMartel Clamps				
Metzenbaum Scissors					Mayo Robson Clamps				
Mayo Scissors (curv)					Payr Pylorus Clamps				
Mayo Scissors (str)					Bakes (dilators)				
Metzenbaum (lg)					Randall Stone				
Mayo (lg str)					Trocar				
Potts Scissors					Heaney				
Needle Holders					Kochers (curv)				
Sponge Sticks					Phaneuf				
Adson Forceps (plain)					Tenaculum				
Adson Forceps (mt)					Uterine Packing				
Forceps (plain)					Pedicle				
Forceps (mt)					Bronchus				
Forceps (plain/long)					Lung Clamps				
Forceps (mt/long)					Bulldog Clamps				
Arterial Forceps					Vascular Clamps				
Rings					Baby Mosquitos				
Suction					Baby Rt. Angles				
Towel Clips					Skin Hooks				
Scalpel Handle #3					Lahey				
Scalpel Handle #7					Hemoclip appliers				
Scalpel Handle #3L					Other				
Rakes									
Army/Navy									
Parker Retractors					COUNTS ARE:				

SCRUB NURSE	RELIEF-SCRUB NURSE	CIRC. NURSE	RELIEF CIRC. NURSE

FORM 996 (9/86) MADISON BUSINESS FORMS

Source: Courtesy of St. Vincent's Medical Center of Richmond, Staten Island, New York.

Exhibit 7-2 Instrument/Sponge/Needle Count Record Instructions Example

General Instructions:

1. Instruments will be counted on all procedures that include invasion of peritoneum and an anticipated incision of more than 3 inches.

2. Instruments will be counted on all other procedures that do not invade the peritoneum but where incision is anticipated to be greater than 3 inches.

3. Sponges and needles will be counted on all procedures.

4. Incorrectly numbered packaged sponges must be isolated and not used during the procedure.

5. Instruments, counted sponges, and needles should never be taken from the OR for any reason during a procedure.

6. Instruments or needles broken or disassembled during a procedure must be accounted for in their entirety.

7. Used needles should be kept on a needle pad to ensure their containment on the table.

Procedure:

1. Before surgery begins, the scrub nurse and circulating nurse count instruments, sponges, and needles together and out loud as each item is separated in the counting procedure.

2. This original count is recorded immediately after being taken by the circulating nurse, on the Instrument/Sponge/Needle Count Record.

3. All instruments, sponges, and needles added to the operative field during surgery are counted together and out loud by the scrub and circulating nurses and recorded immediately by the circulating nurse on Form #998A in the column marked "Added."

4. During the operative procedure, the circulating nurse:
   a) Counts all sponges that are discarded from the operative field together and out loud with the scrub nurse
   b) Separates sponges into units
   c) Places counted sponges by units into plastic bags

5. Before closure of peritoneum begins, the scrub nurse and the circulating nurse count together and out loud:
   a) All instruments, sponges, and needles contained within the operative field that were counted before surgery and that were added during surgery.
   b) All instruments, sponges, and needles that have been discarded from the operative field that were counted before surgery and that were added during surgery.
   c) The circulating nurse records the tally in the column marked "Before Peritoneum Closure."
   d) The circulating nurse reports to the surgeon, out loud, the results of this count.

6. Before skin closure begins the scrub and circulating nurses count out loud and together all instruments that were used after the peritoneum closure and all items included in Section A of the Instrument/Sponge/Needle Count Record Form #998A.
   a) This final count is recorded by the circulating nurse in the column marked "Final Count."
   b) Result of this count (e.g., correct or incorrect) is recorded on Form #998A in the appropriate space.
   c) The scrub nurse and circulating nurse write their name and status in the appropriate space on Form #998A.

Source: Courtesy of F. Zarnick, Director of Nursing Services, St. Vincent's Medical Center of Richmond, Staten Island, New York.

Exhibit 7-3 Instrument Count Sheet Example

Minor Set SMC

Setcode ID/SN: GEN01 / 00010
Department/Speciality:
Packaging: 3/4 Size Container
Remarks:
Comments:

Production No.: 20040513000001
Printed On: 5/13/2004 8:28 PM
User: Joan Spear

Act	Min	Tgt	Catalog	Instrument Name	1st	2nd	Add	Final
				PUT ON STRINGER				
2		2	BH648R	Kocher Forceps Str 1×2 9"				
4		4	BH201R	Adson Delicate Forceps Cvd 7 1/4"				
4		4	BH443R	Rochester-pean Forceps Cvd 6 1/4"				
8		8	BH167R	Crile Forceps Cvd 6 1/4"				
4		4	EA030R	Babcock Tissue Forceps 6"				
4		4	EA016R	Allis Forceps 5×6 6"				
2		2	BH144R	Crile Forceps Str 5 1/2"				
4		4	BF463R	Lorna Towel Clamp Non-perf 5 1/8"				
1		1	BM065R	Tc Mayo-hegar Needle Holder Hvy Serr 6"				
2		2	BM066R	Tc Mayo-hegar Needle Holder Hvy Serr 7"				
1		1	BC242R	Tc Mayo Disect Scis Rnd Bld Str L-6 3/4"				
1		1	BC243R	Tc Mayo Disec Scis Rnd Blds Cvd L-6 3/4"				
1		1	BC261R	Tc Metzenbaum Scissors Cvd 5 3/4"				
1		1	BC263R	Tc Metzenbaum Scissors Cvd 7"				
				LAY IN PAN				
1		1	BF122R	Foerster Sponge Fcps Serr Str 9 1/2"				
2		2	SU3472	Richardson Retractor 9-1/4 32×29mm				
2		2	SU3474	Richardson Retractor 10 38×38mm				
2		2	SU3470	Richardson Retractor 9-1/4 25×19mm				
2		2	BT041R	Usa-army Retractors 8 3/4" 2/set				
1		1	BV200R	Self-retaining Retr 3×4 Sharp 7 3/4"				
1		1	GF862R	Pool Suction Cannula Charr. 30				
2		2	BD512R	Adson Tissue Fcps Fine Serr 4 3/4"				
1		1	BD579R	Tissue Forceps 2×3 6 1/4"				
2		2	BB074R	Scalpel Handle #3 With Measure				
2		2	BD701R	Brown Atraumatic Tissue Forceps 6"				
1		1	US061R	Metal Sponge Bowl 1 Qt				
1		1	US066R	Metal Medicine Cup 2 Oz				
2		2	FB414R	Debakey Atra Fcps 2.8mm Str 6"				
1		1	00107	Cautery Holder				
2		2	BV996R	Gelpi Vaginal Retractor 5 1/4"				

Actual: 64 Target: 64 Assembled By: Joan Spear

instacount PLUS Aesculap 3773 Corporate Parkway; Center Valley PA 18034 800258-1946

Source: Adapted from Aesculap, Inc. Used with permission.

72. Preprinted count sheets are also helpful for those healthcare personnel responsible for set assembly.

73. Some facilities require that the documentation of counts be placed in the patient's intraoperative record.

74. The intraoperative record should document the outcome of the count. Regardless of where the documentation is maintained, it must be retrievable, be traceable to the patient, and include the following information:
    - Types of counts: soft goods, sharps, instruments, miscellaneous items
    - Number of counts
    - Names and titles of personnel involved in the count
    - Results of the counts

- Surgeon who was notified of the count results
- Any adjunct technology used and associated records
- Explanation for any waived counts
- Number and location of any instruments intentionally remaining with the patient or radiopaque soft goods intentionally retained as therapeutic packing
- Unretrieved device fragments left in the wound
- Actions taken when count discrepancies occur
- Rationale for counts not performed or completed according to policy
- Outcome of action taken (AORN, 2012, p. 326)

Section Questions

1. Describe the variety of "soft goods" that must be counted. [Ref 30]
2. How are sponges handled during the counting process? [Ref 31]
3. Why must packages of sponges be counted, even when the number in the package is printed on the label? [Ref 32]
4. How is a package with an incorrect number of sponges managed? [Ref 33]
5. How should the circulating nurse manage the used sponges that the scrub person discards from the field? [Refs 35–37]
6. What determines how sponges are discarded following a procedure? [Refs 38–39]
7. Describe the procedure for counting sponges intraoperatively. [Refs 40–41]
8. What happens when the circulating nurse reports an incorrect count to the surgical team? [Ref 44]
9. At what point is a retained item reportable to The Joint Commission? [Ref 45]
10. Identify some steps to minimize the possibility of a retained surgical item. [Ref 46]
11. If the surgeon packs the wound in the operating room, which type of sponge should be used? [Ref 47]
12. Why should sponges with a radiopaque marker not be used for wound dressing? [Refs 48–49]
13. Describe the items that are considered "sharps." [Ref 51]
14. How does the procedure for counting sharps compare to that for counting sponges? [Ref 52]
15. Why are suture packets kept unopened on the field until the suture is needed? [Ref 54]
16. Must multipacks of sutures delivered to the field be opened immediately to count the individual needles? [Ref 55]
17. When a needle breaks on the surgical field, how is the needle managed for counting purposes? [Refs 56–57]
18. What should be done when a needle is removed from the sterile field? [Ref 58]
19. How are suture packages utilized during a needle count? [Ref 60]

(continues)

Section Questions (continued)

20. How are sharps disposed of following a surgical procedure? [Ref 61]

21. What determines when an instrument count can be omitted? [Ref 62]

22. When are instrument counts done for a surgical procedure? [Refs 63, 65]

23. Besides patient safety, what other value is there in counting instruments? [Ref 64]

24. How are instruments with multiple parts counted? [Ref 66]

25. Identify some practices that make counting instruments more efficient. [Refs 69–72]

● ● ● **References**

American Hospital Association Resource Center Blog (AHA) (2011). *Retained surgical items: incidence and how to avoid*. Chicago: AHA. Available at: http://aharesource center.wordpress.com/2011/03/29/retained-surgical-items -incidence-and-how-to-avoid/. Accessed September 2012.

Association of periOperative Registered Nurses (AORN) (2012). *Perioperative Standards and Recommended Practices*. Denver, CO: AORN.

Association of periOperative Registered Nurses (AORN) (2011). *Perioperative Nursing Data Set*, 3rd ed. Denver, CO: AORN.

Centers for Medicare & Medicaid Services (CMS) (2011). *Evidence-based guidelines for selected and previously considered hospital-acquired conditions*. Baltimore: CMS. Available at: www.cms.gov/Reports/Downloads/LaBresh _EB-GL-HAC-2010.pdf. Accessed September 2012.

Edel E (2012). Surgical count practice variability and the potential for retained surgical items. *AORN J*;95(2):228–238.

Greenberg C, Rogenbogen S, Lipsitz S, et al. (2008). The frequency and significance of discrepancies in the surgical count. *Ann Surg*;248(2):337–341.

Norton E, Martin C (2012). Patients Count on It: an initiative to reduce incorrect counts and prevent retained surgical items. *AORN J*;95(1).

Occupational Safety and Health Administration (OSHA) (2011). *Bloodborne pathogens*. Standard 29CFR, 1910-1030. Washington, DC: OSHA. Available at: www.osha .gov/pls/oshaweb/owadisp.show_document?p_table =standards&p_id=10051. Accessed September 2012.

Peterson C (2002). Rectifying counts; neurostimulators; double gloving; reprocessing single-use devices; simultaneous counting (clinical issues). *AORN J*;76(3):510–515.

Rowlands A, Steeves R (2010). Incorrect surgical counts: a qualitative analysis. *AORN J*;92(4):410–419.

Steelman V, Cullen J (2011). Designing a safer process to prevent retained surgical sponges: a healthcare failure mode and effect analysis. *AORN J*;94(2):132–141.

Post-Test

Read each question carefully. Each question may have more than one correct answer.

1. Surgical counts
   a. ensure that nothing will be left behind in the patient.
   b. are required by regulatory agencies such as TJC.
   c. attempt to reconcile what was delivered to the field with what remains at the end of the procedure.
   d. are governed by facility policy.

2. A "never event" is defined as
   a. an event that is not documented.
   b. an event that never happened.
   c. an unexpected occurrence involving death or serious injury that is reasonably preventable by following evidence-based guidelines.
   d. a procedure that is canceled.

3. A retained surgical item
   a. may cause unnecessary pain and suffering.
   b. often goes undetected until after the patient has been discharged.
   c. can present months or years after surgery with adhesion formation and encapsulation.
   d. is found most frequently in the abdomen or pelvis.

4. Which statement(s) is (are) true about litigation involving retained surgical items?
   a. Cases are usually indefensible because of "res ipsa loquitur."
   b. The operative record always documents the count as "incorrect."
   c. The scrub person is usually the one named in the lawsuit.
   d. The perioperative nurse is legally accountable for counts.

5. Which three themes are identified as challenges to correct counts?
   a. Individual behaviors
   b. Hospital policies
   c. Environmental factors
   d. Communication difficulties

6. Counts should be performed
   a. before the procedure begins.
   b. whenever a counted item is added to the sterile field.
   c. when wound closure begins.
   d. after the dressings have been applied.

7. Which statement(s) is (are) true about counts?
   a. Counts are performed by the scrub person and the circulating nurse.
   b. Both the scrub person and the circulating nurse must be able to visualize each item counted.
   c. If the circulating nurse is busy, the scrub person can count with another member of the surgical team.
   d. The scrub person documents the count.

8. Which statement(s) is (are) true about counts?
   a. A commercially prepared package with an incorrect number of items must be removed from the room so that it does not interfere with the count.

    b. After the procedure begins, the circulating nurse delivers items to the field; the scrub nurse opens and counts them when there is time, and reports the number to the circulating nurse to document.

    c. The circulating nurse counts discarded sponges, and the scrub person verifies the number during the final count.

    d. Never assume that the amount listed on the package accurately reflects the number of items inside.

9. Which statement(s) is (are) true about counts?

    a. The count sequence begins with the items in use on the field.

    b. Count procedures should be consistent, following the same sequence each time.

    c. Sponge counts begin with the largest sponges in use and proceed to the smallest.

    d. Counts include all items opened for the procedure, whether they were used or not.

10. A correct count

    a. should be documented in the operative record.

    b. guarantees that nothing has been left behind in the patient.

    c. should be communicated to the surgeon and the operative team.

    d. is completed when the dressing is placed on the patient.

11. Steps to minimize the possibility of an incorrect sponge count include

    a. waiting until the end of the procedure when the scrub person has time to concentrate to bag and count sponges.

    b. keeping the number and type of sponges used to a minimum.

    c. keeping all sponges in the room until the end of the procedure.

    d. not removing trash and linen until the patient leaves the room.

12. The procedure for counting sharps

    a. is the same as that for counting soft goods.

    b. requires needles to be verified by the scrub nurse and the circulating nurse when suture packages are opened on the field.

    c. involves accounting for all pieces of an item that breaks.

    d. usually allows the surgeon the discretion to leave a needle or piece of a needle in the patient if the risk of removing it is too great.

13. Instrument counts

    a. should be resolved before skin closure.

    b. are also a means of inventory control.

    c. must account for all pieces of an instrument with multiple parts.

    d. are not necessary when the incision is small.

14. Which statement(s) is (are) true about counts?

    a. Instruments are usually counted only twice.

    b. It is helpful when instruments sets are standardized.

    c. Facility policy determines the procedures that do not require instrument counts.

    d. Instruments dropped from the field should be removed from the room.

15. Documentation of counts in the operative records includes

    a. the type of counts.

    b. results of the counts.

    c. the surgeon who was notified of the count results.

    d. the rationale for counts not performed or completed according to policy.

Competency Checklist: Counts in Surgery   www

Under "Observer's Initials," enter initials upon successful achievement of the competency. Enter N/A if the competency is not appropriate for the institution.

Name _____

	Observer's Initials	Date
1. Counts are performed and documented:		
a. Prior to procedure	_____	_____
b. During the procedure when items are added	_____	_____
c. Before closure of a body cavity	_____	_____
d. When closure begins	_____	_____
e. At the time of relief	_____	_____
2. Counts are performed concurrently and aloud by the scrub person and the circulating nurse.	_____	_____
3. Items being counted are separated for visibility and are visible to the scrub person and the circulating nurse.	_____	_____
4. Sharps are maintained on a needle mat (or other device designed for this purpose).	_____	_____
5. Counts are verified when personnel are relieved.	_____	_____
6. Contents of multipack sutures are verified when each package is opened.	_____	_____
7. Sponges that are discarded are counted in units of five or ten and bagged.	_____	_____
8. All sponges, sharps, or instruments opened for the procedure are retained in the room until the procedure is completed.	_____	_____
9. The count begins at the surgical site and progresses to the Mayo tray and the back table.	_____	_____
10. Sponges are handled according to OSHA guidelines.	_____	_____
11. The surgeon is notified of the count results.	_____	_____
12. Names of all persons who performed counts during the procedure are documented.	_____	_____
13. Documentation is complete.	_____	_____

Observer's Signature   Initials   Date

_____

Orientee's Signature

_____

8

Prevention of Injury: Hemostasis, Tourniquets, and Electrosurgical Equipment

---

LEARNER OBJECTIVES

1. Describe the natural process of hemostasis.
2. Explore approaches to artificial hemostasis.
3. Discuss mechanical hemostasis.
4. Identify three potential patient injuries associated with tourniquets.
5. List two criteria for evaluating achievement of the desired patient outcome relative to tourniquets.
6. Describe nursing interventions to prevent patient injury when a tourniquet is used.
7. Identify three potential patient injuries related to electrosurgical equipment.
8. Define terminology associated with electrosurgery.
9. Describe potential injury related to capacitive coupling.
10. Identify the desired patient outcome relative to electrosurgery.
11. List four criteria for evaluating achievement of the desired patient outcome relative to electrosurgery.
12. Describe nursing interventions to prevent patient injury when electrosurgical equipment is used.
13. List information that should be documented when a tourniquet or electrosurgical equipment is used.
14. Discuss use of an ultrasonic energy device (scalpel) and an argon beam coagulator.

WWW

LESSON OUTLINE

I. Hemostasis
  A. Natural Methods of Hemostasis
  B. Artificial Methods of Hemostasis
    1. Chemical Hemostasis
    2. Mechanical Hemostasis
II. Tourniquets
  A. Overview

  B. Nursing Diagnosis: Desired Patient Outcomew
  C. Nursing Interventions

III. Electrical Hemostasis: Electrosurgery
  A. Overview
  B. Electrosurgical Components
    1. Generator
    2. Active Electrode

Hemostasis

1. Hemostasis is the arrest or control of bleeding. Historically, attempts to achieve hemostasis have included applications of egg yolk, dust, cobwebs, hot oil, cautery with hot irons, and use of crude sutures made from materials such as cotton or harp strings derived from sheep intestine. Until the advent of modern hemostatic methods, blood loss made surgery difficult and was a serious surgical complication.

2. Modern hemostatic methods, including electrosurgery and tourniquet application, have greatly enhanced the surgeon's ability to perform slow, deliberate surgery and to operate in a field where control of bleeding permits excellent visualization of anatomical structures.

3. Hemostasis may be achieved by natural or artificial methods.

Natural Methods of Hemostasis

4. When an injury occurs to a blood vessel, a roughened surface is created. Platelets adhere to this surface, and when several layers accumulate, a platelet plug is formed. A platelet plug is often sufficient to seal small injuries. As the platelets break down, they release thromboplastin into the blood. Thromboplastin is necessary for coagulation to occur.

5. Platelet plug formation is not the same as coagulation. In coagulation, a fibrin clot is formed. Coagulation is a complex mechanism involving multiple clotting factors and a series of reactions. During coagulation, prothrombin, which is present in blood, reacts with thromboplastin, which is released when tissues are injured and platelets break down. Prothrombin, thromboplastin, and calcium ions in the blood form thrombin. Thrombin then unites with fibrinogen, a blood plasma, to form fibrin. Fibrin is the basic structure of the clot and reinforces the platelet plug. Initially this fibrin is white. As platelets, white cells, and red cells become entangled in the fibrin, however, the clot becomes red, taking on the appearance we recognize as a blood clot. The process of coagulation is self-regulated; as blood loss is controlled, coagulation ceases.

6. In spite of the complexity of the coagulation process, it is rapid and sufficient to prevent blood loss from most small wounds.

Artificial Methods of Hemostasis

7. Natural hemostasis is not sufficient to control the gross bleeding and oozing that occur during surgery. Artificial hemostatic methods—chemical, mechanical, or thermal—may be used in such a case. These methods include thrombin, absorbable gelatin, oxidized cellulose, microfibrillar collagen, collagen pads, styptics, pressure, instruments, ties, suture ligatures, ligating clips, staples, bonewax, tourniquets, and electrosurgery. Tourniquets and electrosurgery have significant patient safety implications and are addressed in depth in this chapter.

Chemical Hemostasis

Thrombin

8. Thrombin is an enzyme that combines with fibrinogen and accelerates the coagulation process. It is useful in controlling capillary bleeding.

9. Thrombin is supplied as a dry white powder that may be sprinkled on an oozing site, but is more frequently mixed with water or saline to form a solution that is used in conjunction with a gelatin sponge. This combination is particularly useful in vascular surgery for controlling capillary bleeding at the site of a vascular graft.

10. Thrombin will lose its potency within 3 hours and should be mixed just prior to use.

11. Thrombin is for topical use only; it must never be injected.

12. Thrombin has traditionally been made from dried cow's blood. Bovine thrombin preparations have occasionally been associated with abnormalities in hemostasis, ranging from asymptomatic alterations in laboratory tests such as prothrombin time (PT) and partial thromboplastin time (PTT), to severe bleeding or thrombosis. These abnormalities have rarely been fatal. Repeated clinical applications of topical bovine thrombin increase the likelihood that antibodies against thrombin and/or factor V may be formed.

13. Thrombin derived from human plasma is now available. Recombinant thrombin is less immunogenic, and it is expected that products using this technology will be used more frequently.

Absorbable Gelatin

14. Absorbable gelatin is made from a purified gelatin solution and is available as a powder, a compressed pad (Gelfoam), and beads. In the compressed form, it resembles Styrofoam.

15. When placed on an area of capillary bleeding, fibrin is deposited in the interstices of the pad; the pad swells, and clot formation progresses. Gelfoam pads are available in a variety of sizes and may be cut to the desired size.

16. Gelfoam may be used alone, but is frequently soaked in a thrombin solution. Gelfoam may also be soaked in epinephrine before application. In the powder form, gelatin is mixed with sterile saline to form a paste.

17. Gelfoam absorbs 45 times its weight in blood. It is not soluble; when left in the body, however, it will be absorbed in 20 to 40 days. Once hemostasis has been achieved, it is common practice to remove gelatin to prevent compression of adjacent anatomic structures.

Oxidized Cellulose

18. Oxidized regenerated cellulose (Oxycel, Surgicel, Surgicel Nu-Knit) is a specially treated knitted gauze or cotton product applied directly to an oozing surface to control bleeding.

19. When oxidized cellulose contacts whole blood, it increases in size, forms a gel, and promotes clot formation. It absorbs seven to eight times its own weight.

20. Oxidized cellulose starts working within minutes, swelling to create a pseudo-clot, which puts pressure on the wound, thereby helping to speed up the normal clotting process and preventing further blood loss. The pseudo-clot can be left in situ, where it is fully absorbed after 1 to 2 weeks.

21. Oxidized cellulose must be removed when used around the optic nerve or spinal cord, because swelling of the cellulose can exert harmful pressure on these structures.

Microfibrillar Collagen

22. Microfibrillar collagen (Avitene, Instat) is a fluffy, white, absorbable material made from purified bovine dermis. It is applied as a dry product that is placed directly over the source of bleeding. It is often used in crevices and areas of irregular contour. Hemostasis is achieved when platelets and fibrin adhere to the collagen and clot formation progresses.

23. Microfibrillar collagen is useful where tissue is friable. Although it is absorbable, excess material is removed once hemostasis has been achieved.

24. Collagen pads, sponges, and felt are also available and are applied directly to a bleeding surface.

Styptic

25. Styptics are agents that cause blood vessel constriction. Epinephrine is a frequently used styptic; it is often added to a local anesthetic such as lidocaine to constrict blood vessels and decrease bleeding.

26. Silver nitrate, in the form of a stick or pencil with a silver nitrate crystal head, is another form of styptic applied topically to small vessels.

Mechanical Hemostasis

Instruments, Ties, Suture Ligatures, and Ligating Clips

27. A hemostatic clamp may be used to occlude the end of a bleeding vessel. As long as the clamp remains in place, bleeding will not occur. Clamping is a temporary means of hemostasis and is followed by the application of a tie, a suture ligature, a ligating clip, electrosurgery, or electrocautery.

28. A tie is a strand of material tied around the vessel to occlude the lumen. A suture ligature is a tie with an attached needle that is used to

anchor the tie through the vessel. A ligating clip (Hemoclip, Ligaclip, Surgiclip) is a stainless steel, tantalum, or titanium clip used to permanently close off a vessel. Except for clips made from synthetic absorbable suture, ligating clips remain permanently within the patient.

Bonewax

29. Bonewax is made from beeswax and is used to stop bleeding from bone. This material is rolled into a ball and rubbed over a cut bone surface to control bleeding. Bonewax is used most often in neurosurgery and orthopedic surgery.

Pressure

30. Manual pressure applied directly to small vessels may delay bleeding long enough for clot formation to begin. Pressure is applied with sponges to blot areas of bleeding. When the sponge is removed, it is possible to identify the area of bleeding and to use additional methods of hemostasis.

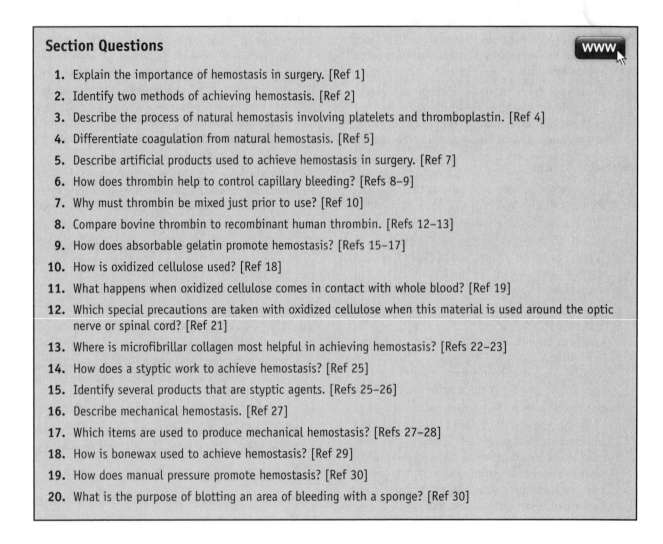

Section Questions

1. Explain the importance of hemostasis in surgery. [Ref 1]
2. Identify two methods of achieving hemostasis. [Ref 2]
3. Describe the process of natural hemostasis involving platelets and thromboplastin. [Ref 4]
4. Differentiate coagulation from natural hemostasis. [Ref 5]
5. Describe artificial products used to achieve hemostasis in surgery. [Ref 7]
6. How does thrombin help to control capillary bleeding? [Refs 8–9]
7. Why must thrombin be mixed just prior to use? [Ref 10]
8. Compare bovine thrombin to recombinant human thrombin. [Refs 12–13]
9. How does absorbable gelatin promote hemostasis? [Refs 15–17]
10. How is oxidized cellulose used? [Ref 18]
11. What happens when oxidized cellulose comes in contact with whole blood? [Ref 19]
12. Which special precautions are taken with oxidized cellulose when this material is used around the optic nerve or spinal cord? [Ref 21]
13. Where is microfibrillar collagen most helpful in achieving hemostasis? [Refs 22–23]
14. How does a styptic work to achieve hemostasis? [Ref 25]
15. Identify several products that are styptic agents. [Refs 25–26]
16. Describe mechanical hemostasis. [Ref 27]
17. Which items are used to produce mechanical hemostasis? [Refs 27–28]
18. How is bonewax used to achieve hemostasis? [Ref 29]
19. How does manual pressure promote hemostasis? [Ref 30]
20. What is the purpose of blotting an area of bleeding with a sponge? [Ref 30]

Tourniquets

Overview

31. Application of a tourniquet prior to surgery provides a bloodless surgical field. A pneumatic tourniquet is often used for surgery on an extremity. Tourniquets are most frequently used in orthopedic, podiatric, and plastic surgery procedures. The resultant bloodless field enhances the surgeon's ability to complete the surgery and prevents blood loss for the patient. Once the tourniquet is released, the severed vessels will bleed, and cauterization or ligation will be necessary to stop bleeding.

32. Tourniquet cuffs of various shapes and sizes are available. Tourniquet cuffs may be either reusable or designed for a single use. The simplest tourniquet is a piece of rubber tubing, such as a Penrose drain, that is placed around an extremity in preparation for a venipuncture.

33. An Esmarch bandage is a long piece of rolled latex that is wrapped tightly around an extremity from the distal end toward the proximal end to exsanguinate the extremity. Before application of a tourniquet, the extremity is raised to permit gravity to drain blood from the extremity. The Esmarch bandage compresses superficial blood vessels and further forces the blood from the extremity. The Esmarch bandage is removed, and while the limb is raised to prevent blood from returning to the extremity, the pneumatic tourniquet is applied.

34. Pneumatic tourniquets are inflated and maintained at a specified pressure required for the surgery and requested by the surgeon. They contain an internal bladder housed in a pressure cuff. The bladder is inflated with either ambient air or compressed gas from a cartridge, tank, or compressed-air line.

35. A cuff with a double bladder is used when the extremity will be anesthetized with a regional block (Bier block).

Nursing Diagnosis: Desired Patient Outcome

36. Nursing diagnosis: high risk for injury related to use of tourniquet. Injuries from a tourniquet can include skin injury, such as a chemical burn from prep solutions soaked in the padding under the tourniquet; abrasion, bruise or blister formation; and swelling, pain, or nerve injury, including paralysis.

37. The Association of periOperative Registered Nurses (AORN) outcome standard states, "The patient is free from signs and symptoms of injury caused by extraneous objects" (2011, p. 165). The patient should not experience an injury as a result of tourniquet use.

Nursing Interventions

38. Nursing interventions to prevent injury from tourniquet application require knowledge of equipment use and appropriate safety precautions. Institutional policy and practice may dictate who has responsibility for tourniquet application. Regardless of who actually applies the tourniquet, the nurse, surgeon, and anesthesia personnel all share responsibility for patient safety with regard to its use.

39. The perioperative nurse must be able to select a tourniquet of the appropriate size and shape in good working condition, must be knowledgeable of the principles underlying use of the tourniquet, and must be competent in its application.

40. Prior to tourniquet application, the patient's skin should be assessed for integrity and turgor, and the extremity size should be evaluated to select a tourniquet cuff of appropriate size.

41. The perioperative nurse should assess the patient's condition for possible contraindications—for example, diabetes mellitus, vascular graft, compromised circulation, vascular disease, deep vein thrombosis (DVT), increased intracranial pressure, severe crush injury, open fracture, and infection (AORN, 2012, pp. 178–179).

42. Because tourniquet use can lead to circulatory stasis, acidosis, hypoxemia, and sickle cell anemia can be contraindications to this hemostasis method. The decision to use a tourniquet on a patient with sickle cell anemia is made by the anesthesiologist, who will take into consideration the patient's hemoglobin type and level (McEwen, 2012a).

43. Medications such as prophylactic antibiotics that must be infused prior to incision should be completely infused before a tourniquet is applied.

44. The pneumatic tourniquet should be tested and inspected for integrity, cleanliness, and function prior to use. Most automated systems contain a microprocessor that performs a self-test and self-calibration upon activation. Newer tourniquet systems have the following characteristics:
    - Recommend a limb occlusion pressure based on a reading from a sensor that is placed on the patient's toe or finger prior to surgery.
    - Include an audible indicator that reports cuff status, changes in pressure, and passage of a specified amount of time.
    - Contain a battery backup.

45. The tourniquet system should be tested according to the manufacturer's written instructions and healthcare facility policy prior to use. All tourniquet systems are not alike, and it is critical that testing is performed according to the specific manufacturer's instructions. Substitute tubing or gas should never be used.

- The perioperative nurse should check for compatibility of the cuff, tubing, and regulator.

- Audible alarms and indicators should be set to a level that can be heard above other sounds in the operating room.

- The cuff and tubing should be clean and free of cracks or holes. Cuffs may be punctured if a towel clip is used to hold it in place. Cracks can result in unintentional pressure loss.

- Close inspection of the cuff for cleanliness is important. Velcro fasteners are areas where microorganisms can proliferate and other debris can collect. Water left in a tourniquet cuff port can cause microbial growth, with the potential for entry of microorganisms into the tourniquet-regulating mechanism when the cuff is deflated (AORN, 2012, p. 184). Tourniquet cuffs and bladders should be cleaned, rinsed, and dried between patient uses. An Environmental Protection Agency (EPA)–registered tuberculocidal germicide should be used to clean this equipment, and the manufacturer's instructions for use strictly followed. It is important to adequately rinse the equipment so as to remove any germicide residue that might cause skin irritation. The gauges and pressure source should also be inspected for cleanliness and cleaned as needed.

- Connections should be secure, and electrical cords should be intact.

- Inspection should include a check of the last inspection of the device by biomedical engineering personnel. A sticker indicating inspection by biomedical engineering personnel within the last 12 months should be present.

- When nitrogen gas is used to inflate the cuff, the level of gas in the tank should be checked before each use to ensure that the tank contains an adequate amount for the duration of the intended surgery.

46. The selection of a tourniquet cuff should take into consideration the surgical site and the size of the patient's extremity. Contour cuffs are appropriate in situations where the circumference of the distal tourniquet site is significantly different from the circumference of the proximal edge. For example, the distal circumference of the calf may be significantly less than the proximal circumference. In this situation, the use of a straight (rather than contoured) tourniquet could result in excess tourniquet at the distal site. A significant difference in the distal and proximal circumferences is not unusual in obese patients (AORN, 2012, p. 486).

47. The cuff should allow a snug fit at both the distal and proximal edges. The tourniquet cuff should be wider than half the limb diameter. As wide a cuff as possible should be selected. A wide cuff can reduce the risk of injury to underlying vessels, muscles, and nerves by reducing the pressure required to obtain a bloodless field. The length of the cuff should permit an overlap of at least 3 inches but not more than 6 inches (AORN, 2012, p. 486). Too much overlap can cause increased pressure in the area of the overlap.

48. The tourniquet should fit snugly. In general, a snug fit allows two fingers under the cuff. If only one finger fits under the cuff, the cuff is too tight; if three fingers fit, it is too loose (McEwen, 2012b).

49. Except where the manufacturer specifies in writing that padding is not required, the tourniquet should not be applied to unprotected skin. A stockinette material should be wrapped around the extremity where the tourniquet will be applied. Webril is sometimes used for this purpose; although it does protect the skin, the fibers can become embedded in the Velcro fasteners and are difficult to remove. Take care to prevent bunching or wrinkling of the material, which can cause uneven pressure against the skin with the potential for impairing skin integrity.

50. When a patient is extremely obese, an assistant should apply traction to the excess skin until the tourniquet is applied to prevent overlapping of skin and possible pressure or shearing injury.

51. The operative limb should be verified by the surgical team. Tourniquets placed on the upper arm or thigh should be placed on the limb at the point most proximal to the surgery and at the point of maximum circumference, according to the manufacturer's written instructions.

52. Calf tourniquets should be placed with the proximal edge of the cuff at the area of largest circumference (AORN, 2012, p. 180). When a tourniquet is applied to the calf, take care not to compromise the head of the fibula, as this problem can result in damage to superficial nerves in the area.

53. Protect the area of tourniquet application from any potential or actual pooling or collection

of fluids that can irritate the skin. Prepping agents, if allowed to pool and soak into the padding under the cuff, can cause a chemical burn to the skin. Protect the area from pooling of fluids during surgery by applying a protective fluid barrier—one might be included as part of the extremity drape and will be applied during the draping procedure.

54. The tourniquet should be set at the lowest pressure needed to create a bloodless field. Excessive inflation pressure can damage underlying tissue, whereas too low a pressure can cause passive congestion of the limb, shock, and hemorrhagic infiltration of a nerve (AORN, 2012, p. 181).

55. The tourniquet is customarily set at a standard pressure depending on the limb (e.g., 250 mm Hg for arms; 350 mm Hg for legs) and adjusted based on the patient's mean arterial pressure.

56. Patient age, extremity size, systolic blood pressure, and tourniquet cuff size are factors that determine inflation pressures.

57. Inflation times should be kept to a minimum. Excessive inflation times can damage underlying tissue and cause injury as severe as permanent paralysis. For an adult, 1 hour for an upper extremity and 1.5 to 2 hours for a lower extremity are the usual maximum inflation times. A lower pressure is used for children and for patients in whom blood supply to the extremity is diminished. Insufficient pressure and subsequent prolonged venous congestion can also result in nerve injury.

58. During the surgery, the nurse should periodically report to the surgeon the length of time that the tourniquet has been inflated. Most tourniquet systems automatically display pressure readings and inflation time and will sound an alarm when a predetermined time is reached. Intervals for reporting inflation times should be agreed upon between the surgeon and the nurse and may be indicated in the facility policy for tourniquet application. Anesthesia personnel also monitor inflation times. All team members must work in concert to ensure adequate and appropriate communication regarding the tourniquet.

59. Throughout the surgery, the nurse should refer to the tourniquet gauge to determine fluctuations in pressure that might indicate a tourniquet failure.

60. In the case of inadvertent loss of pressure, the tourniquet should be totally deflated, and the extremity allowed to reperfuse.

61. The tourniquet should be deflated upon instructions from the surgeon. When bilateral tourniquets are used, as in the case of bilateral arthroscopies, the cuffs should be deflated individually, with a 30-minute minimum time frame between extremities. This will prevent excessive metabolites from entering the bloodstream too rapidly.

62. Core body temperature is gradually increased after tourniquet inflation due to the decreased heat loss from the affected limb. Deflation leads to a transient decline in core temperature owing to the redistribution of body heat. Hypothermic blood from the ischemic limb exacerbates this drop in core temperature (Raju, 2010). The patient's temperature should be monitored and measures taken as needed. Take care to prevent overheating, especially in children.

63. AORN-recommended practices for use of the pneumatic tourniquet state that the perioperative nurse should document the following information:
    - Tourniquet system and identification (serial) number
    - Calibrations
    - Cuff pressure
    - Skin protection
    - Location of the tourniquet
    - The assessment of skin and tissue integrity under the cuff before and after tourniquet use
    - Time of inflation and deflation
    - Identification of the person who applied the cuff
    - Assessment of the entire extremity (AORN, 2012, p. 185)

    Documentation should also include an evaluation of the achievement of desired outcome.

Section Questions

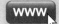

1. What is the purpose of a tourniquet used for surgery on extremities? [Ref 31]
2. What purpose does the Esmarch bandage serve in preparing for the use of a tourniquet? [Ref 33]

(continues)

Section Questions (continued)

3. Which types of patient injury can occur with the use of a tourniquet? [Ref 36]

4. What are nursing responsibilities associated with the choice of a tourniquet? [Refs 39–40, 44, 46]

5. What are some contraindications for using a tourniquet? [Refs 41–42]

6. How is the administration of prophylactic antibiotics coordinated with the use of a tourniquet? [Ref 43]

7. What is involved in testing a tourniquet? [Ref 45]

8. What is one challenge in selecting an appropriate tourniquet cuff for an obese patient? [Ref 46]

9. What are some criteria for assessing the fit of a tourniquet cuff? [Refs 47–48]

10. How is padding used in conjunction with a tourniquet? [Ref 49]

11. What is one method for avoiding skin damage when placing a tourniquet cuff on an obese patient? [Ref 50]

12. Where on the operative extremity should the tourniquet be placed? [Refs 51–52]

13. What can happen to the patient if the tourniquet is not protected from fluids? [Ref 53]

14. Which dangers are associated with setting the tourniquet pressure too high or too low? [Ref 54]

15. Which patient factors affect the adjustment of tourniquet inflation pressure? [Ref 56]

16. What are the customary inflation times for the upper and lower extremities? [Refs 57–58]

17. Who is responsible for monitoring and communicating inflation times? [Ref 58]

18. Why should bilateral cuffs not be deflated at the same time? [Ref 61]

19. How does using a tourniquet contribute to an increase in the patient's core temperature? [Ref 62]

20. Which information should the perioperative nurse document related to tourniquet use? [Ref 63]

Electrical Hemostasis: Electrosurgery

Overview

64. Electrosurgery is used routinely in most surgical procedures for providing hemostasis and dissecting tissue.

65. As radio-frequency electrical current passes through tissue, heat is generated in sufficient amounts to produce tissue vaporization–cutting or fulguration–coagulation.

66. There are two basic types of electrosurgery: bipolar and monopolar.

Electrosurgical Components

67. Monopolar electrosurgery involves three components:

   • An electrosurgical unit (ESU) or generator

   • An active electrode

   • A dispersive electrode

Bipolar electrosurgery requires:

   • A generator

   • A bipolar active-electrode hand piece that delivers current through the forceps utilizing the patient tissue, with the current returning through the forceps back to the generator

Generator

68. The unit that supplies the current is referred to as an electrosurgical unit or generator (Figure 8-1).

69. In the 1920s, Dr. William Bovie was instrumental in the development of one of the first spark-gap vacuum-tube generators that produced cutting with hemostasis. Bovie's design remained the basis for electrosurgical units until the 1970s, when solid-state electrosurgical units were introduced. Solid-state units with small printed circuit boards and transistors replaced the much larger vacuum-tube

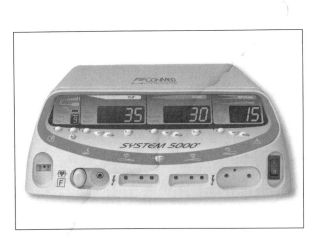

Figure 8-1 Electrosurgical generator
Source: Courtesy of ConMed Corporation.

machines. Nevertheless, the term "Bovie" continues to be synonymous with the electrosurgery unit regardless of the style of the unit.

70. Current is produced by the generator and flows through the active electrode accessory that delivers the current into the patient. The dispersive electrode is an accessory that is in contact with the patient and returns the current from the patient to the electrosurgical generator.

71. Early electrosurgical units presented significant risk for a burn or shock injury. Early generators were the ground-referenced units, meaning they used the ground to complete the electrosurgery circuit. If the patient came in contact with something else that was also grounded, the current could seek an alternate pathway to ground. Such alternate sites might include electrocardiogram electrodes and sites where the patient touched a grounded metal item. Because alternate pathways to ground were usually smaller than the dispersive electrode, the current was concentrated and could cause a burn. Burns could also occur at the patient return electrode site. Ground-referenced systems have been replaced with isolated systems in most modern operating rooms.

72. Generators today are available as both solid-state and isolated systems and have dramatically reduced the risk of injury. However, electrosurgery use can create a high risk for fire.

73. Isolated systems represent a significant improvement over ground-referenced systems and provide for increased patient safety. In an isolated system, a transformer within the generator isolates the current from the ground. Current is restricted to pathways to and from the generator. In addition to isolated circuits, systems used today include a patient-return electrode-monitoring system. With this type of system, the current that enters the patient is measured and compared with the current returning through the dispersive electrode. If the current is not sufficiently balanced, the unit will sound an alarm and become deactivated. These systems have virtually eliminated burns under the dispersive electrode and alternate sites ("Bovie burns").

74. Electrosurgical units are designed to deliver current that will cut, coagulate, or both cut and coagulate. The type of waveform that is selected determines whether cutting, coagulation, or a combination of the two will occur.

75. A continuous low-frequency waveform will cause cutting to occur. In the cutting mode, tissue is severed as intense heat is delivered from the active electrode and focused on tissue to be severed. The active electrode is held slightly above the tissue.

76. An interrupted or dampened waveform results in coagulation. In the coagulation mode, when the active electrode is in direct contact with the tissue, the ends of small- to moderate-sized vessels are seared and bleeding is controlled—a process referred to as desiccation. When the active electrode is slightly above the tissue, a spark is produced and tissue is coagulated.

77. When a combination of the cut and coagulation waveform is selected, cutting and coagulation occur simultaneously.

78. The amount of power and the type of current are regulated by controls on the electrosurgical unit and the accessories.

79. The surgeon selects the type of current (waveform) and the amount of power based on the procedure and the surgeon's preference.

Active Electrode

80. The active electrode delivers current from the generator to the operative site. Active electrodes may be disposable or reusable, although single-use electrodes are more common. Most active electrodes are handheld devices with interchangeable tips and a cord that attaches to the electrosurgical generator. Active electrode tips may be shaped as a blade, ball, loop, hook,

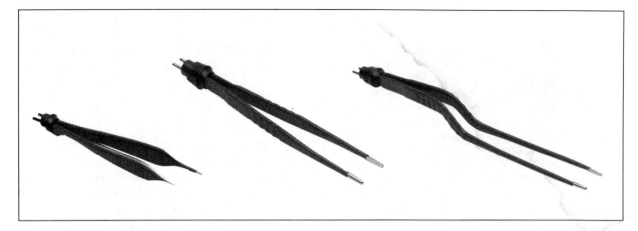

Figure 8-2 Active electrodes: Bipolar forceps
Source: Courtesy of ConMed Corporation.

or needle that fits into the pencil-shaped handle or other device (Figure 8-2). Active electrodes may also be combined with a suction catheter.

81. Active electrodes are activated by either a foot control or a control on the hand piece.

82. Active electrodes may be bipolar or monopolar. A monopolar electrode has one active pole or tip. This tip delivers concentrated current to the target tissue. The current is then dissipated through the patient's body to the dispersive electrode, and then returned to the generator.

83. Bipolar electrodes are shaped to resemble forceps with two poles or tips (bipolar forceps). One tip acts as the active electrode, and the other tip acts as the return or dispersive electrode. Current flows from the generator down one tine of the forceps, through the tissue between the forceps' tips, and returns to the generator through the other tine of the forceps. Because the current flows only between the tips of the forceps, lower voltages are required. Bipolar forceps provide precise hemostasis, and current is not dispersed throughout the patient. Bipolar electrosurgery does not require a dispersive electrode, as current passes between the tines of the forceps and does not travel through the patient's body.

Dispersive Electrode

84. Dispersive electrodes are referred to by many names—for example, grounding pad, inactive electrode, patient plate, Bovie pad, and return electrode.

85. Current enters the patient via the active electrode, where it is concentrated at the operative

site to achieve the desired tissue effect. Current is then dissipated through the patient to the dispersive electrode and returned to the generator (Figure 8-3).

86. The dispersive electrode is much larger than the active electrode, so current density is low at this site and burns do not normally occur.

87. Reusable metal dispersive electrodes have been replaced with products that incorporate a patient-return electrode with a pressure-reduction pad and have current-limiting abilities to protect the patient from pad-site burns.

88. The most commonly used dispersive electrode is a disposable adhesive foil pad covered with foam and impregnated with electrolyte gel. The dispersive electrode is placed in direct contact with the patient's skin in a muscular area, avoiding bone and any implanted prostheses. It has a cord that attaches to the generator. The pad easily conforms to the patient's body contour and provides uniform contact with the patient; the adhesive promotes good conductivity. Modern electrosurgical systems employ a dispersive electrode that works with the

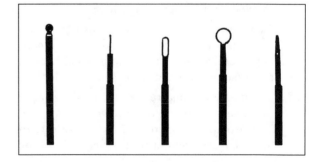

Figure 8-3 Active electrode tips

generator to identify potential current concentration at the dispersive electrode site sufficient to cause a burn. When such an event occurs, the machine will sound an alarm and be deactivated. A scenario in which this might occur is if the attachment of the dispersive electrode loosens from the patient so that the electrode is only partially in contact with the patient's skin.

89. One commonly used pad (MEGA 2000 Soft) measures 920 square inches in area. This type of pad (referred to as a capacitive pad) is placed on the operating room table to maximize contact with the patient. The patient lies directly on the pad, or a sheet can be placed between the patient and the pad. Unlike a disposable dispersive electrode, the pad does not adhere or stick to the patient. A cord connects the pad to the generator. Reusable dispersive electrodes may have patient weight minimums and requirements for placement. The pad must be used according to the manufacturer's instructions. It is important to note that return-electrode monitoring systems may not function with large capacitive electrodes (Figure 8-4).

Application

90. Many surgeons prefer electrosurgery to other methods of hemostasis that involve cutting and tying tissue. Use of electrosurgery permits rapid cutting and coagulation and may reduce surgical time. However, coagulated tissue produces a foreign-body reaction and must be absorbed during the healing process. If an excessive amount of coagulated tissue is present in the wound, sloughing may occur, inhibiting healing by first intention.

91. A single power setting is not appropriate for all surgeries. Differences in generator performance, surgical technique, active electrode size, patient size, and location of the patient return electrode affect power settings. Generally, low power is used in neurosurgery, dermatology procedures, and oral and plastic surgery.

92. Fulguration and desiccation are two types of coagulation. Fulguration relies on sparking

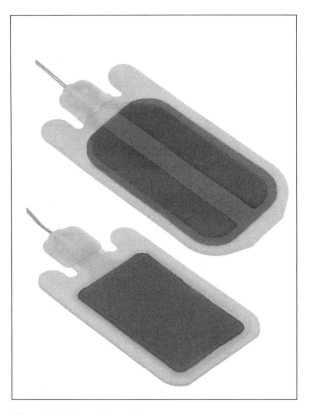

Figure 8-4 Grounding pads
Source: Courtesy of ConMed Corporation.

to coagulate large bleeders and to char tissue. The active electrode does not actually contact the tissue. As sparks contact tissue, superficial coagulation initially results. As the sparking continues, superficial coagulation is followed by necrosis. Fulguration is frequently used by urologists in transurethral resections where the intent is to cause necrosis and destroy tissue.

93. Desiccation—a technique used in most surgeries—refers to coagulation produced by direct contact of the active electrode with the tissue. Desiccation results in hemostasis but does not always result in necrosis. It slowly drives the water content out of the cells. Most surgeons will use coagulation current, which actually cuts and coagulates tissue.

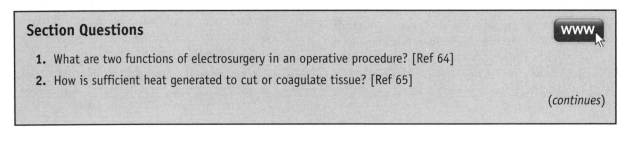

Section Questions

1. What are two functions of electrosurgery in an operative procedure? [Ref 64]
2. How is sufficient heat generated to cut or coagulate tissue? [Ref 65]

(continues)

Section Questions (continued)

3. Which three components must be in place for effective and safe monopolar electrosurgery? [Ref 67]

4. Which component used with monopolar electrosurgery is unnecessary when bipolar electrosurgery is used? [Ref 67]

5. What is the significance of the term "Bovie"? [Ref 69]

6. How does a dispersive electrode work? [Ref 70]

7. Explain how a patient could get an "alternate-site burn" when ground-referenced generators were used. [Ref 71]

8. What risk does electrosurgery present besides electrical injury to the patient? [Ref 72]

9. Explain how modern generators have reduced the risk of electrical injury to the patient. [Ref 73]

10. Differentiate between cutting tissue and coagulation using electrosurgery. [Refs 74–77]

11. Describe the active electrode. [Refs 80–81]

12. Differentiate between monopolar and bipolar active electrodes. [Refs 82–83]

13. Explain the purpose of a dispersive electrode. [Refs 84–85]

14. Why is the dispersive electrode much larger than the active electrode? [Ref 86]

15. Describe the most commonly used dispersive electrode. [Ref 88]

16. What happens when the dispersive electrode loosens from the patient? [Ref 88]

17. How does a capacitive pad differ from a dispersive electrode? [Ref 89]

18. Which adverse patient outcome can be related to excessive amounts of coagulated tissue? [Ref 90]

19. Which factors affect the power setting on the electrosurgical generator? [Ref 91]

20. Contrast fulguration and desiccation. [Refs 92–93]

Nursing Diagnosis: Desired Patient Outcomes

94. Nursing diagnosis for patients on whom electrosurgery is used: high risk for injury related to use of electrosurgery. Although improvements in electrosurgical equipment have minimized the risk of alternate-site burns, electrosurgery still carries a risk for impaired skin integrity. Not all facilities have the most modern equipment, and even modern machines do not eliminate the potential for injury. Older dispersive electrode pads can allow concentration of current and subsequent burn if there is poor contact (i.e., poor electrical connection between the patient and the dispersive electrode). Poor contact can also be caused by incorrect placement of the pad.

95. A patient burn can occur if the active electrode touches the patient at an unintended site, or if the generator is accidentally activated and the active electrode is not housed in a protective receptacle.

96. There is an increased risk of burn injury from electrosurgery in the context of minimally invasive endoscopic surgery.

97. In laparoscopic surgery, the active electrode is introduced into the patient through the abdominal wall via a cannula. The internal view is limited, and the shaft of the laparoscope and the cannula are not visualized. Unintended transfer of energy along the laparoscope or cannula shaft, or along the active electrode shaft, can result in an internal burn that might go unnoticed. Inadvertent activation of the active electrode outside the visible field can also cause an internal burn. The result may be an undiagnosed burn that perforates the bowel and results in postoperative peritonitis—a life-threatening complication because of the time lapse between the patient's discharge and diagnosis of the infection.

98. Electrosurgical complications in laparoscopic surgery can result from the following sources:

- Insulation failure on the active electrode
- Direct coupling between the active electrode and other metal instruments or with tissue
- Capacitive coupling

99. Insulation failure means the insulation of an active electrode is not intact and allows current to flow to an unintended area, where it may contact tissue and burn the abdominal viscera. For instance, faulty insulation on a suction cannula can cause the tip of the suction cannula to act as an active electrode that can burn through abdominal viscera and cause life-threatening injury.

100. Insulation defects may be so small as to go unnoticed during routine instrument examination.

101. Injury will occur if the current is directed to the cannula in which the electrode is housed. Energy can be transferred through the entire shaft of the cannula, burning the abdominal wall, skin, or adjacent structures touching or in near contact with the cannula.

102. In direct coupling, the tip of the active electrode touches another metal instrument. The current is transferred to that instrument, which in turn acts as an active electrode, causing a burn at the contact site. This type of injury is within the surgeon's view, and repair can be attempted before the completion of surgery.

103. Capacitive coupling is the transfer of electrical current from the monopolar active electrode through coupling of stray current into other conductive surgical equipment. When radio-frequency current flows through an electrode, the flow induces stray currents in other nearby conductors. Currents can be induced onto the nearby conductors even though the insulation on the active electrode is intact. The current may be passed on to a metal cannula or working channel of a laparoscope or other metal instrument through which the electrode is passed. This creates the potential for a burn, most likely at the abdominal wall or on external skin. The current transfers to the second metal surface through intact insulation, which in turn electrifies the entire instrument. This can result in an intra-abdominal burn, which in turn creates a risk of peritonitis for the patient.

104. The risk for capacitive coupling injury increases when high voltage and fulguration are used and the mix of instrumentation does not account for the dynamics of capacitive coupling.

105. Recent advances in endoscopic instrumentation include laparoscopic bipolar active electrodes and shielded monopolar active electrodes with monitors designed to detect insulation failure. Active electrode monitoring (AEM) detects insulation failure and capacitive coupling and will deactivate the electrosurgical system from delivering current. Shielded monopolar monitoring systems detect insulation failure and will automatically deactivate the current. Bipolar electrodes localize current. These systems offer safety advantages and protect the patient from insulation failure and capacitively coupled electrosurgical current.

106. Two other risks associated with the use of electrosurgery are fire and plume inhalation (Ball, 2010).

107. Fire in the operating room from electrosurgical equipment is not unknown. Patient injuries and deaths from this hazard have been reported.

108. An active electrode that has been engaged and is in contact with a flammable item, such as a drape, a piece of gauze, or linen, has the potential to start a fire. The operating room is an oxygen-enriched environment that quickly helps to spread fire, which can become intense in just a few minutes.

109. Plume or surgical smoke resulting from electrosurgical application remains a concern. The National Institute for Occupational Safety and Health (NIOSH) has detected chemicals in surgical smoke that may be harmful and has identified electrosurgical smoke as a potential health hazard. Adverse effects of surgical smoke include eye irritation, headache, nausea, acute or chronic inflammatory respiratory changes, asthma, chronic bronchitis, light-headedness, nasopharyngeal lesions, throat irritation, and weakness and fatigue (Ball, 2010 p. e2).

110. NIOSH, the American National Standards Institute (ANSI), and AORN recommend evacuation and filtration of surgical smoke. In the absence of a dedicated smoke evacuator, wall suction with an inline ULPA filter can be used, but only during surgeries in which a small amount of smoke is generated and only when the flow rate of the wall suction is adequate.

111. High-filtration surgical masks should not be considered a first line of protection but only

adjunct protection (ANSI, 2011; AORN, 2012, p. 131).

Desired Patient Outcome/Criteria

112. Desired patient outcome: the patient will experience no injury as a result of the use of electrosurgery.

113. Criteria to evaluate successful achievement of the desired outcome include no evidence of the following complications:

    - Impaired skin integrity (burn) at the dispersive electrode site or alternate current path such as electrocardiograph monitoring leads
    - A burn at an unintended site
    - A burn at the entrance site of laparoscopic instrumentation
    - Fever or abdominal pain associated with peritonitis

Nursing Interventions: Patient and Staff Safety

114. Although electrosurgery is performed by the surgeon and/or assistants, perioperative nursing interventions are critical to a safe patient outcome.

115. Prior to surgery, the patient's skin should be assessed for the placement of the dispersive electrode. The electrode should not be positioned over scar tissue, excessive adipose tissue, metal prosthetic implant, pacemaker, or automatic implantable cardioverter-defibrillator device (ICD).

116. The following guidelines and safety measures will minimize the risk of electrosurgical burn. The scrub person will implement some of the measures; the circulating nurse will implement others.

    ### Before the procedure

    - Use only those dispersive and active electrodes that are compatible with the generator.
    - Prior to use, inspect the generator for frayed cords and loose connections.
    - Ensure the alarm system is intact and activated.
    - Test the alarm, and set it loud enough to be heard during surgery.
    - Turn the generator off between cases.

- Use only equipment that has been inspected by biomedical engineering personnel. Inspection stickers should be visible and must not be expired.
- Do not use reusable active electrodes beyond their intended life. Refer to the manufacturer's guidelines for the permitted number of uses.
- In some older generators, two electrodes can be attached a single generator. With this type of setup, when one active electrode is activated, the other is automatically activated. These generators should not be used when it is anticipated that two electrodes will be required.
- Select a dispersive electrode appropriate to the patient's size and in accordance with the manufacturer's guidelines. Never cut the dispersive electrode to modify its size or shape.
- Check the dispersive electrode to ensure that there is adequate adhesive and gel, that cord connections are secure, and the expiration date has not been exceeded.
- Place the dispersive electrode on the patient over clean, dry skin that covers a large muscle mass and as close to the operative site as possible. Such placement will help ensure good contact with the patient's skin, ensure sufficient current dispersal, and minimize current through the patient's body.
- Avoid placing the dispersive electrode over the following areas:
    - Bony prominences and scar tissue, as they are less conductive and higher in resistance, which can slow the passage of electrosurgical current and concentrate the current. Areas with implants contain scar tissue.
    - Excessive hair and areas where fluids can accumulate and compromise the adhesive. If necessary to ensure adherence, hair should be clipped at the dispersive electrode site.
    - Excess adipose tissue, as this poorly vascularized tissue can impede conductivity of electrical current and dissipation of heat. Muscular areas generally have adequate blood circulation and promote conductivity of the electrical current. Suitable areas of placement include the anterior and posterior thigh, the calf, the upper arm, the midback, and the abdomen.

- Areas close to electrocardiograph electrodes, because current may be attracted to these electrodes and cause an alternative-site burn.
- Tattoos, many of which contain metallic dyes that, at least theoretically, can cause a burn.
- Between the patient and a warming device. The combination of heat at the dispersive electrode site and heat from a warming device can affect how the dispersive electrode adheres to the skin (AORN, 2012, pp. 105–106).
- Metal implants should not be in the circuit path between the active electrode and the dispersive electrode.

- Ensure that there is no point of contact between the patient and any metal surfaces, such as the operating room table.
- Ask the patient to remove any metal jewelry that is near where the active electrode will be used. Should the active electrode contact the jewelry, it could result in a burn.
- If two dispersive electrodes are used, the manufacturer's instructions must be followed for their placement and application.
- Avoid tenting of surgical drapes, which can result in an accumulation of oxygen. Oxygen will enrich a fire.

During the procedure

- Place the generator close enough to the patient to prevent cords from being pulled taut, creating tension at the connection sites. Electrical cords should be free of bends and kinks.
- Verbally confirm the power settings with the surgeon. Power settings should be kept as low as possible. If a request is made to increase power because the present setting is no longer adequate, check for loose connections and generator malfunction. In older equipment, this may signal that the current is seeking an alternate path. Replace the generator if a malfunction is discovered or suspected.
- Do not place liquids on the generator; spilled liquids may cause the equipment to malfunction. Placing the foot pedal into a plastic bag will keep it clean and dry.
- Prior to surgery, inspect the active electrodes for insulation defects. If a defect is noted, the device must not be used.

- Position the active electrode on the sterile field, close to the operative site, and in a protective container or holster so that accidental activation will not cause incidental burns to the patient or ignite drapes.
- Keep the active electrode clean during surgery by periodically removing charred tissue. Eschar creates impedance that may result in a request for a higher power setting. Clean the tip with a moist sponge or a scratch pad intended for this purpose. Do not clean it with a dry sponge. An active electrode inadvertently activated and in contact with a dry sponge (gauze pad) can start a fire.
- Do not use electrosurgery in the presence of flammable agents. Prep solutions containing flammable agents must be allowed to dry before using electrosurgery, according to the manufacturer's instructions. Other factors, such as pooling onto drapes, towels, and body hair, can alter the drying time of the prep solution.
- Open suture packages containing alcohol should be kept away from the area of the active electrode.
- Sponges are flammable; use moistened sponges in the area of the active electrode.
- Be diligent when using electrosurgery in oxygen-enriched environments—including around a nasal cannula, when the patient is receiving oxygen via an oxygen mask, and when the anesthesia provider is using an uncuffed endotracheal tube.
- Methane gas, which can be present in the intestinal tract, is flammable. The active electrode should not be activated in the presence of methane gas.
- Evacuate electrosurgical smoke from the field.
- In the event of the failure of any of the electrosurgical components, retain the defective items for follow-up with biomedical personnel and for reporting of medical instrumentation failure as required.
- During lengthy procedures, or when the patient is repositioned during surgery, verify that the dispersive electrode continues to maintain good contact with the patient.

Section Questions

www

1. With improvements in electrosurgery equipment, what accounts for the continued risk for impaired skin integrity? [Refs 94–95]

2. Describe the minimally invasive surgery environment that creates risk for burn injury. [Ref 97]

3. How can insulation failure result in a burn injury? [Refs 99–100]

4. What happens if current is directed to the cannula in which the electrode is housed? [Ref 101]

5. What is direct coupling and how can it result in patient injury? [Ref 102]

6. Describe capacitive coupling and the patient injuries that could result from it. [Refs 103–104]

7. Describe the new developments in endoscopic instruments that minimize the risk of burn injuries. [Ref 105]

8. Explain how electrosurgery can cause a fire in the operating room. [Ref 108]

9. Which interventions can protect personnel from surgical smoke or plume? [Refs 109–110]

10. Which criteria are used to evaluate successful achievement of preventing harm from electrosurgery? [Ref 113]

11. Prior to the surgical procedure, describe the process of ensuring the safe use of the electrosurgery generator. [Ref 116]

12. Describe the ideal site for placement of the dispersive electrode. [Ref 116]

13. Explain why certain sites should be avoided when placing the dispersive electrode. [Ref 116]

14. How might tenting of the drapes affect fire safety during a surgical procedure? [Ref 116]

15. What should the perioperative nurse do when the surgeon continually asks that the power setting be increased on the electrosurgical unit? [Ref 116]

16. Where should the active electrode be positioned on the sterile field? [Ref 116]

17. How can eschar on the active electrode interfere with safe electrosurgery? [Ref 116]

18. Which flammable materials might be found on a sterile field that could be ignited by an active electrode? [Ref 116]

19. Describe three oxygen-rich environments that would be high-risk areas for the use of electrosurgery? [Ref 116]

20. Why would you not discard a defective active electrode? [Ref 116]

Electrosurgical Use During Endoscopic Surgery: Special Precautions

117. The following additional precautions are appropriate when using electrosurgery during endoscopic surgery:

- Prior to surgery, inspect the active electrodes for insulation defects. If a defect is noted, the electrode must not be used. If a defect is noted during the surgery or following the procedure, inform the surgeon that the patient might have potentially sustained an inadvertent internal burn. Some laparoscopic instruments have a double-sheathed shaft of insulation of different colors that can help to identify an insulation defect.

- Active electrode monitoring equipment is used to detect insulation failures and capacitive coupling on active electrode instrumentation in use during endoscopic surgery. Active electrode monitoring equipment should be used whenever available.

- Use all-metal trocar cannula systems. All-metal trocar systems help reduce the risk of capacitive coupling. Should electrical current build up on the metal cannula, the current will be absorbed into the abdominal wall. All-plastic trocar cannula systems are acceptable but are not preferable to all-metal systems. Trocar cannula systems consisting of a combination of plastic and metal should not be used.

118. The patient who has an internal cardioverter-defibrillator device (ICD) should have the device deactivated prior to surgery; the ICD should then be reactivated following the procedure. The facility should have a procedure in place for deactivation and reactivation of the ICD. Presence of an ICD should be documented and the facility's policy for deactivation and reactivation followed. Regardless of who has the responsibility for activation and deactivation, the perioperative nurse must ensure that the ICD and appropriate actions related to it are documented. As an alternative, bipolar electrosurgery should be used when possible, as it does not interfere with the ICD.

119. A pacemaker presents a potential electrical hazard with electrosurgery as electrosurgery can interfere with the operation of some pacemakers. To prevent current from passing near the heart or pacemaker, the tip of the active electrode should be kept as far from the pacemaker as possible. The dispersive electrode should not be placed near the pacemaker. Instead, it should be placed as close as possible to where the active electrode will be used and in such a way that the pacemaker is not in the circuit path between active and dispersive electrodes. Safety guidelines for patients with a pacemaker should be prepared in advance of surgery based on the pacemaker manufacturer's instructions. A bipolar energy source is the preferred option.

120. Patients with a pacemaker or ICD should have continuous electrocardiogram monitoring during procedures where electrosurgery is used, and a defibrillator and a pacemaker magnet or programming unit should be readily available.

121. Following surgery, the dispersive electrode should be removed slowly and carefully to avoid denuding the skin. The placement area should be inspected for injury. The patient's skin should be checked for integrity.

122. Documentation of electrosurgical use should include the following information:
    - Assessment of the skin preoperatively
    - Identification of electrosurgical equipment and settings
    - Site of dispersive electrode placement
    - Name of person who applied electrode
    - Assessment of skin postoperatively

Ultrasonic Energy Devices

Overview

123. With an ultrasonic energy device, ultrasonic motion is used to cut and coagulate tissue. The ultrasonic scalpel generator is a microprocessor that uses controlled high-frequency power to drive an acoustic system within a hand piece. Electrical energy is converted into mechanical energy or ultrasonic waveforms. The energy is transmitted to the hand piece through a blade that vibrates.

124. The mechanical vibrations move at a speed of 55,500 vibrations per second. They are transferred to the blade, which, when in contact with tissue, denatures protein and creates a sticky coagulum, thereby sealing blood vessels. Cutting and coagulation occur simultaneously.

System Components

125. Ultrasonic system components include a generator, a hand piece, and a foot pedal. The generator is a microprocessor that converts electrical energy into mechanical energy. A cable attaches the hand piece to the generator.

126. Variously configured blades and accessories permit use of this technology in both open and endoscopic surgery.

Tissue Effects

127. Ultrasonic technology balances cutting and coagulation. It cuts and coagulates at temperatures lower than those needed for electrosurgery. The cutting speed and the coagulation effects are inversely related. Four factors control the effect upon tissue:
    - Tissue tension:
        - More tension leads to faster cutting and less hemostasis.
        - Less tension leads to slower cutting and more hemostasis.
    - Blade sharpness:
        - The shear mode cuts faster than the blunt mode.
        - The blunt mode provides more coagulation when vascular structures are encountered.
    - Power:

– Increasing the power on the generator increases the cutting speed and decreases the coagulation.

– Decreasing the power results in slower cutting and increased coagulation.

- Time:

– With shorter tissue application, there is faster cutting and less hemostasis.

– With longer tissue application, there is slower cutting and more hemostasis.

Technology Characteristics

128. The ultrasonic scalpel may be used as an adjunct to or a substitute for electrosurgery.

129. Because mechanical motion is the basis for this technology, no electrical energy is required and no energy is transferred through the patient. Therefore, a dispersive electrode is not required.

130. Because minimal thermal damage is inflicted, precise dissection near vital structures is possible.

131. The controlled coagulation effect results in minimal char and tissue desiccation. Ultrasonic energy coagulates at temperatures up to 100°C (212°F) versus electrosurgery temperatures of 150°C (302°F) or higher. The ultrasonic scalpel also creates less plume than electrosurgery.

Applications

132. The ultrasonic scalpel is intended for soft tissue where bleeding control and minimal thermal damage is desired.

Argon Beam-Enhanced Electrosurgery

Overview

133. Argon beam-enhanced electrosurgery technology uses a beam of ionized argon to achieve rapid hemostasis by coagulation. Argon gas combined with an electrosurgical pencil delivers radio-frequency energy to tissue in a white-light beam of ionized argon. The flow of the argon gas clears the tissue of liquid blood and other fluid, and the energy from the ionized argon beam creates a superficial eschar directly on the tissue that helps to prevent further bleeding. Coagulation occurs from the arcing effect of electrical energy, not from the argon gas.

134. Argon is an inert gas and is noncombustible. Plume, odor, and tissue damage are decreased when this technology is used.

System Components

135. System components include a generator, a multifunction hand piece that may be used for open or endoscopic surgery, and a dispersive electrode. Active electrodes include blade and needle tips for open procedures and a variety of electrode tips for endoscopic surgery. Flexible coagulation electrodes are available in a variety of lengths.

136. The dispersive electrode functions in the same manner as the dispersive electrode used with a monopolar electrosurgical system.

137. The clinical benefits of argon beam coagulation include rapid, efficient coagulation; formation of a thin, flexible eschar; less charring; and less tissue damage than with traditional electrosurgical coagulation.

Application

138. Argon beam coagulation is used for open and endoscopic procedures in which coagulation and low tissue penetration are desired. It is used to control bleeding from vascular structures where large areas of coagulation are needed and to control surface bleeding of organs such as the liver.

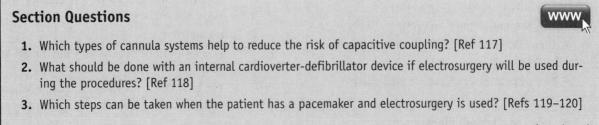

Section Questions

1. Which types of cannula systems help to reduce the risk of capacitive coupling? [Ref 117]

2. What should be done with an internal cardioverter-defibrillator device if electrosurgery will be used during the procedures? [Ref 118]

3. Which steps can be taken when the patient has a pacemaker and electrosurgery is used? [Refs 119–120]

(continues)

Section Questions (continued)

4. How is the dispersive electrode removed following surgery? [Ref 121]

5. Which information should be documented in the medical record when electrosurgery is used? [Ref 122]

6. Describe how an ultrasonic device cuts and coagulates tissues. [Refs 123–124]

7. Describe how each of the four factors controls the effect of ultrasonic energy on tissue. [Ref 127]

8. Describe three benefits of ultrasonic energy. [Refs 130–131]

9. What are the clinical benefits of argon beam-enhanced electrosurgery? [Ref 137]

10. In which situations is argon beam coagulation most appropriately used? [Ref 138]

● ● ● References

American National Standards Institute (ANSI) (2011). *ANSI Z136.3: American National Standard for Safe Use of Lasers in Health Care Facilities.* Orlando, FL: Laser Institute of America.

American National Standards Institute (ANSI) (1996). *ANSI Z136.3: American National Standard for Safe Use of Lasers in Health Care Facilities*, p. 15. Orlando, FL: Laser Institute of America.

Association of periOperative Registered Nurses (AORN) (2012). *Perioperative Standards and Recommended Practices.* Denver, CO: AORN.

Association of periOperative Registered Nurses (AORN) (2011). *Perioperative Nursing Data Set.* Denver, CO: AORN.

Ball K (2010). Surgical smoke evacuation guidelines: compliance among perioperative nurses. *AORN J*;92(2):e1–e23.

McEwen J (2012a). *Contraindications to tourniquet use.* Available at: www.tourniquets.org/clinical_applications .php#contraindications. Accessed September 2012.

McEwen J (2012b). *Tourniquet use and care.* Available at: www.tourniquets.org/use_care.php#appropriate_pressure. Accessed September 2012.

Moss CE, Bryant C, Stewart J, et al. (1990). *NIOSH Health Hazard Evaluation Report*, University of Utah Health Sciences Center. HETA 88-101-2008. Atlanta: NIOSH.

Raju P (2010). *Arterial tourniquets: anaesthesia tutorial of the week 200.* Available at: http://totw.anaesthesiologists .org/wp-content/uploads/2010/10/200-Arterial-Tourniquets .pdf. Accessed September 2012.

• •

Post-Test

WWW

Read each question carefully. Each question may have more than one correct answer.

1. Hemostasis
   a. is the arrest or control of bleeding.
   b. is accomplished both by natural and artificial means.
   c. is sometimes achieved with the formation of a platelet plug.
   d. requires that coagulation occur.

2. Which statement(s) is (are) true about coagulation?
   a. As platelets from a platelet plug break down, thromboplastin is released into the blood.
   b. Coagulation is a complex process that begins with the interaction of prothrombin and thromboplastin.
   c. Potassium ions are part of the coagulation process.
   d. Fibrin is the basic structure of a clot.

3. Which additional statement(s) is (are) true about coagulation?
   a. It is self-regulating; the process will stop on its own when bleeding stops.
   b. It is a slow process, and even small wounds need prompt attention.
   c. The clot becomes red as platelets, white blood cells, and red blood cells become entangled in the fibrin.
   d. Thromboplastic is released when tissues are injured and platelets break down.

4. Which statement(s) is (are) true about thrombin?
   a. Thrombin is useful in controlling major artery bleeding.
   b. Thrombin is a hormone that combines with fibrin to form a clot.
   c. Thrombin is for topical use only.
   d. Thrombin made from human plasma has fewer side effects than bovine thrombin.

5. Which statement(s) is (are) true about absorbable gelatin?
   a. Absorbable gelatin is available in a compressed pad (Gelfoam), powder, or beads.
   b. Fibrin is deposited into the interstices of Gelfoam, which swells and promotes clot formation.
   c. Gelatin is sometimes used with thrombin or epinephrine.
   d. Gelfoam is soluble and is usually left in the wound.

6. Which statement(s) is (are) true about oxidized cellulose?
   a. Oxidized cellulose is placed directly on an oozing surface.
   b. When it comes in contact with blood, oxidized cellulose swells, forms a gel, and promotes clot formation.
   c. Oxidized cellulose forms a pseudo-clot that puts pressure on the wound to speed up the clotting process.
   d. Oxidized cellulose can be left in place and will be fully absorbed in a week or two.

7. Which statement(s) is (are) true?
   a. Microfibrillar collagen is often used in crevices and sites of irregular contour.
   b. Styptics cause blood vessels to dilate.
   c. Hemostatic clamps must be replaced with a ligature or ligating clip for permanent hemostasis.
   d. Manual pressure is a form of temporary hemostasis.

8. Which statement(s) is (are) true about tourniquets?

    a. A tourniquet is used to create a bloodless field for surgery.

    b. Tourniquets create hemostasis so that when they are deflated, there is no further bleeding.

    c. An Esmarch bandage is wrapped around the extremity to force blood out and remains in place during surgery.

    d. Tourniquet pressures are preset by the manufacturer.

9. Which of the following might be contraindications for tourniquet use?

    a. Hypertension

    b. Open fracture

    c. DVT

    d. Sickle cell anemia

10. Which of the following are appropriate nursing interventions related to tourniquets?

    a. Choosing the size of tourniquet to use

    b. Ensuring that prophylactic antibiotics are not infused until the cuff has been inflated

    c. Testing the cuff and the tourniquet

    d. Assessing the patient's skin integrity and potential for complications

11. Which statement(s) is (are) true about tourniquet cuffs?

    a. A contoured cuff is useful when the distal circumference of the extremity is very different from the proximal circumference.

    b. The cuff selected should be as narrow as possible.

    c. The cuff should overlap at least 3 to 6 inches.

    d. Padding under the cuff is necessary to prevent damage to the skin.

12. Which statement(s) is (are) true about tourniquet management?

    a. The nurse should remind the surgeon periodically how long the tourniquet has been inflated.

    b. If the tourniquet's pressure drops, it should be inflated immediately to the desired pressure setting.

    c. Bilateral tourniquets should be deflated simultaneously.

    d. Deflating the tourniquet results in an increase in core body temperature.

13. Which statement(s) is (are) true about electrosurgery?

    a. Electrosurgery generates enough heat to vaporize tissue.

    b. In an isolated system, current is restricted to pathways to and from the generator.

    c. Both monopolar and bipolar electrosurgery require an active electrode and a dispersive electrode.

    d. Cutting tissue requires a continuous waveform; coagulating tissue requires an interrupted or dampened waveform.

14. Which statement(s) is (are) true about active electrodes?

    a. Active electrodes are usually handheld devices that deliver current from the generator to the operative site.

    b. The current from a monopolar electrode passes from the tip, through the patient, to the dispersive electrode.

    c. The current from a bipolar electrode passes through the tissue between the tips of the forceps.

    d. Bipolar electrosurgery requires higher voltage than monopolar electrosurgery.

15. Which statement(s) is (are) true about dispersive electrodes?
    a. The dispersive electrode is also called a grounding pad or Bovie pad.
    b. The active electrode delivers current to the operative site, which is then concentrated at the dispersive electrode.
    c. The dispersive electrode is much larger than the active electrode, and current density at the dispersive electrode is high.
    d. The dispersive electrode must make good contact with the patient to work properly.

16. Which statement(s) is (are) true about coagulation?
    a. A single power setting is appropriate for most surgery.
    b. Coagulated tissue produces a foreign-body reaction and must be absorbed during the healing process.
    c. Fulguration and desiccation are two types of coagulation.
    d. Fulguration is more commonly used than desiccation.

17. Which statement(s) is (are) true?
    a. Capacitive coupling occurs when the tip of an electrode touches another metal instrument.
    b. Insulation defects are easily seen and defective instruments are replaced.
    c. Adverse effects of plume, or surgical smoke, include eye irritation, respiratory changes, throat irritation, and fatigue.
    d. High-filtration surgical masks are not a first line of defense relative to surgical smoke.

18. Which of the following nursing interventions promote electrosurgical safety?
    a. Attach two electrodes to the generator if two people will be using them simultaneously during the procedure.
    b. If the dispersive electrode is too large, trim it to fit snugly on the area you have selected.
    c. Check for frayed cords, test the alarm of the electrosurgical unit, and be sure that the alarm is loud enough to be heard during surgery.
    d. Avoid placing the dispersive electrode over scar tissue, a bony prominence, or in the vicinity of an implant.

19. Which of the following nursing interventions promote electrosurgical safety?
    a. The electrosurgical generator is a handy place to put saline to be delivered to the back table.
    b. Store the active electrode in a protective receptacle on the surgical field.
    c. The eschar that builds up on the active electrode tip helps to disperse the current effectively.
    d. Use the suction catheter to remove surgical smoke from the field.

20. Which statement(s) is (are) true about ultrasonic energy devices?
    a. An ultrasonic device has both cutting and coagulation settings.
    b. Ultrasonic devices cut and coagulate at higher temperatures than needed for electrosurgery.
    c. The effect of the ultrasonic device is affected by tissue tension, blade sharpness, generator power, and time.
    d. Ultrasonic devices and electrosurgery cannot be used at the same time.

Competency Checklist: Hemostasis—Tourniquet www

Under "Observer's Initials," enter initials upon successful achievement of the competency. Enter N/A if the competency is not appropriate for the institution.

Name _____

	Observer's Initials	Date
1. Equipment assembled:		
a. Webril	_____	_____
b. Tourniquet	_____	_____
c. Esmarch	_____	_____
d. Other	_____	_____
2. Skin condition on extremity assessed	_____	_____
3. Appropriate size cuff selected	_____	_____
4. Tourniquet inspected and tested:		
a. Cuff	_____	_____
b. Console	_____	_____
c. Tubing	_____	_____
d. Connections	_____	_____
e. Electrical cords	_____	_____
f. Power source/amount of gas in tank	_____	_____
g. Cleanliness	_____	_____
5. Cuff applied:		
a. Over padding	_____	_____
b. At the proximal point of the limb selected (at the maximum circumference)	_____	_____
c. Tourniquet covers the intended area only—nothing unintended under the cuff	_____	_____
6. Tourniquet inflated and deflated upon surgeon instructions	_____	_____
7. Length of inflation reported at agreed-upon intervals	_____	_____
8. Pressure gauge checked during procedure for fluctuations in pressure	_____	_____
9. Documentation:		
a. Skin assessment under cuff before and after tourniquet application	_____	_____
b. Location of cuff	_____	_____
c. Time of inflation and deflation	_____	_____
d. Tourniquet identification number	_____	_____
e. Identification of person who applied the cuff	_____	_____

Observer's Signature   Initials   Date

_____

Orientee's Signature

_____

· ·

Competency Checklist: Electrosurgical Equipment

www

Under "Observer's Initials," enter initials upon successful achievement of the competency. Enter N/A if the competency is not appropriate for the institution.

Name _____

	Observer's Initials	Date

1. Equipment assembled:
   a. Electrosurgical generator   _____ _____
   b. Active and dispersive electrode   _____ _____
   c. Foot pedal   _____ _____
2. Generator:
   a. Inspected for frayed cords and loose connections   _____ _____
   b. Alarm checked and setting is audible   _____ _____
   c. Inspected for biomedical inspection   _____ _____
   d. No liquids placed on top of the generator   _____ _____
3. Skin assessed for integrity prior to application of dispersive electrode   _____ _____
4. Dispersive electrode:
   a. Appropriate size chosen   _____ _____
   b. Inspected for adequate adhesive/gel   _____ _____
   c. Positioned over a large muscle mass (not positioned over a bony   _____ _____
      prominence, excessively hairy site, large metal prosthetic implant,
      or pacemaker)
   d. Skin contacted uniformly   _____ _____
   e. Areas close to electrocardiographic electrodes avoided   _____ _____
   f. Pad used/placed according to the manufacturer's instructions for use   _____ _____
5. Active electrode:
   a. Inspected for insulation defects (equipment for testing insulation used)   _____ _____
   b. Inspected for loose connections   _____ _____
   c. Housed in protective container/holster on the field   _____ _____
6. Power settings confirmed with surgeon   _____ _____
7. Equipment positioned so as not to cause tension at connection sites   _____ _____
   (generator is close to patient)
8. Troubleshooting:
   a. Surgeon repeatedly requests higher settings   _____ _____
      • All connections checked   _____ _____
      • Adherence of dispersive electrode checked   _____ _____
   b. Alarm sounds
      • All connections checked   _____ _____
      • Adherence of dispersive electrode checked   _____ _____
9. Dispersive pad removed slowly   _____ _____

	Observer's Initials	Date

10. Documentation:
    a. Assessment of skin preoperatively and postoperatively   _____ _____
    b. Identification of electrosurgical equipment and settings   _____ _____
    c. Site of dispersive electrode placement and person who applied electrode   _____ _____
    d. Assessment of skin   _____ _____

Observer's Signature   Initials   Date

_____

Orientee's Signature

_____

Prevention of Injury: Use and Care of Basic Surgical Instrumentation

Nursing Diagnosis: Desired Patient Outcome

1. The patient undergoing surgery is at risk for injury and infection related to use of surgical instrumentation.

2. Potential injury can include tearing of tissue caused by an instrument that does not perform as expected or the retention of a foreign body caused by a portion of an instrument that breaks or falls off inside the patient and is not retrieved.

3. A patient may also incur an infection or a foreign-body reaction from an improperly cleaned or sterilized instrument (Pyrek, 2012; Tosh et al., 2011, p. 1180). An instrument

that is inappropriately processed may have a retained toxic residue that can harm a patient (Association for the Advancement of Medical Instrumentation [AAMI], 2011, p. 61). An improperly processed instrument or one that malfunctions can delay a patient's surgery, increasing the patient's anxiety and interfering with the flow of the operative schedule.

4. Following surgery, the patient should be free from signs and symptoms of injury caused by extraneous objects (Association of peri-Operative Registered Nurses [AORN], 2011, p. 165) and should be free of signs and symptoms of infection (AORN, 2012, p. 255) related to improperly processed or malfunctioning instruments.

5. When a patient sustains an injury or an infection during surgery, it is sometimes difficult or impossible to identify the exact cause. For example, a postoperative infection may result from poor aseptic technique, poor surgical technique, inadequate skin preparation, improperly cleaned and processed instrumentation, the patient's state of health, or a combination of any of these factors.

6. If an instrument was inadequately processed and a toxic residue results, the effect of that residue may not be measurable for some time, and a cause-and-effect relationship may never be established. This inability to assign causality does not negate the necessity to take all requisite steps to protect the patient from injury related to instrumentation.

7. Meticulous aseptic technique, coupled with proper use and care of surgical instruments, provides the best insurance against an injury or infection related to surgical instrumentation.

8. Desired outcomes related to surgical instruments include absence of excessive swelling or discoloration at the surgical site, minimal pain (excluding the incision site), no sign of infection, and no evidence of retained instrument or instrument part upon instrument count or subsequent X ray.

Overview

Evolution of Surgical Instrumentation

9. Surgical instrumentation dates back to 10,000 B.C., when stone knives were used to perform surgery. Trephined skulls dating to the Neolithic era provide evidence that surgery was performed long before sophisticated surgical instrumentation was developed. Some early surgical implements included sharpened flints used for circumcision and sharpened animal teeth used for blood-letting.

10. Until the 1700s, instruments were made by blacksmiths, cutlers, and armorers. In the 1700s and 1800s, when surgery gained recognition as a scientific discipline, skilled craftsmen—silversmiths, wood turners, coppersmiths, and steel workers—began to make surgical instruments.

11. Instruments were made to individual specifications and often incorporated ornate, finely carved wooden or ivory handles. They were often cased in velvet-lined boxes.

12. The advent of anesthesia in the 1840s enabled surgeons to work slowly and deliberately and also generated the need for more precise and varied surgical instrumentation. With the concurrent acceptance of instrument sterilization, wooden and ivory handles were replaced by all-metal instruments that could withstand repeated sterilization.

13. The development of stainless steel in the 1900s further enhanced manufacturers' ability to make precise surgical instruments, and instrument-making evolved into a highly skilled occupation. Many craftsmen from Europe, especially Germany, came to the United States to instruct apprentices. Germany is often considered the home of high-quality surgical instruments, and many instruments used in the United States today are manufactured in Germany.

14. The majority of surgical instruments are manufactured from stainless steel, although titanium, vitallium, and other metals are also used.

15. Recent advances in surgery, especially in minimally invasive endoscopic surgery, combined with the discoveries of new materials, has led to the development of many new, precise, sophisticated, complex, delicate, and very expensive surgical instruments, scopes, and cameras.

Proper Care and Handling: Departmental Impact

16. A large portion of the operating room budget is devoted to the purchase and repair of surgical instruments.

17. Proper instrument care and handling can preserve inventory and reduce expenditures for

repair. Instruments that do not function properly, are out for repair, or are processed incorrectly can cause delays in surgery—a source of frustration for both the surgical team and the patient.

18. Proper care and handling of surgical instruments requires knowledgeable personnel with critical thinking skills who understand the processes necessary to prepare a variety of instruments for surgery and who have demonstrated competence in instrument care.

Manufacture of Surgical Instruments

19. The majority of basic instruments are made from stainless steel, which is composed of iron ore and varying amounts of carbon and chromium. Carbon provides the necessary hardness to the steel, and chromium provides a stainless, corrosion-resistant quality. Most stainless-steel instruments are made from alloys that are high in carbon and low in chromium.

20. There are more than 80 different types of stainless steel. The quality of stainless steel varies according to its composition. The American Iron and Steel Institute grades steel using a three-digit number, based on various qualities and on the amount of carbon and chromium it contains.

21. Stainless steel series 300 and 400 are commonly used for the manufacture of surgical instruments. The 300 series is used primarily for noncutting instruments, while the 400 series is used for both cutting and noncutting instruments.

22. Both the 300 and 400 series comprise high-quality stainless steel that resists rust and corrosion, has good tensile strength, and maintains a keen edge. The specific stainless steel selected for instrument manufacture is determined by the intended use and desired flexibility and malleability of the instrument.

23. The initial step in instrument manufacture is the conversion of raw steel into sheets that are milled, ground, or lathed into instrument blanks. These blanks are then forged, die-cast, molded, or machined into specific instrument pieces of various shapes and sizes. Excess metal is trimmed, and the component parts are hand-assembled, ground, and buffed.

24. Each instrument is then heat-treated, or tempered, to achieve the desired spring, temper, and balance. Balance and temper provide the flexibility that is necessary to withstand the stress of repeated use.

25. After an inspection that may include X ray or fluoroscopy to expose defects, the instrument is subjected to a finishing process, called passivation, to protect the surface and to minimize corrosion. During passivation, the instrument is immersed in a nitric acid bath that removes carbon steel particles and promotes the formation of a chromium oxide surface coating. Removal of the carbon particles may leave behind tiny pits that must be polished away.

26. The final step is polishing, which creates a smooth surface on which a continuous layer of chromium oxide forms. Passivation and polishing essentially close the instrument pores and retard corrosion. The chromium oxide layer continues to form when the instrument is exposed to the atmosphere and when it is subjected to the oxidizing agents contained in cleaning agents.

27. There are three types of instrument finish: bright, highly polished; satin or dull; and ebony. The highly polished finish resists surface corrosion. It is shiny and reflects light, which, on occasion, may distract the surgeon or obscure visibility. The majority of instruments have this finish. The scrubbed person can minimize this distraction with careful placement of the overhead lights.

28. The satin finish eliminates glare and is slightly more susceptible to corrosion.

29. The least common finish is ebony, which is black and eliminates glare. The black surface is useful in laser surgery to prevent reflection of the laser beam.

30. Stainless steel is not completely stainless. The chemical composition and the final heat and rinsing processes during manufacture determine the degree to which an instrument resists staining. Although stainless steel resists corrosion and staining, with repeated use, some spotting or staining may occur.

31. The degree of spotting, staining, or corrosion of stainless steel instruments also depends on the quality of water and chemicals used for processing. The way in which instruments are used, cleaned, processed, and maintained also affect the extent of corrosion and spotting.

32. Titanium instruments have a bluish finish. Titanium is stronger and lighter than stainless steel and more corrosion resistant. Titanium is

used primarily for the delicate, precise instruments used in microsurgical and neurosurgical procedures.

33. Three types of joints are used in the manufacture of instruments that consist of two halves: screw, box lock, and semi-box. The screw joint, which is seen most often in older instruments, uses a screw to secure the two halves of the instrument. Jointed instruments with box locks articulate with a box on one half fitted into a slot in the other half. This joint is more common than the semi-box joint, which allows the two halves of an instrument to be separated.

34. Instrument names are not consistent. Various manufacturers, facilities, and individuals may identify the same instrument by different names. There are some recognizable patterns in the nomenclature of surgical instruments. An instrument can be named in the following ways:

    • By function: clamp, scissors, needle holder, pickups

    • By visual description: rake, hook, ribbon (retractors); knife

    • For the inventor: DeBakey forceps, Bookwalter retractor, Bishop forceps, Balfour retractor, Weitlaner retractor, Gelpi retractor, Satinski clamp

    • Scientifically by its function in Latin, French, or another language: osteotome (Latin: bone knife), rongeur (French: gnawer); tracheotome (Latin: tracheal knife), scalpel (Latin: scraper/scratcher); speculum (Latin: mirror)

Nursing Responsibilities Related to Surgical Instrumentation

35. Operating room and sterile processing department (SPD) personnel share the responsibility for the care and handling of instruments. Instruments are usually purchased by the operating room and processed in the SPD. Perioperative nurses are responsible for knowing how to care for instruments properly, even if they do not participate in the cleaning and sterilization process.

36. Perioperative nursing personnel responsible for setting up for a surgical procedure, and nurses or technicians who function in the scrub role, should be able to determine whether instruments are adequately prepared, function properly, and are ready for use. In addition to the inspection of instruments in the SPD prior to packaging and sterilization, instruments should be inspected during setup for surgery so only functional instruments are handed to the surgeon.

Loaner Instrumentation

37. In some instances, the hospital does not own the instruments needed for a particular procedure. Instead, it borrows a "loaner set" of instruments from the manufacturer. This is particularly true of orthopedic instruments used for joint surgery, where the healthcare facility purchases the implant but borrows the instrumentation necessary for an implantation procedure. There may be a fee for this service. Borrowing a "loaner set" is also common with instruments for a new procedure that is just being introduced.

38. The perioperative nurse's ultimate responsibility is to provide for patient safety. Proper care and handling of instruments are deterrents to patient injury.

39. Loaner instrumentation should always be inspected, inventoried, cleaned, packaged, and sterilized in-house before use.

40. The "loaner set" should be delivered to the healthcare facility the day before the surgery so that it can be processed appropriately. The perioperative nurse should not accept instruments from a vendor without sending them to the SPD for processing.

41. Sets that have been packaged and sterilized in another healthcare facility should be sent to the SPD and cleaned, inspected, packaged, and sterilized in-house before use in surgery.

42. The complexity and high cost of instrumentation, diversity of materials, and potential for patient injury require that the nurse know what special handling is required, which cleaning and sterilization methods are appropriate, and how to determine whether an instrument is functioning properly and, therefore, safe for use in surgery.

43. When an instrument or instrument set is needed urgently, the nurse must implement or direct the cleaning and sterilization process. SPD personnel are the experts in instrument processing;

when a question arises about cleaning or processing, they should be consulted.

44. The exception to accepting instruments that have been processed elsewhere is when instruments have been processed by a company whose business is instrument processing and with which the healthcare facility has a contract. Such businesses have processes in place to ensure appropriate processing and aseptic transportation of instrumentation.

Section Questions

www

1. Which types of patient injury can be related to instruments? [Refs 1–3]

2. How can such injuries be prevented? [Ref 7]

3. Which recent advance in surgery has led to the development of a whole new array of surgical instruments? [Ref 15]

4. Aside from preventing injury, which positive outcomes are associated with the proper care and handling of surgical instruments? [Ref 17]

5. Which characteristics of the 300 and 400 series of stainless steel make them ideal for surgical instruments? [Ref 22]

6. What is the purpose of heat-treating or tempering surgical instruments? [Ref 24]

7. What do passivation and polishing accomplish? [Refs 25–26]

8. What is the purpose of the three different types of finishes found on surgical instrument? [Refs 27–29]

9. Which factors affect spotting, staining, and corrosion of stainless steel instruments? [Refs 30–31]

10. What advantages does titanium have over stainless steel? [Ref 32]

11. What are some of the naming patterns for surgical instruments? [Ref 34]

12. Who is responsible for the care and handling of surgical instruments? [Refs 35–36]

13. In which instances might a facility use a "loaner set" of instruments? [Ref 37]

14. Where should the loaner set of instruments be processed? [Ref 41]

15. What is the exception to in-house processing of borrowed instruments? [Ref 44]

Categories of Instruments

45. Surgical instruments can be organized into five categories:
    - Cutting—such as scalpels, scissors, osteotomes, curettes, and rongeurs
    - Grasping—such as clamps, forceps, and needle holders
    - Retracting—such as hand-held and self-retaining retractors, and specula
    - Suctioning—such as suction tips
    - Miscellaneous instruments—such as cannulas, probes, dilators, and calipers

Cutting Instruments

46. Cutting instruments, such as scalpels and scissors, are sharp. It is the scrubbed person's responsibility to ensure that sharp instruments are, indeed, sharp. Dull instruments can cause patient injury, and replacing instruments can cause increase the length of a procedure.

47. Scalpels consist of a handle and a disposable blade. The handle has a groove at the tip for attaching the blade. Blades are changed as needed during the procedure. Scalpel handles are available in a variety of lengths and sizes; scalpel blades are available in a variety of sizes and shapes (Figure 9-1).

48. Blades are commercially prepackaged and are sterile. They may have a rounded, tapered, or hooked cutting edge. These instruments are delivered to the sterile field by the circulating nurse and contained on a magnetic mat or other receptacle designed to prevent accidental injury. At the end of surgery, all blades are placed on the needle mat, and the mat is disposed of in a designated sharps container.

49. To prevent accidental injury when attaching or changing blades, the scrub person should grasp the blade firmly with a needle holder and

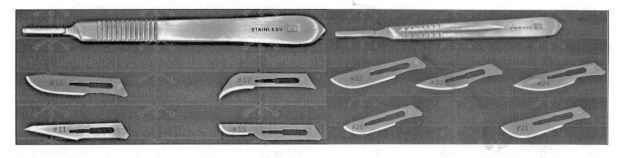

Figure 9-1 Scalpel handle with associated blades
Source: Courtesy of Indigo Instruments: www.indigo.com.

attach it to the knife handle. Blades must not be hand-held during attachment to or removal from the handle.

50. The scrubbed person hands the scalpel to the surgeon with the cutting edge facing away from the surgeon's palm.

51. The hands-free technique is the safest approach to passing a scalpel: only one person touches the instrument at a time. The scrubbed person places the scalpel (or any sharp instrument) on a magnetic pad or in an emesis basin on the field, and the surgeon retrieves the item from there. A safe or neutral zone on the field between the scrubbed person and surgeon may be identified, and sharp instruments placed there for retrieval.

52. Another technique to prevent injury is to verbalize the transfer each time a scalpel is passed. For example, the surgeon may say, "Blade back," indicating to the scrub person that a scalpel is being returned.

53. As a result of the 2000 Needlestick Safety and Prevention Act, the Occupational Safety and Health Administration (OSHA, 2012a) amended the bloodborne pathogen standard to require the use of safer devices to protect healthcare workers from sharps injury. In response, many facilities have converted to products that offer shielded scalpel blades and no longer permit use of the traditional scalpel handle that requires the blade to be loaded manually.

54. Policies for safe handling of scalpels and other sharps may vary according to the institution; however, all facilities should have a sharps policy that is strictly enforced.

55. Scissors are manufactured in many different sizes and styles. Mayo and Metzenbaum scissors

are used often and are included in most general surgery instrument sets (Figure 9-2).

56. Mayo scissors are sturdy and have either a straight or curved tip. Curved Mayo scissors are used to cut heavy, tough tissue. Straight-tipped Mayo scissors are used for cutting sutures and may be used to cut gauze or disposable drapes as needed.

57. Metzenbaum scissors have a rounded tip, are more delicate than Mayo scissors, and are used to cut or dissect delicate tissue. All of these scissors open and close in the same manner as household scissors.

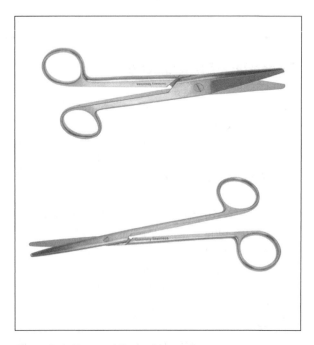

Figure 9-2 Mayo and Metzenbaum scissors
Source: Courtesy of Symmetry Surgical, Nashville, TN. Used with permission.

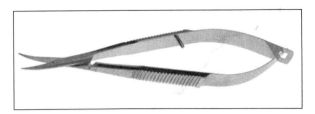

Figure 9-3 Castroviejo scissors

Source: Courtesy of Symmetry Surgical, Nashville, TN. Used with permission.

58. Spring-action scissors in which the jaws are held open are designed for more delicate surgeries, such as plastic, micro, or eye surgery. A single movement of the thumb and forefinger presses the spring together, closing the jaws. Releasing the pressure opens the jaws (Figure 9-3).

59. Examples of other sharp dissectors are osteotomes and chisels used for cutting bone; curettes and rongeurs, used for cutting bone and soft tissue; and periosteal elevators, used for separating tissue from bone or from other tissue (Figure 9-4).

60. Examples of blunt dissectors are the back end of a knife handle, a small peanut-shaped sponge, or a folded 4¾-inch gauze (Raytec) clamped firmly in the jaws of an instrument. Blunt curettes and elevators are also available.

Clamps

61. Clamps are instruments designed to hold tissue or other materials. They are manufactured in a wide variety of shapes and sizes, with tips that may be straight, curved, or angled. Some clamps are fine and delicate; others are more substantial.

62. The overall design is similar for all clamps: finger rings for holding the instrument, shafts of varying length, a joint (a screw or box lock) that joins the two halves of the instrument and permits opening and closing, a ratchet at the proximal end for locking the instrument in a closed or partially closed position, and a distal tip or jaw. The design of the jaw determines the instrument's use (Figure 9-5).

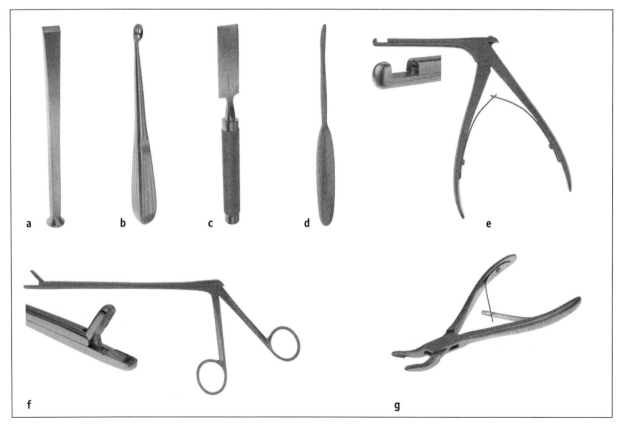

Figure 9-4 Other cutting instruments: a) chisel, b) curette, c) osteotome, d) periosteal elevator, e) Kerrison bone rongeur, f) Spurling soft tissue rongeur, g) Lambert bone rongeur

Source: Courtesy of Symmetry Surgical, Nashville, TN. Used with permission.

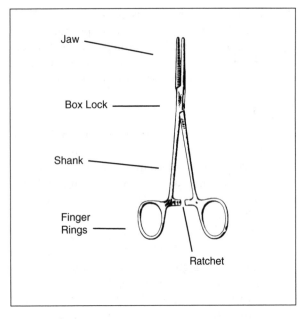

Figure 9-5 Clamp

Source: Courtesy of Jarit Instrument Company, Hawthorne, NY.

Hemostatic Clamps

63. Hemostatic clamps, commonly referred to as hemostats, are used to control bleeding. The clamping jaws of the instrument are horizontally serrated. This design allows the clamp to compress the vessel with enough force to stop bleeding. The serrations also prevent the clamp from slipping off the tissue. The scrubbed person passes clamps by holding the shaft and placing the finger rings in the surgeon's hand.

64. Common hemostats include the mosquito, Crile, Kelly (Rochester Pean), tonsil (Schnidt), and mixter (Figure 9-6).

65. Mosquitoes are small clamps that may be either curved or straight. They are most often used to clamp small bleeders in the superficial layers of tissue.

66. Criles are curved and slightly longer and heavier than mosquitoes.

67. Tonsil clamps are curved and longer than Criles. They are used where additional length is needed.

68. Kellys are straight or curved and are heavier than Crile or tonsil clamps.

69. The mixter has a right-angle tip that can be passed under a vessel to capture a suture tie. Longer mixters are useful for clamping and separating tissue in the abdominal cavity. Shorter mixters are often used to separate tissue during surgery on vasculature that is not deep within the body.

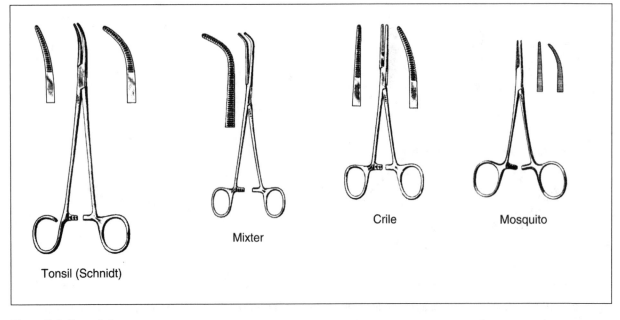

Figure 9-6 Hemostats

Source: Courtesy of Jarit Instrument Company, Hawthorne, NY.

Noncrushing Vascular Clamps

70. The jaws of vascular clamps have opposing rows of fine serrations designed to occlude a vessel without crushing it. The jaws may be straight, curved, rounded, or angled.

Occluding Clamps

71. Occluding clamps are used to clamp tissue, such as bowel or blood vessels, where prevention of leakage and minimization of tissue trauma are desired. The serrations on occluding clamps are vertical, close together, and arranged in multiple rows.

Grasping and Holding Clamps

72. Grasping or holding clamps have a variety of tip shapes. They are used for retracting tissue and to facilitate dissection and suturing. The surgeon can grasp the tissue with one hand and suture or dissect it with the other hand. Some grasping clamps are used to hold sponges, suture needles, or suture ties.

73. Common grasping clamps include Allises, Babcocks, Kochers (Ochsners), sponge forceps, towel clips, tenacula, and needle holders (Figure 9-7).

74. The tips of an Allis clamp have multiple blunt teeth that do not crush or damage tissue. Allis clamps are used on delicate tissue.

75. Babcock clamps have a curved and fenestrated tip with no teeth. A Babcock can be used to grip or enclose delicate structures such as a fallopian tube or a ureter.

76. A Kocher clamp has transverse serrations and a single heavy tooth at its tip and is useful for grasping tough tissue. Sponge forceps (ring forceps) can be used to hold tissue, but most often are used to hold a folded 4¾ -inch gauze sponge that can be used to blot or sponge fluids or blood or to retract tissue.

77. Towel clips are used to secure towels around the operative site and to hold drapes in place. Towel clips may have sharp tips that penetrate drapes or blunt tips that do not. When towel clips that penetrate the drapes are used, the points are considered contaminated; they cannot be removed and repositioned (Figure 9-8).

78. Needle holders are designed to hold a needle securely in place so that the needle does not rotate or slip. Needle holders may or may not have a locking ratchet. The surface of the jaws may be smooth, diamond-cut made from tungsten carbide, or cross-hatched (Figure 9-9). Tungsten carbide diamond-cut jaws are designed to prevent the needle from twisting and turning. Needle holders with tungsten carbide jaws are identified by their gold-plated ring handles.

79. Needle holders used for very fine sutures have a spring action rather than a ratchet action. The needle is held in place when the surgeon presses the spring together between the thumb and forefinger. When the pressure is released, the jaws open and the needle is released.

Grasping Forceps

80. Grasping and holding instruments that are not shaped as clamps are referred to as forceps or pickups (Figure 9-10). Forceps are similar to tweezers, with two arms and a spring action. They lift and hold tissue with a single movement that presses the arms together and approximates the tips; releasing the pressure separates the tips.

81. The surgeon frequently holds forceps in one hand to grasp the tissue while cutting, coagulating, separating, or suturing tissue with the other hand.

82. Forceps vary in length and sturdiness, may have vertical or horizontal serrations, and may have one or more teeth at the tips. Toothed forceps are used to hold thick tissue, such as skin that may require extra grip. Nontoothed forceps hold more delicate tissue and cause minimal trauma.

Retractors

83. Retractors are designed to facilitate visualization of the operative field while preventing trauma to the surrounding tissue.

84. Retractors are available in many sizes and shapes. Some retractors require that the surgeon or assistant exert pressure to retract tissue from the operative site; other retractors are self-retaining.

85. Common non-self-retaining retractors include rakes, Richardsons, Deavers, Army-Navys, Parkers, and malleables (ribbons) (Figure 9-11). Slender, colored, radiopaque silicon bands (vessel loops) can be used to retract delicate structure.

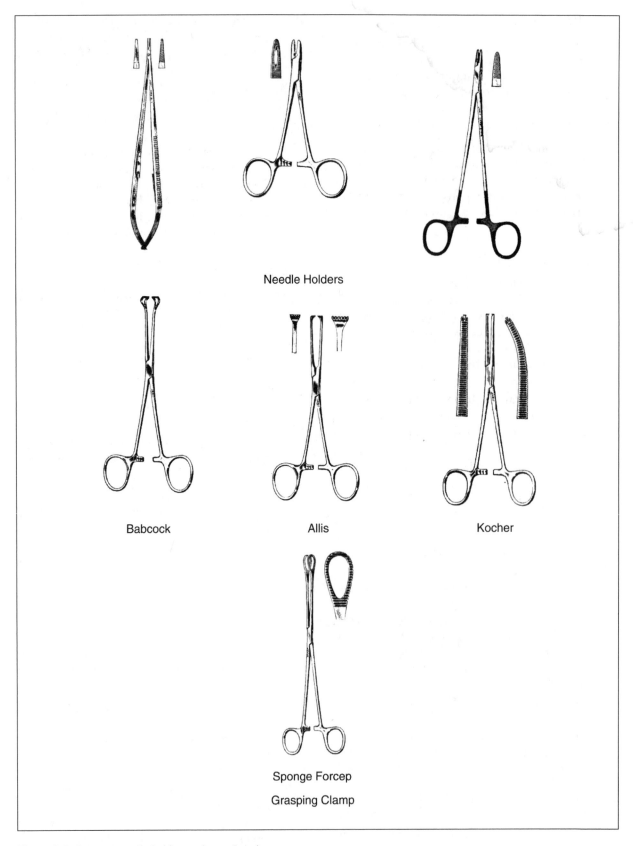

Figure 9-7 Common needle holders and grasping clamps

Source: Courtesy of Jarit Instrument Company, Hawthorne, NY.

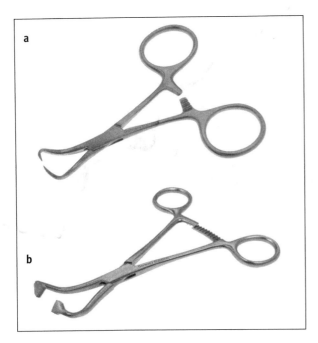

Figure 9-8 Towel clips: a) sharp tips, b) blunt tips
Source: Courtesy of Symmetry Surgical, Nashville, TN. Used with permission.

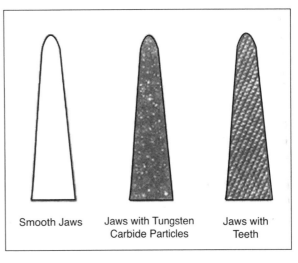

Figure 9-9 Needle holder jaws
Source: Courtesy of Ethicon, Inc., Somerville, NJ.

Smooth Jaws   Jaws with Tungsten Carbide Particles   Jaws with Teeth

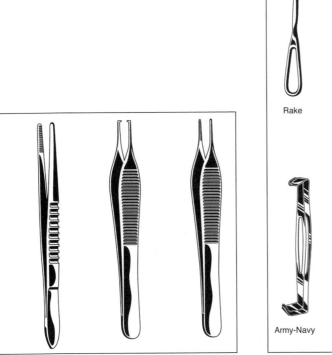

Figure 9-10 Tissue forceps with and without teeth
Source: Courtesy of Jarit Instrument Company, Hawthorne, NY.

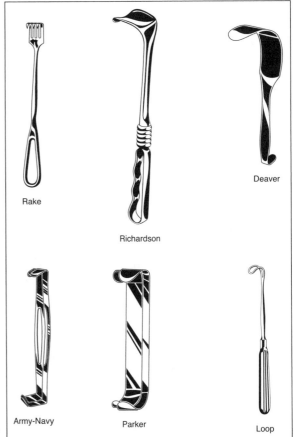

Rake   Richardson   Deaver

Army-Navy   Parker   Loop

Figure 9-11 Handheld retractors
Source: Courtesy of Jarit Instrument Company, Hawthorne, NY.

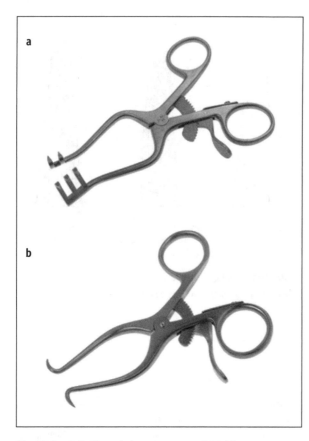

Figure 9-12 Self-retaining retractors: a) Weitlaner retractor, b) Gelpi retractor

Source: Courtesy of Symmetry Surgical, Nashville, TN. Used with permission.

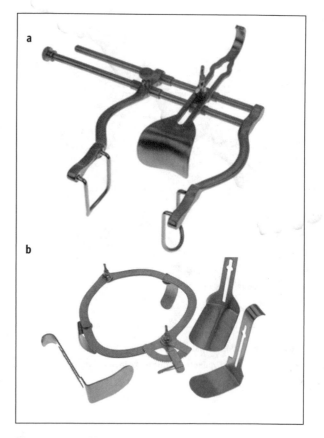

Figure 9-13 Self-retaining abdominal retractors with assorted blades: a) Balfour abdominal retractor, b) O'Sullivan-O'Connor abdominal retractor

Source: Courtesy of Symmetry Surgical, Nashville, TN. Used with permission.

86. Weitlaners and Gelpis are self-retaining retractors (Figure 9-12). A Balfour is an abdominal self-retaining retractor with a blade to hold back internal structures (Figure 9-13). Some self-retaining retractors, such as the Bookwalter and Thompson retractors, can be attached to the operating table and support blades of various lengths and configurations (Figure 9-14).

Suction

87. Suction instruments are used to remove blood and other fluids from the operative field.

88. Frazier, Yankauer, and Poole suction devices may be included in a basic instrument set (Figure 9-15).

89. A Frazier-tip suction is an angled tube that comes in a variety of diameters. A small-diameter Frazier suction is used where capillary bleeding and small amounts of fluid are

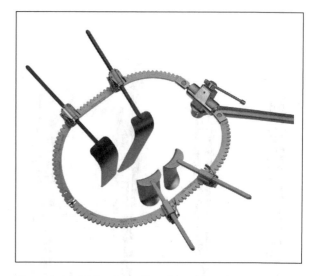

Figure 9-14 Bookwalter adjustable self-retaining retractor (attaches to the OR table)

Source: Courtesy of Symmetry Surgical, Nashville, TN. Used with permission.

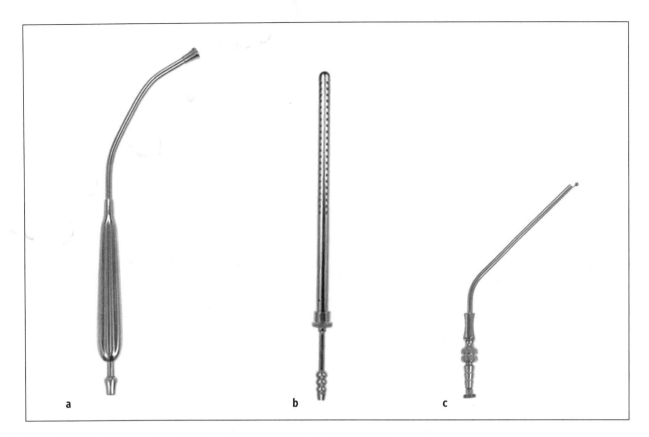

Figure 9-15 Suction cannulas: a) Yankauer, b) Poole, c) Frazier (with stylet)
Source: Courtesy of Symmetry Surgical, Nashville, TN. Used with permission.

encountered so as to maintain a dry field without the use of sponges. Some Frazier suction devices incorporate an active electrode into the tip so they may be used to coagulate tissue as well as suction fluid.

90. A Yankauer suction is a slightly angled tube that is used in most general surgeries, and in procedures involving the mouth and throat.

91. A Poole suction is a straight tube with an outer perforated shield that acts as a filter. It is useful where large amounts of blood or fluid collect and where the surgical area is deep, such as a body cavity.

Other

92. Thousands of instruments have been designed for specific surgical specialties. For example, each manufacturer of joint implants has developed a set of instruments specific to that implant.

93. Many powered instruments have also been developed. Drills and saws of various types are

available for orthopedic, neurologic, and ear, nose, and throat (ENT) surgery.

94. The phenomenal growth in minimally invasive surgery has led to the development of a wide variety of rigid and flexible fiber-optic endoscopes and accessory instruments.

95. Rigid scopes have become commonplace in the operating room and are used in every surgical specialty. Cystoscopes, hysteroscopes, arthroscopes, and laparoscopes are the most widely used rigid endoscopes.

96. An increasing number of small-diameter semi-rigid and flexible fiber-optic endoscopes, such as sinus scopes, ureteroscopes, and cholenephroscopes, are available as well.

97. Large-diameter flexible fiber-optic endoscopes are more commonly used in endoscopy units for gastrointestinal procedures.

98. In the early days of minimally invasive surgery, the surgeon inserted a rigid endoscope attached to a light source into the patient's body and

observed the internal organ or site by looking though the endoscope eyepiece (Figure 9-16). Today, the endoscope is more likely to be coupled to a camera, or the camera may be incorporated into the endoscope; in both cases, the image is displayed on a video monitor.

99. Accessory instruments for minimally invasive surgery are designed to dissect, cut, grasp, cauterize, clip, suction, or suture tissue. The typical design includes a ring handle for holding the instrument; a long, small-diameter, insulated shaft for insertion into the patient; and a tip or jaw engineered for a specific purpose (Figure 9-17). Scissors, cautery, grasping devices, ligating clip holder, and suction tips are commonly used.

100. With the advent of robotic surgery, another set of specialized instruments has been developed.

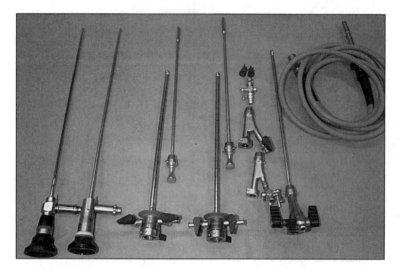

Figure 9-16 Scopes
Source: Courtesy of Spivey Station Surgery Center, Jonesboro, GA.

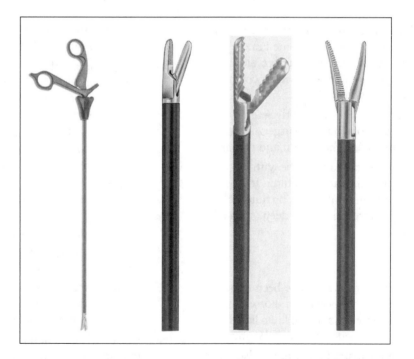

Figure 9-17 Laparoscopic scissors, laparoscopic instrument tip examples
Source: Courtesy of Aesculap, Inc., Center Valley, PA. Used with permission.

Section Questions

<image name="www button" />

1. Which negative outcomes can occur when cutting instruments are not sharp? [Ref 46]

2. How does the scrubbed person prevent injury when attaching or detaching a scalpel blade from the handle? [Ref 49]

3. Describe safe techniques for passing sharp instruments among scrubbed personnel. [Refs 51–52]

4. What are the primary functions of the two most commonly used surgical scissors? [Refs 55–57]

5. Beside scalpels and scissors, which other instruments are considered "sharp"? [Ref 59]

6. What do surgeons use for blunt dissection? [Ref 60]

7. Describe the overall design of a clamp. [Ref 62]

8. What is the purpose of the horizontal serrations on hemostatic clamps? [Ref 63]

9. What distinguishes a vascular clamp? [Ref 70]

10. Describe the various uses for grasping and holding clamps. [Ref 72]

11. Name six different grasping/holding clamps and explain how they differ. [Refs 73–79]

12. What is the purpose of a forceps or pickup? [Refs 80–81]

13. Why are there both forceps with teeth and forceps without teeth? [Ref 82]

14. What is the purpose of using a retractor during a surgical procedure? [Ref 83]

15. Which type of retractor does not require an assistant to hold it in position? [Ref 84]

16. What is the purpose of suction instruments? [Ref 87]

17. Describe some uses for semi-rigid and fiber-optic endoscopes. [Ref 96]

18. Describe the relationship of instruments and camera in minimally invasive surgery as currently practiced [Ref 98]

19. Which types of instruments have been developed to support minimally invasive surgery? [Ref 99]

20. Which other types of surgery might require specialized surgical instrumentation? [Ref 100]

Care and Handling

Cleaning

101. Instruments contaminated with blood, body fluids, or tissue should be rinsed during and immediately following the procedure. When blood or other debris is permitted to dry on an instrument, it can harden and become trapped in joints, lumens, and serrations, or between scissor blades, causing malfunction, facilitating rusting and pitting, and making final cleaning more difficult.

102. Debris and organic material should not be permitted to dry on instruments. Material that has dried within lumens is very difficult to remove and may remain attached to the lumen during washing and sterilization, interfering with the sterilization process.

103. Dead organisms in organic debris can cause pyrogenic or foreign-body reactions (AAMI, 2011, p. 64). Improperly processed flexible endoscopes have also been responsible for contaminated specimens.

104. During the procedure, instruments should be kept free of gross soil by wiping with a sponge/lap pad moistened with sterile water. Instruments with a lumen are kept open and free of debris by irrigating the lumen with sterile water, using a syringe and irrigating below the surface of water to prevent aerosolization of debris.

105. Tenacious biofilms can form on the surface of instruments that remain in contaminated water or when debris is allowed to dry. Instruments should be cleaned as soon as possible.

106. Instruments should be cleaned as soon as possible after surgery. When a delay is necessary,

instruments should be treated with an enzymatic solution, foam, or gel spray that prevents adherence of debris. Instruments should be transported to the decontamination area in leak-proof containers, covered trays, or specially designed carts. These should be labeled to indicate the presence of biohazardous contents (AAMI, 2011 pp. 47–48).

107. AAMI recommends washing instruments in an automated washer-disinfector or washer-decontaminator. In the absence of an automated system, instruments may be cleaned manually (AAMI, 2011, p. 57).

108. In the presence of gross or dried-on debris, some precleaning may be necessary. Instruments that can tolerate immersion may be presoaked in a proteolytic enzymatic detergent according to the instrument manufacturer's and the detergent manufacturer's recommendations.

109. Personnel who are responsible for washing instruments should be attired in protective gloves, waterproof aprons, and face shields.

110. Ultrasonic cleaners may also be used to remove debris; however, gross debris should be removed prior to ultrasonic cleaning.

111. Ultrasonic cleaning uses sound waves in a process called cavitation to remove debris from all parts of the instrument. Ultrasonic waves generate tiny bubbles that collapse or implode, creating tiny vacuums that pull soil from the instrument.

112. Ultrasonic cleaning is not appropriate for all instruments, and an instrument's compatibility with the ultrasonic cleaning process must be determined before its use. For example, ultrasonic cleaning will destroy the seal on lensed instruments.

113. Following ultrasonic cleaning, rinse instruments to remove loose debris, and lubricate instruments with movable parts with an antimicrobial water-soluble lubricant. The lubricant should be used according to the manufacturer's instructions.

114. Automated cleaning systems are designed to wash, rinse, sonicate (use ultrasound), disinfect, and lubricate instruments.

115. Lensed instruments, flexible scopes, powered drills, and instruments that cannot tolerate high temperatures or immersion in water cannot be processed in an automated washing system. These devices must be cleaned manually according to the manufacturer's instructions. For some specialized instruments, such as flexible endoscopes, specialized cleaning equipment is available.

General Guidelines for Care and Cleaning

116. All instruments should be handled and cleaned according to the manufacturer's instructions. General guidelines for care and cleaning of instruments include the following points:

- Instruments should be used only for the purpose for which they were designed. Misuse can result in improper alignment, dulling of sharp edges, and cracking of joints or tips.
- During use, instruments may be kept clean by wiping and frequent rinsing in sterile distilled water (immersion).
- Instruments should be handled gently and individually or in small lots.
- Instruments should be placed carefully, not tossed, into the splash basin. Entangled instruments can become misshapen or damaged.
- Lighter, more delicate instruments should be placed on top of heavy, sturdier instruments. Delicate instruments can be damaged easily by the weight of heavier instruments.
- Following a surgical procedure, instruments should be cleaned promptly. Instruments are washed and rinsed in water, not in saline. Prolonged exposure to blood and saline can cause corrosion and pitting of stainless steel. To reduce the potential for spotting caused by alkaline mineral deposits, demineralized or distilled rinse water is preferred.
- All instruments opened for a surgical procedure, whether or not they were actually used, are considered contaminated and must be decontaminated and cleaned prior to resterilization. Decontamination is the process that renders instruments safe to handle. In some circumstances, cleaning alone may be sufficient to achieve decontamination; however, a wash cycle followed by a thermal or chemical disinfection cycle is programmed into most automated cleaning systems.
- In preparation for cleaning, all hinges and joints should be opened to expose box locks and serrations where blood and debris may be concealed.

- Some automated cleaning systems provide special attachments for instruments with lumens. Lumened instruments should be attached to irrigating ports within the washer when available.

- Some instrument sets, especially those intended for orthopedic surgery, are housed in specialty trays imprinted with a template inscribed with the name of each instrument and where in the set the instrument should be placed. The instruments fit snugly into the outlined slots. The template makes it easy for the scrubbed person to select the instruments that the surgeon requests, and it helps SPD personnel reassemble the set correctly. While it is tempting to keep instruments in their slots throughout processing, best practice requires that the instruments be removed from their slots, washed, and then returned to their indicated slots.

- All instruments with removable parts should be disassembled for cleaning.

- Instruments should be washed with a noncorrosive, low-sudsing, free-rinsing detergent, with as neutral a pH as possible. Rinsing may not completely remove a high-sudsing detergent, which could cause spotting and staining.

- Alkaline detergent is an excellent choice for cleaning organic soil, and acid detergent is a good option for removing inorganic soil. However, a neutral pH is recommended because alkaline detergents can stain and corrode instruments and acid detergents can cause pitting.

- Enzyme detergents consist of a detergent and one or more enzymes that break down organic debris. Enzyme detergents may be designed to remove fats or protein and should be selected accordingly.

- During manual cleaning, use only soft brushes to clean serrations and joints. Steel wool, scouring powder, and other abrasives can cause scratches and remove protective finishes.

- Instruments should be held below the surface of the water and washed in a manner that prevents splashing and aerosolization of debris.

- Use only water-soluble lubricants. Oil-based lubricants leave a residue that can compromise the sterilization process by preventing steam contact during the steam sterilization process (AAMI, 2011, p. 59).

Inspection

117. Inspect instruments prior to, during, and after surgery. Inspection is an ongoing process, the majority of which occurs after decontamination and prior to the assembly of sets in preparation for sterilization. Instruments are inspected to ensure that they are clean and in proper working condition. Instruments that fail inspection should be removed and sent for repair. If instruments need sharpening, they should not be put back into sets.

118. Instruments should be inspected by the scrubbed person just prior to surgery. Although time may permit only a cursory inspection, this check is sometimes sufficient to detect a defective instrument that could result in a delay in surgery or cause a patient injury.

119. During surgery, the surgeon may detect an instrument malfunction that is not immediately visible and can be observed only when the instrument is used. For instance, tissue scissors should not be tested on other materials. When this occurs, the instrument should be set aside and marked clearly for repair.

120. Inspection should include the following steps:

    - Clamps, scissors, and forceps are checked to ensure that tips are even and that they approximate properly. Tips should be in alignment and should not overlap.

    - To be in perfect alignment, the serrations on the jaws of the clamps must mesh perfectly. To test how well the serrations mesh, clamps are fully closed and held up to a light. If the serrations mesh perfectly, no light will be visible between the jaws. Misuse of clamps often results in misalignment.

    - Instruments that feature a tooth or teeth at the tips are checked to ensure that they approximate and open freely. Tips that are not aligned properly will stick together. Release will be sluggish and can result in torn tissue.

    - Ratchets and hinges must close easily and hold firmly. If the jaws of clamps spring open during use, they may be misaligned, the ratchet teeth may be worn, or the shanks may be bent or have insufficient tension. To test the ratchet, the instrument is closed on the first ratchet tooth and held by the box lock; the ratchet portion is then tapped against a solid surface. If the instrument springs open, the ratchets are faulty. A clamp that springs open when clamped on a blood vessel can cause injury to the patient.

- Joints and hinges should move easily. Stiff joints may indicate inadequate cleaning, a need for lubrication, or a defective instrument.

- Box locks are inspected for cracks and looseness. Excessive play in the box lock indicates an alignment problem. Clamps with loose box locks will not hold tissue securely. Cracked box locks are an indication of impending breakage. Broken instruments have the potential for causing patient injury.

- Scissor cutting edges must be smooth and sharp. Blades are inspected for burrs and chips. Scissor blades with burrs and chips will not cut cleanly and can cause trauma to tissue. Tips of Mayo and Metzenbaum scissors should cut through four layers of gauze with little resistance.

- Inspect the edges of sharp instruments, such as osteotomes, chisels, and rongeurs, for chips, nicks, or dents.

- Needle holders should hold a needle securely without slipping or rotation. Test this by securing a needle in the jaws and locking the instrument in the second ratchet tooth. If the needle can be easily moved by hand, the holder is worn and needs repair or replacement.

- If plated instruments are in use, they must be inspected for chips that can harbor microorganisms and for worn spots that can rust during autoclaving. (Although most instruments are made of stainless steel, a few older plated instruments remain in use. Plated instruments are made by putting a chromium, cadmium, nickel, or silver coating directly on forged steel.)

- Because rigid endoscopes may become damaged during repeated sterilization, the scrubbed person may do a quick check for clarity prior to surgery by holding the scope toward light and looking through the eyepiece, holding the scope far enough away from the eye so as not to risk contamination. A cloudy lens may indicate a leak in the lens seal with a subsequent accumulation of moisture inside. A partially blocked view or black spots in the field of vision may indicate a crack in one or more of the internal glass lenses or rods.

- More sophisticated tests that assess the resolution, clarity, and projected image of rigid endoscopes are typically conducted by SPD personnel just prior to packaging. Testing should also be done at the time of purchase and after repairs.

- Repairs that are poorly made will result in expensive repeated repairs. The ability to compare scope quality after repair with baseline data will allow the person responsible for managing scopes to evaluate repair services. The cost of repairing rigid endoscopes can consume more of the annual operating-room instrument budget than the purchase of new endoscopes.

- Inspect flexible fiber-optic endoscopes for obvious external defects to the outer sheath. Rotate positioning controls to ensure they move smoothly and easily. Hold the lens to the light while observing the distal end for tiny black spots. Black spots indicate a broken fiber, and broken fibers result in decreased light transmission.

- Inspect fiber-optic cords for nicks. Attach a cord to a light source and observe the distal end for tiny black spots that indicate broken fibers that will result in diminished illumination.

- Connect the camera to a video monitor and observe the picture. The coupler and the controls should move easily.

- Determine that all parts of a multipart instrument are present and that instruments are assembled correctly. Loose pins and screws can cause an instrument to malfunction, and a part can be lost inside a patient.

- Inspect instruments with insulation to verify that all insulation is intact. Insulation cracks or flaws can cause a patient burn that could lead to serious injury such as peritonitis, or even death.

Section Questions

www

1. Why is rinsing debris immediately from instruments important? [Refs 101–103]

2. How are instruments kept clean during a surgical procedure? [Ref 104]

3. What can happen to instruments that remain in contaminated water? [Ref 105]

4. When instruments cannot be cleaned immediately following a procedure, how should they be managed? [Ref 106]

5. Which type of equipment does AAMI recommend as an alternative for manual cleaning for removing debris from instruments? [Ref 107]

6. Which protective equipment should be worn by the personnel responsible for washing instruments? [Ref 109]

7. Explain how the process of cavitation removes debris from instruments. [Ref 111]

8. Why is ultrasonic cleaning inappropriate for lensed instruments? [Ref 112]

9. What is done with instruments following ultrasonic cleaning? [Ref 113]

10. Besides lensed instruments, which other instruments cannot tolerate high temperatures or immersion in water? [Ref 115]

11. Who is the final authority for how any instrument should be handled and cleaned? [Ref 116]

12. When layering instruments in a pan, which instruments should be placed on the bottom and which on top? [Ref 116]

13. Which fluids can cause corrosion and pitting of stainless steel? [Ref 116]

14. In what should instruments be soaked to reduce the potential for spotting from alkaline mineral deposits? [Ref 116]

15. Following a surgical procedure, how are the instruments that were opened but not used during the procedure handled? [Ref 116]

16. How can you ensure that all surfaces of an instrument are exposed so that blood and debris is not concealed? [Ref 116]

17. When instruments come in trays with specific slots for each instrument, how are cleaning and decontamination of the instruments handled? [Ref 116]

18. How do you prepare an instrument with multiple parts for cleaning and disinfection? [Ref 116]

19. Why must instruments be held below the surface of the water while being washed? [Ref 116]

20. Why is water-soluble lubricant used for surgical instruments? [Ref 116]

21. When does the process of inspecting instruments occur? [Refs 117–118]

22. What should you look for when inspecting clamps, scissors, and forceps? [Ref 120]

23. What makes the teeth of forceps stick together? [Ref 120]

24. How can you test the ratchet of a clamp to be sure that it is functioning properly? [Ref 120]

25. How can you test the sharpness of Mayo and Metzenbaum scissors? [Ref 120]

26. How do you test a needle holder to see if it holds needles securely? [Ref 120]

27. What is the significance of a cloudy endoscope lens? [Ref 120]

28. What is the significance of a partially blocked view or black spots in the field of an endoscope lens? [Ref 120]

29. What do tiny black spots in a fiber-optic cord signify? [Ref 120]

30. Which serious outcome can result from faulty insulation on an instrument? [Ref 120]

● ● ● **References**

Association for the Advancement of Medical Instrumentation (AAMI) (2011). *Comprehensive Guide to Steam Sterilization and Sterility Assurance in Health Care Facilities.* ANSI/AAMI ST79:2011. Arlington, VA: AAMI.

Association of periOperative Registered Nurses (AORN) (2012). *Perioperative Standards and Recommended Practices.* Denver, CO: AORN.

Association of periOperative Registered Nurses (AORN) (2011). *Perioperative Nursing Data Set.* Denver, CO: AORN.

Occupational Safety and Health Administration (OSHA) (2012a). *Bloodborne Pathogens* 1910.1030 (d)(4)(iii)(b). 56 Fed. Reg. 64004 (2011, December). Washington, DC: OSHA.

Occupational Safety and Health Administration (OSHA) (2012b). *Enforcement procedures for the occupational exposure to bloodborne pathogens,* Directive CPL 02-02-069. Washington, DC: OSHA. Available at: www.osha.gov/pls/oshaweb/owadisp.show_document?p_table=DIRECTIVES&p_id=2570. Accessed June 2012.

Pyrek K (2012). FDA, AAMI examine medical device reporting issues. *Infection Control Today* (January 6, 2012). Available at: www.infectioncontroltoday.com/articles/2012/01/fda-aami-examine-medical-device-reprocessing-issues.aspx. Accessed June 2012.

Tosh P, Disbot M, Duffy J, et al. (2011). Outbreak of *Pseudomonas aeruginosa* surgical site infections after arthroscopic procedures: Texas, 2009. *Infect Control Hosp Epidemiol*;32(12):1179–1186.

Post-Test

Read each question carefully. Each question may have more than one correct answer.

1. Name one important infection control issue related to surgical instruments.
   a. Improperly cleaned instruments can cause infection.
   b. TASS is the result of poorly cleaned instruments.
   c. Dirty instruments can cause a delay in the surgical procedure.
   d. Improperly cleaned instruments can cause a foreign-body reaction.

2. The majority of surgical instruments are made of which material?
   a. Titanium
   b. Vitallium
   c. Steel
   d. Plastic

3. Passivation is the process during instrument manufacture that
   a. puts an ebony finish on the instrument to reduce glare.
   b. protects the surface and minimizes corrosion.
   c. hardens the metal and ensures that the instrument will retain its shape.
   d. removes spots and stains from the instrument.

4. Rake, hook, and ribbon retractors are examples of instruments named
   a. scientifically.
   b. for the inventor.
   c. by visual description.
   d. by function.

5. Nursing responsibilities related to surgical instrumentation include
   a. familiarity with all names by which an instrument can be called.
   b. the ability to determine whether an instrument has been adequately prepared for use.
   c. cleaning and disinfecting all instruments used during a surgical procedure.
   d. recognizing the material from which each instrument on the sterile field is made.

6. When instruments for a procedure have been borrowed from the vendor or another facility, the perioperative nurse must ensure that the instruments
   a. are sterile when they arrive.
   b. are delivered to the facility in time for the procedure.
   c. are accompanied by the vendor's representative in case questions about the instruments arise.
   d. have been inspected, inventoried, cleaned, packaged, and sterilized in-house.

7. Which of the following promotes safety in the handling of scalpels and blades?
   a. The scrubbed person loads the blade onto the scalpel handle by hand.
   b. The surgeon loads the scalpel blade himself or herself.
   c. The blade is loaded onto the scalpel handle using an instrument such as a needle holder.
   d. The Needlestick Safety and Preventions Act (2000) requires that only disposable, preassembled scalpels can be used.

8. Which of the following measures most effectively promotes safety in the passing of sharp instruments to the surgeon?

   a. The surgeon and the scrubbed person hold the instrument at the same time.

   b. The scrubbed person places the sharp instrument in a neutral zone and surgeon retrieves it himself or herself.

   c. The scrubbed person passes the scalpel with the blade facing the surgeon's palm.

   d. The scrubbed person and the surgeon announce their intention to pass a sharp instrument.

9. The overall design that is similar for all clamps includes the following components:

   a. finger rings, a joint, a ratchet, and a distal tip or jaw.

   b. finger rings, a screw joint, and serrated jaws.

   c. finger rings, a ratchet, and jaws with teeth.

   d. finger rings, a box lock, and jaws that cannot damage tissue.

10. For which purposes are hemostatic clamps used?

    a. Grasp tissue.

    b. Control bleeding.

    c. Approximate tissue.

    d. Hold sponges for blotting tissue.

11. Babcock and Allis clamps have which characteristics in common?

    a. They are vascular clamps.

    b. They are utility clamps used in many different ways.

    c. They are used on delicate tissues.

    d. They are heavy-duty clamps.

12. Another name for grasping forceps is

    a. tweezers.

    b. clamp.

    c. retractor.

    d. pickups.

13. What is the purpose of a retractor?

    a. Facilitate visualization of the operative field.

    b. Hold the suture in place during wound closure.

    c. Give the surgical assistant something to do.

    d. Keep the assistant's hands out of the operative field.

14. Frazier, Yankauer, and Poole are three types of

    a. hemostatic clamps.

    b. retractors.

    c. needle holders.

    d. suction devices.

15. Cystoscopes, hysteroscopes, and arthroscopes are examples of

    a. jointed instruments.

    b. rigid endoscopes.

    c. flexible endoscopes.

    d. powered endoscopes.

16. The typical design of accessory instrumentation for minimally invasive surgical procedures includes the following elements:

   a. ring handle; long, small-diameter, insulated shaft; and tip or jaw.

   b. grip handle, long shaft, fiber-optic cable, and atraumatic tip.

   c. ring handle; long, large-diameter shaft; and insulated tip or jaw.

   d. grip handle, long insulated shaft, and fiber-optic tip or jaw.

17. Instruments should be rinsed during and immediately following procedures because

   a. debris causes infection.

   b. dried debris makes final cleaning more difficult.

   c. debris dried in box locks cannot be removed.

   d. debris dried on cutting surfaces dulls the blades.

18. Cavitation used by ultrasonic cleaners involves

   a. sound waves that create bubbles that float debris to the surface.

   b. ultrasonic waves that enhance the efficacy of the detergent.

   c. sound waves that generate tiny bubbles that implode, pulling soil from the instrument.

   d. heating the detergent so that it dissolves soil more effectively.

19. The scrub person keeps instruments clean during the procedure by wiping and frequent rinsing in

   a. saline.

   b. detergent solution.

   c. enzymatic solution.

   d. sterile water.

20. To test the function of a ratchet,

   a. close the ratchet to the first tooth, grasp the box lock, and tap against a solid surface.

   b. close the ratchet tightly, grasp the box lock, and tap against a solid surface.

   c. close the ratchet to the first tooth, grasp the rings, and tap against a solid surface.

   d. close the ratchet tightly, grasp the rings, and tap against a solid surface.

• •

Competency Checklist: Instrumentation—Care and Handling

Under "Observer's Initials," enter initials upon successful achievement of the competency. Enter N/A if the competency is not appropriate for the institution.

Name _____

	Observer's Initials	Date
1. Instrument inspection, prior to procedure:		
a. Tips approximate	_____	_____
b. Serrations mesh	_____	_____
c. Ratchets hold securely	_____	_____
d. Jaws open and close easily	_____	_____
e. Cutting instruments are sharp	_____	_____
f. Needle holders hold needle securely	_____	_____
g. Scopes are clear	_____	_____
h. Electrode insulation intact	_____	_____
i. Camera relays image to monitor	_____	_____
2. Scalpel loaded and passed safely	_____	_____
3. Instruments handled carefully (placed, not tossed into basin)	_____	_____
4. Instruments cleaned periodically during procedure (rinsed, wiped, irrigated with water)	_____	_____
5. Instruments used only as intended (e.g., does not open medication vial with a Kocher clamp)	_____	_____
6. Instruments contained/covered in preparation for transport to the decontamination area	_____	_____
7. Instruments awaiting washing are moistened with enzymatic instrument spray	_____	_____
8. Wears personal protective equipment when washing instrument	_____	_____
9. Washes instrument(s) below the surface of the water	_____	_____
10. Operates ultrasonic cleaner correctly	_____	_____

Observer's Signature   Initials   Date

_____

Orientee's Signature

_____

10

Prevention of Injury: Wound Management

Nursing Diagnoses: Desired Patient Outcomes

Potential Injury

1. Patients undergoing surgery are at risk for compromised or interrupted wound healing and infection.

2. Wound dehiscence is the partial or complete separation of the wound edges after wound closure.

3. Wound evisceration is the actual protrusion of the abdominal viscera through the incision.

4. Both wound dehiscence and evisceration are relatively uncommon; however, patients who undergo abdominal and pelvic surgery are at highest risk of these complications.

5. The incidence of wound dehiscence is lowest in patients younger than 44 years of age and highest in patients older than age 75 (Agency for Healthcare Research and Quality [AHRQ], 2010).

6. Many factors determine the patient's risk for injury related to wound closure.

   - Dehiscence or evisceration that occurs on days 1 to 3 postoperatively is usually the result of inadequate wound closure.

   - Occurrences after the third postoperative day are often the result of excessive vomiting or coughing, infection, distention, or dehydration.

   - Patients with preexisting conditions, such as obesity, diabetes, malignancy, immunocompromise, dehydration, or malnourishment with hypoproteinemia, may experience delayed or complicated wound healing, which usually accounts for wound separation that occurs 2 or more weeks postoperatively.

7. Aseptic technique, suture materials, and surgical technique also influence wound healing. The majority of surgical wound infections are initiated along or adjacent to suture lines (Berry & Kohn, 2013, p. 553). A break in aseptic technique as well as poor surgical technique can contribute to wound infection. Suture materials vary in their ability to avoid infection.

Desired Patient Outcomes/Criteria

8. The desired outcomes for the patient who undergoes surgery are freedom from injury and infection related to wound closure.

9. Evaluation criteria include absence of the following conditions:

   - Dehiscence or evisceration

   - Excessive scar formation

   - Wound-site infection, including abscess, serous drainage, cellulitis, fever 72 hours postoperatively, redness, and pain or swelling 72 hours postoperatively

Surgical Wounds

Surgical Wound Classification

10. Surgical wound classifications used by the Centers for Disease Control and Prevention (CDC) were introduced by the National Academy of Sciences in 1964 (Table 10-1).
    Class I: clean
    Class II: clean contaminated
    Class III: contaminated
    Class IV: dirty or infected

11. *Clean wound* (Class I):

    - The gastrointestinal (GI), genitourinary, and respiratory tracts are not entered.

    - No inflammation is encountered.

    - There has been no break in aseptic technique.

12. Examples of clean surgical procedures include hernia repair, carpal tunnel repair, total joint replacement, and cataract extraction.

13. Class I wounds usually do not have a drain and are closed by primary union. The wound edges are brought together, and healing occurs with minimal edema or discharge with no localized infection.

14. The majority of surgical wounds are Class I. Most are elective surgeries and are not predisposed to infection (Ethicon, 2007, p. 6).

15. *Clean contaminated wound* (Class II):

    - The GI, genitourinary, or respiratory tract is entered under planned, controlled means.

    - Surgeries involving the biliary tract, appendix, vagina, and oropharynx are included in this category provided there is no major break in aseptic technique, no spillage occurs, and no infection is present.

16. Examples of clean contaminated procedures include cholecystectomy, cystoscopy, hysterectomy, bronchoscopy, and intestinal resection when done under controlled circumstances.

17. *Contaminated wound* (Class III):

    - Gross contamination is present without obvious infection.

    - Incisions in which acute, nonpurulent inflammation or gross spillage from the GI tract is present.

    - A major break in aseptic technique occurs.

    - Open fresh accidental wounds are included in this category.

Table 10-1	Surgical Wound Classification			
Class	Class I—Clean	Class II Clean— contaminated	Class III contaminated	Class IV Dirty—infected
Description	• Non traumatic • No infection • No break in technique • No involvement of respiratory, gastrointestinal, or genitourinary tract • Elective C-section without rupture of membranes or trial of labor	• Non-traumatic wound • Inflamed • Minor break in technique • Involves gastrointestinal, respiratory, or genitor urinary tracts (without significant spillage)	• Fresh traumatic wound • Major break in technique • Gross spillage from the gastrointestinal tract • Genito urinary or biliary tracts entered • Acute non-purulent inflammation	• Dirty operative or traumatic wound • Delayed treatment of traumatic wound • Fecal contamination • Foreign body • Retained devitalized tissue • Acute bacterial inflammation or perforated viscus
Examples	• Vascular procedures • Neurological procedures (not inflamed or infected) • Endocrine procedures • Eye surgery (not inflamed, infected, no foreign body) • Orthopedic procedures • Penile prosthesis • Exploratory lap without bowel involvement • Placement of central venous access catheter • Scheduled Caesarian section	• Exploratory lap with bowel involvement • Transection of appendix or cholecystic duct (no infected bile or urine) • Replacement of central venous access catheter • Thoracic procedures • Amputation • Laparoscopy • Colonoscopy • gastroscopy • GU procedures • Ear surgery • Nose/oropharynx procedures • GYN procedures • Hysterectomy • Emergency Caesarean section	• Inflammation • Gross spillage • Fresh accidental wound	• Infected • I&D abscess • Wound debridement
Notes		Any wound open for drainage II (except total hip/knee) Removing old implants (wires, pins, etc...) Re-operation at the same site	Foreign bodies in a wound (bullets, etc...)	

Source: Adapted from University of Connecticut Health Center Department of Surgery: Surgical Wound Classification. Available at: http://nursing.uchc.edu/unit_manuals/perioperative/or/docs/Surgical%20Wound%20Classification.pdf .

18. Examples of contaminated procedures include gunshot wounds, colon resection with GI spillage, and rectal procedures.

19. *Dirty or infected wound* (Class IV):
    - An old traumatic wound with dead tissue exists.
    - An infectious process is present.

20. Examples of dirty or infected procedures include colon resection for ruptured diverticulitis, appendectomy for ruptured appendix, and amputation of a gangrenous appendage.

21. The wound classification system is an important predictor of postoperative outcomes. Surgical site infection (SSI) rates increase as wounds progress from clean to dirty. A large analysis of SSIs based on wound classification (Ortega et al., 2012) demonstrated that infection rates were lower than those reported over the last 60 years, particularly in contaminated and dirty wounds. The overall rates for SSIs were 2.6% in clean wounds, 6.7% in clean contaminated wounds, 8.6% in contaminated wounds, and 11.8% in dirty wounds.

Wound Healing

Primary, Secondary, and Tertiary Intention or Delayed Primary Closure

22. Surgical wounds may heal by primary, secondary, or tertiary intention.

23. The preferred method of wound healing is by primary intention, involving tissue that is handled gently with minimal tissue damage, no breaks in aseptic technique, and all layers of the wound are approximated. The wound generally heals quickly with minimal scarring.

24. Wounds heal by secondary intention when the wound cannot be sutured and is left open. An example is an ulcer where the edges cannot be approximated. The wound heals from the bottom upward and is characterized by a red beefy appearance. Granulation tissue forms in the wound and gradually fills in the defect. The wound heals slowly, and considerable scarring results. Because the wound is open, there is a greater risk for infection than if the wound were healing by primary intention.

25. Wounds heal by tertiary intention or delayed primary closure when the wound is not sutured until several days after the initial surgery. Extensive tissue loss from injury, or debridement of dirty or infected tissue, may result in a wound that cannot be closed at the time of the procedure. The open wound is packed with gauze that is typically changed twice a day. If there is no sign of wound infection within 3 to 5 days and if granulation tissue is present, the wound is closed.

Process of Wound Healing

26. Wound healing is generally divided into three overlapping stages: inflammatory, proliferation, and maturation.

27. The first phase—the *inflammatory stage*—begins when the incision is made and extends through the fourth or fifth postoperative day. The "inflammatory stage" should not to be confused with the "inflammatory response" that includes redness, swelling, and pain.

28. The inflammatory stage is characterized by hemostasis and phagocytosis. Platelets form a clot; fibrin is deposited in the clot; and new blood vessels develop across the sutured wound. A thin layer of epithelial cells bridge and seal the wound.

29. The inflammatory stage is followed by the *proliferation stage*, in which the epithelial cells are regenerated, collagen is synthesized, and new blood vessels form. The new highly vascular tissue is referred to as granulation tissue.

30. The proliferation stage generally lasts 3 to 20 days. Toward the end of this stage, the wound begins to take on a raised pinkish scar and will have gained enough strength to permit suture removal.

31. The final stage of wound healing is the *maturation or remodeling stage*, which can last more than a year. Collagen continues to be deposited and is remodeled; the wound shrinks and contracts; and the thick reddish scar matures to a thin white line (Figure 10-1).

32. Tissue edges generally knit together within 48 hours but initially have little tensile strength. Collagen deposition and remodeling contribute to increased tensile strength, reaching 20% within 3 weeks and gradually achieving a maximum of 70–80% over the ensuing months (Baronoski, 2012, p. 90). Wound healing will take longer in patients who are immunocompromised, taking steroids, or otherwise debilitated.

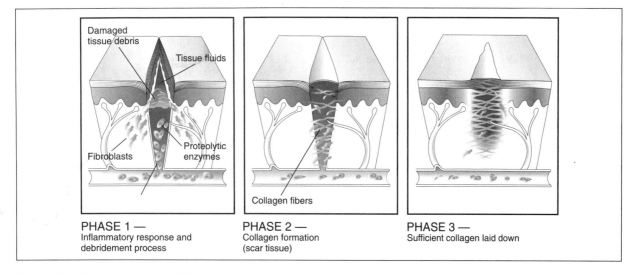

PHASE 1 —
Inflammatory response and
debridement process

PHASE 2 —
Collagen formation
(scar tissue)

PHASE 3 —
Sufficient collagen laid down

Figure 10-1 Tissue response to injury

Source: Reprinted with permission from Ethicon, Inc. (1996), Somerville, NJ.

Section Questions

1. Which adverse outcomes related to a surgical incision do all patients risk? [Ref 1]
2. Contrast wound dehiscence and wound evisceration. [Refs 2–4]
3. Which patient population is at highest risk for wound dehiscence and evisceration? [Ref 5]
4. Discuss the various causes of wound dehiscence, evisceration, and infection. [Refs 6–7]
5. What are the evaluation criteria for desired outcomes for patients who undergo surgery? [Ref 9]
6. What are the criteria for Class I (*clean*) wounds? [Ref 11]
7. List some procedures that are considered *clean* cases. [Ref 12]
8. What are some of the characteristics of *clean* cases? [Refs 13–14]
9. What are the criteria for Class II (*clean contaminated*) wounds? [Ref 15]
10. List some procedures that are considered *clean* cases. [Ref 16]
11. Which criteria indicate that a wound is *contaminated* (Class III)? [Ref 17]
12. Identify some surgical procedures that are considered *contaminated* cases. [Ref 18]
13. Which wounds make up Class IV (*dirty*)? [Ref 19]
14. List some surgical procedures that are considered *dirty* cases. [Ref 20]
15. Describe healing by primary intention. [Ref 23]
16. Describe the process of healing by secondary intention. [Ref 24]
17. Why is there a greater risk for infection with healing by secondary intention than by primary intention? [Ref 24]
18. Which types of wounds heal by tertiary intention? [Ref 25]
19. What characterizes the inflammatory stage of wound healing? [Ref 28]

(continues)

Section Questions (continued)

20. Physiologically, what occurs in the wound during phase 1 of wound healing? [Ref 28]
21. What happens in the wound during the proliferation stage? [Ref 29]
22. What is granulation tissue? [Ref 29]
23. During which phase are the sutures removed from the wound? [Ref 30]
24. What is the primary physiologic activity that occurs during *maturation* or *remodeling*? [Ref 31]
25. Which patient conditions retard wound healing? [Ref 32]

Suture Material

33. The word *suture* as a noun refers to a strand of material used to tie (ligate) a blood vessel (occlude the lumen) or a stitch or row of stitches holding together the edges of a wound or surgical incision.

34. As a verb, *suture* refers to sewing tissue together. The process of *suturing* uses *sutures* to close wounds by approximating tissue edges and holding them in anatomical alignment until healing takes place.

35. Desired characteristics of all sutures include sterility, pliability and ease of handling, consistent tensile strength appropriate to the suture size, ability to maintain the tissue layers in approximation during the healing process, and minimal resultant reactivity in tissue.

36. Tensile strength is the amount of tension or "pull" that a suture will withstand before it breaks. The tension or pull is expressed in pounds. Tensile strength determines the amount of wound support that the suture provides during the healing process. The tensile strength of any suture material should be as strong as the tensile strength (ability to withstand stress) of the tissue in which it is placed. As suture diameter decreases, suture tensile strength decreases.

37. Suture materials must be sterile when they are placed inside the patient's body. This requires packaging that permits sterile presentation to the field.

38. Suture material should be pliable and elicit minimal drag, meaning the material will slide easily through tissue. The material must tie easily, and hold a knot securely.

39. Because suture material is a foreign body, some tissue reaction is inevitable. The foreign-body reaction will persist until the suture is absorbed by the body, encapsulated, or removed. Suture selection includes material that offers the least potential for tissue reaction.

40. Many factors influence the surgeon's choice of suture. These factors include the surgeon's familiarity with the product; physical and biological characteristics of the suture material; suture coatings; healing characteristics of the tissue in which the suture will be placed; presence of infection or contamination; patient characteristics such as age, weight, and state of health; and expected postoperative course of the patient.

41. Although suture selection is the surgeon's responsibility, the perioperative nurse must be familiar with suture material, its unique characteristics, and its appropriate uses to plan for surgical procedures and to respond to unanticipated events, such as surgical complications, emergencies, and suture substitutions.

Classification of Suture Material

42. Standards and classification of suture are set by the United States Pharmacopeia (USP). Sutures are classified as monofilament or multifilament, absorbable or nonabsorbable, and coated or uncoated. Some sutures are supplied both dyed and undyed.

Monofilament and Multifilament Sutures

43. Monofilament sutures comprise a single strand of material. These sutures incur little resistance (drag) as they are drawn through tissue and as they are tied. However, knots made with monofilament suture have a tendency to loosen. Additional throws are needed to secure the knot. Monofilament sutures do not harbor bacteria and, therefore, reduce the potential for a suture-line infection.

44. Multifilament sutures comprise several strands twisted or braided together. They handle and tie securely and provide greater tensile strength than monofilament sutures. Knots in multifilament sutures are also secure without additional throws; however, they exhibit more drag as they are pulled through tissue than monofilament sutures.

45. Multifilament sutures have a certain amount of capillarity—a process that allows tissue fluid to be absorbed into the suture and travel along the strand. Any microorganisms contained in tissue fluid can be carried along the strand into the wound and cause an infection. Multifilament sutures may be coated to improve their handling characteristics and to reduce capillarity.

Section Questions

`www`

1. Identify the desirable characteristics of all sutures. [Ref 35]

2. How does the tensile strength of suture affect wound healing? [Ref 36]

3. What does it mean for a suture to have "minimal drag"? [Ref 38]

4. Why is some tissue reaction to suture inevitable? [Ref 39]

5. Which factors influence the surgeon's choice of suture? [Ref 40]

6. Why is it important for the nurse to know the unique characteristics of different suture options? [Ref 41]

7. Differentiate monofilament from multifilament suture. [Refs 43–44]

8. Which suture (monofilament or multifilament) requires extra throws to keep the knot from loosening? [Ref 43]

9. Which benefits do multifilament sutures have over monofilament? [Ref 44]

10. What is the challenge posed by the capillarity of multifilament sutures? [Ref 45]

Absorbable Suture

46. Absorbable suture is considered temporary, as it is assimilated by the body during the healing process. The assimilation time varies with the type of suture material and patient factors that may accelerate absorption. As the suture is absorbed, its tensile strength decreases.

47. Absorbable suture is made of material that is digested by body enzymes or is hydrolyzed (broken down by water in tissue fluids).

48. Absorbable suture may be either natural or synthetic. Natural absorbable sutures consist of highly purified collagen and are made from the submucosal layer of sheep intestine or the serosa layer of beef.

49. The most common natural absorbable suture is plain or chromatic surgical gut.

50. Plain surgical gut is natural suture with limited use. Its tensile strength decreases rapidly; hence the suture provides support for the wound for only 7 to 10 days. Plain gut suture is used primarily to ligate superficial blood vessels and to suture the subcutaneous tissue layer where tensile strength is not an issue.

51. Surgical gut that has been treated with a chromium salt solution is referred to as chromic gut. Chromatization makes the gut more resistant to absorption.

52. Chromic gut provides more support for healing tissues than plain gut. It retains tensile strength for 10 to 14 days, and is absorbed in approximately 90 days.

53. Plain gut, chromic gut, and collagen sutures are digested by body enzymes through phagocytosis, which results in varying degrees of inflammatory reaction.

54. The rate of decline in tensile strength and absorption of surgical gut is influenced by the type of tissue in which the suture is used, the condition of the tissue, and the state of health of the patient. If the patient is anemic, malnourished, protein deficient, or debilitated, or has an infection, the rate of absorption and the loss of tensile strength may be accelerated.

55. Surgical gut sutures are packaged in a conditioning fluid of alcohol and water that prevents drying and keeps the suture pliable. Surgical gut should be handled only when

moist; therefore, it should be used immediately upon removal from the package. Gut suture that is removed from the package and allowed to dry will lose its pliability. Moistening it with sterile saline just prior to use will restore pliability. Gut suture should not be immersed or permitted to remain in saline or water, because excessive moisture will reduce tensile strength.

56. Synthetic absorbable sutures are made from synthetic polymers of lactic and glycolic acid and polyester. They are absorbed through hydrolysis, which causes the polymer chain to break down. Hydrolysis results in less tissue reaction than enzymatic suture absorption.

57. Synthetic suture's absorption time and loss of tensile strength are predictable, and this material is affected only minimally by the presence of infection, the type of tissue, or the patient's state of health.

58. The tensile strength of synthetic absorbable sutures is greater than that of natural materials and varies from several weeks to several months. For some sutures, a 25% tensile strength remains after 6 weeks; for others, all tensile strength is lost in 2 weeks.

59. The selection of suture must be based on knowledge of the rate of tensile strength, the rate of degradation of the suture material, and the time required for wound healing.

60. Synthetic absorbable sutures that provide the longest wound support times are appropriate for patients who heal slowly, such as the elderly, or patients with acquired immunodeficiency syndrome (AIDS), or those receiving radiation therapy.

61. Synthetic absorbable sutures are packed dry and should not be immersed in solutions, as this treatment can reduce tensile strength.

62. Examples of synthetic absorbable sutures include Dexon (polyglycolic acid), Vicryl (polyglactin 910), PDS (polydioxanone), Maxon (polyglyconate), Monocryl (poliglecaprone), Panacryl (lactide and glycolide), and Biosyn (synthetic polyester).

63. Absorbable suture coated with the antibacterial agent triclosan (Vicryl Plus) is also available. This suture is useful in preventing bacterial colonization.

Nonabsorbable Suture

64. Nonabsorbable suture is made of either natural or synthetic material, is not assimilated by the body, and is considered permanent once it is placed within tissue.

65. Silk and cotton are natural nonabsorbable sutures. Cotton suture is made from cotton fibers that have been combed, aligned, and twisted into a multifilament strand. Because it is somewhat reactive in tissue, this type of suture is used infrequently. Moisture enhances the tensile strength of cotton.

66. Surgical silk is a natural material made from thread spun by silkworms while making cocoons. The silk strands are twisted or braided and are usually dyed black. Silk also comes undyed.

67. Silk loses its tensile strength within 1 year after implantation and cannot be used where very long-term support is needed, such as in a heart valve. Silk is not totally nonabsorbable and may dissolve after several years. On occasion, a silk suture will migrate to the wound surface—a process referred to as "spitting."

68. Silk is one of the most widely used nonabsorbable sutures; it is often used in the gastrointestinal tract. It is pliable and holds a knot securely. Because of its capillarity, silk is treated to resist absorption of body fluids.

69. Nylon, polyester, polyethylene, polybutester, and polypropylene are some of the synthetic polymers used to manufacture synthetic nonabsorbable sutures. Synthetic fibers cause less tissue irritation, retain their strength longer, and have a higher tensile strength than do natural fibers.

70. Nylon suture (e.g., Ethilon, Dermalon, Nurolon, and Surgilon) has high tensile strength and is inert in the body. It is smooth and slides easily through tissue. Additional throws in the knot and square ties are necessary to provide knot security.

71. Nylon is often used for skin closure and, because it can be manufactured into very fine strands, is suitable for ophthalmic surgery, microsurgery, and neurosurgery.

72. Nylon suture used on the face and neck is removed in 2 to 5 days. On other skin areas, suture removal is typically within 8 days.

73. Polyester suture (e.g., Dacron, Mersiline, Ethibond, Tevdek, Bondek, and TiCron) is closely braided, is available in a variety of sizes, and is usually coated with a specially designed lubricant that reduces drag as the suture passes through tissue. Polyester suture is often used in cardiac surgery and neurosurgery

74. Polybutester suture (Novafil) is a monofilament suture with more flexibility and elasticity than other synthetic polymers, is more easily stretched, and may produce more compliant anastomoses.

75. Polypropylene suture (e.g., Prolene, Pronova, Surgilene, Surgidac) is an inert monofilament, has good tensile strength, and slides smoothly through tissue. It is available in a variety of sizes, including very fine strands. Its use is standard in cardiovascular surgery and other surgeries where prolonged healing is anticipated. Additional throws and square ties are necessary to ensure knot security.

76. Polypropylene suture should be gently stretched before use to eliminate memory and prevent kinking.

77. Stainless steel suture has the highest tensile strength and is the most inert of all sutures. It is particularly useful where strong permanent wound security is needed, such as for approximating the sternum following cardiovascular surgery. Metallic suture is difficult to handle and requires an exacting suture technique. It has very limited application.

Suture Diameter

78. Suture diameter ranges from a heavy size 7 to a very fine size 11-0. In decreasing thickness, suture sizing begins with 7 and decreases as the numbers fall to 0. Then, as the number of zeros increases (2-0, 3-0, 4-0, . . .), the diameter of the suture continues to become smaller (Figure 10-2).

79. Tensile strength decreases as suture diameter decreases. Sutures of size 5-0 through 11-0 are finer than a human hair and are often used in microsurgery. They are fragile and must be handled with the utmost care.

80. Generally, the most appropriate suture is one with the smallest diameter that will hold the wound during healing. The majority of sutures used in general surgery have diameters in the 1 to 4-0 range.

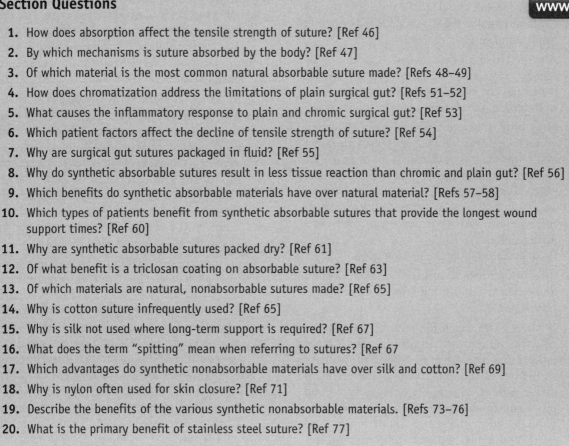

Section Questions   www

1. How does absorption affect the tensile strength of suture? [Ref 46]
2. By which mechanisms is suture absorbed by the body? [Ref 47]
3. Of which material is the most common natural absorbable suture made? [Refs 48–49]
4. How does chromatization address the limitations of plain surgical gut? [Refs 51–52]
5. What causes the inflammatory response to plain and chromic surgical gut? [Ref 53]
6. Which patient factors affect the decline of tensile strength of suture? [Ref 54]
7. Why are surgical gut sutures packaged in fluid? [Ref 55]
8. Why do synthetic absorbable sutures result in less tissue reaction than chromic and plain gut? [Ref 56]
9. Which benefits do synthetic absorbable materials have over natural material? [Refs 57–58]
10. Which types of patients benefit from synthetic absorbable sutures that provide the longest wound support times? [Ref 60]
11. Why are synthetic absorbable sutures packed dry? [Ref 61]
12. Of what benefit is a triclosan coating on absorbable suture? [Ref 63]
13. Of which materials are natural, nonabsorbable sutures made? [Ref 65]
14. Why is cotton suture infrequently used? [Ref 65]
15. Why is silk not used where long-term support is required? [Ref 67]
16. What does the term "spitting" mean when referring to sutures? [Ref 67
17. Which advantages do synthetic nonabsorbable materials have over silk and cotton? [Ref 69]
18. Why is nylon often used for skin closure? [Ref 71]
19. Describe the benefits of the various synthetic nonabsorbable materials. [Refs 73–76]
20. What is the primary benefit of stainless steel suture? [Ref 77]

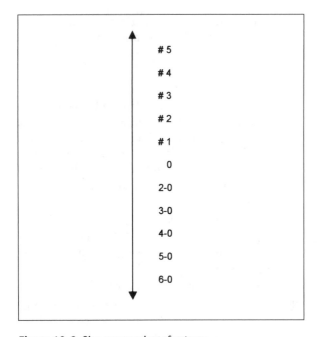

Figure 10-2 Size progression of sutures

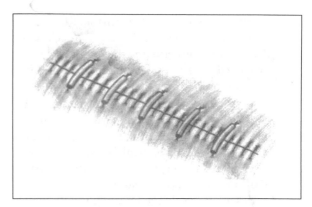

Figure 10-3 Retention suture bolster
Source: Reprinted with permission from Ethicon, Inc. (1996), Somerville, NJ.

Suture Selection: Considerations

81. Many factors influence suture selection, such as expected length of time for healing, presence of contamination in the wound, desired cosmetic results, and surgeon preference.

82. Absorbable sutures are used in tissue that heals rapidly. Typical applications include subcutaneous fat, the stomach, the submucosal layer of the colon, the bladder, and the biliary tract.

83. Nonabsorbable suture is used where extended wound support is needed, such as with fascia and tendons. It is routinely used in vascular, cardiac, and neurosurgery. However, absorbable suture with long-lasting tensile strength, such as polydioxanone (PDS II), is used where further tissue growth is expected, as in pediatric patients.

84. Nonabsorbable suture that will be removed is used in ophthalmic surgery, for skin closure, and when temporary additional wound support is needed.

85. In some cases, retention sutures are used to provide temporary additional abdominal wound support, such as to support the primary suture line in abdominal wound closure in an obese patient, to support healing by second intention, to eliminate dead space within the wound, and to prevent accumulation of fluid in an abdominal wound. Retention sutures

are nonabsorbable materials placed approximately 2 inches beyond the edge of the primary suture line and pass through all layers of the abdominal wall. Once it is ascertained that the primary wound has healed sufficiently, the retention sutures are removed (Figure 10-3).

Suture Package Information

86. Sutures are supplied sterile from the manufacturer in a double envelope package. The inner sterile package contains the sterile suture(s). The outer package is a peel package designed to permit aseptic delivery of the inner suture package to the sterile field.

87. Information required by the USP is printed on each suture package. This information includes the type of material; trade name; generic name; product number; size; length; color; number of needles in the package if more than one; description of the needle; braided or monofilament, absorbable or nonabsorbable; coating material if used; manufacturer; date manufactured; expiration date; and a statement of compliance with USP standards (Figures 10-4 and 10-5).

88. Sutures are supplied in boxes containing multiple packages. They are commercially sterilized with ethylene oxide or ionizing radiation. Sutures are not intended to be resterilized. The suture manufacturer does not supply reprocessing guidelines. Unused sutures should not be resterilized because product integrity cannot be guaranteed using hospital sterilization processes and cycles, and use characteristics of resterilized suture are no longer predictable. Using reprocessed sutures could jeopardize patient safety.

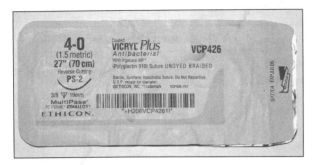

Figure 10-4 Suture package

Source: Reprinted with permission from Ethicon, Inc. (1996), Somerville, NJ.

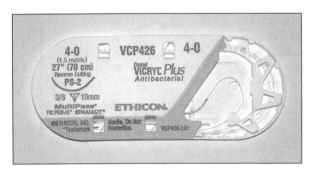

Figure 10-5 Suture package

Source: Reprinted with permission from Ethicon, Inc. (1996), Somerville, NJ.

Surgical Needles

Needle Characteristics

89. Surgical needles are designed to carry suture material through tissue with minimum trauma. They are precision made to provide some flexibility without breaking. Surgical needles are characterized by their shape, type of point, size, and means by which the suture material is attached.

90. The three basic parts of the needle are the point, shaft or body, and eye. The eye is the point where the suture material joins the needle (Figure 10-6).

91. Needle points may be tapered, cutting, or blunt (Figure 10-7).

92. Tapered needles are used in tissue that offers little resistance to the needle as it passes through, such as peritoneum or intestine. A taper-point needle is designed with the shaft gradually tapering to a sharp point so as to make the smallest possible hole in the tissue.

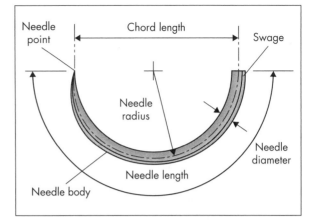

Figure 10-6 Anatomy of a suture needle

Source: Reprinted with permission from Ethicon, Inc. (1996), Somerville, NJ.

93. A cutting-point needle is designed with a razor-sharp tip and is used for tissue that is difficult to penetrate, such as skin or tendon.

94. Cutting needles have cutting edges that extend along the shaft. Variations of the cutting needle are used according to surgical preference in selected tissue.

95. Blunt-tip needles have a rounded end and are used in friable tissue, such as the liver or kidney, when neither piercing nor cutting is appropriate. Blunt needles are also used for safety purposes to reduce risk of exposure to blood-borne pathogens. They are especially useful for suturing in a deep cavity where visualization is difficult, as in gynecological surgery.

96. The shaft of the needle may be straight or curved. Possible curvatures are $^1/_4$, $^3/_8$, $^1/_2$, and $^5/_8$ circle (Figure 10-8). Selection of needle shape and size is determined by the size and properties of the suture material, the nature of the surgery, and the surgeon's preference.

Needle Attachment

97. The needle may be attached to the suture during manufacture, or the suture may be threaded through the needle at the time of surgery.

98. Needles with suture attached are referred to as swaged, and the suture is referred to as swaged or atraumatic. In such a case, the needle and suture strand are a continuous unit in which needle diameter and suture diameter are matched as closely as possible, thereby minimizing tissue trauma. Almost all sutures used in surgery are atraumatic.

POINT/BODY SHAPE	APPLICATIONS
Conventional Cutting	ligament nasal cavity oral cavity pharynx skin tendon
Reverse Cutting	fascia ligament nasal cavity oral mucosa pharynx skin tendon sheath
MICRO-POINT Reverse Cutting Needle	eye
Precision Point Cutting	skin (plastic or cosmetic)
Side-cutting Spatula	eye (primary application) microsurgery ophthalmic (reconstructive)

Figure 10-7a Needle points and body shapes with typical applications.

Source: Reprinted with permission from Ethicon, Inc. (1996), Somerville, NJ.

POINT/BODY SHAPE	APPLICATIONS	
TAPERCUT Surgical Needle	bronchus calcified tissue fascia ligament nasal cavity oral cavity ovary perichondrium periosteum	pharynx tendon trachea uterus vessels (sclerotic)
Taper	aponeurosis biliary tract dura fascia gastrointestinal tract muscle myocardium nerve peritoneum	pleura subcutaneous fat urogenital tract vessels
Blunt	blunt dissection (friable tissue) fascia intestine kidney liver spleen cervix (ligating incompetent cervix)	
CS ULTIMA Ophthalmic Needle	eye (primary application)	
PC PRIME Needle	skin (plastic or cosmetic)	

Figure 10-7b Needle points and body shapes with typical applications.

Source: Reprinted with permission from Ethicon, Inc. (1996), Somerville, NJ.

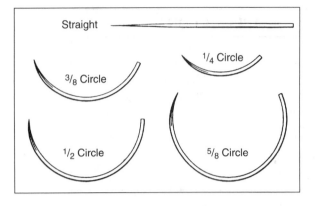

Figure 10-8 Needle shapes. Surgical needles vary in shape, size, type of point, body and how suture is attached (swaged or threaded)

Source: Reprinted with permission from *Perspectives on Sutures*, p. 52, 1978, Davis and Geck.

99. A modification of the permanently swaged suture is the controlled-release suture, sometimes referred to as a "pop-off." In this type of attachment, the needle and suture are one continuous unit; however, they are easily separated with a light tug. Controlled-release sutures facilitate rapid, interrupted suturing techniques.

100. Suture strands may be threaded through a needle with a round, oval, or square eye in much the same manner as a household needle (Figure 10-9).

101. A French-eyed needle has a slit from the inside of the eye to the proximal end of the needle. The suture is forced, rather than threaded, through this slit (Figure 10-9).

102. Threaded needles require additional time to prepare for use, making them less efficient than atraumatic suture.

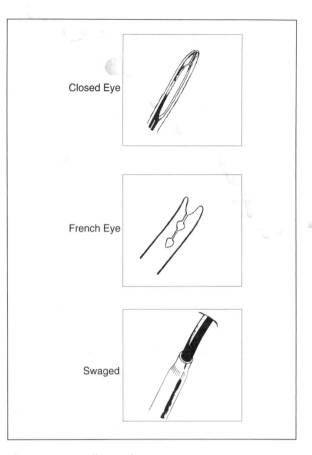

Figure 10-9 Needle attachments

Source: Reprinted with permission from Ethicon, Inc. (1996), Somerville, NJ.

103. Using a threaded needle necessitates two strands of suture being pulled through tissue. This bulk causes additional tissue trauma, which explains why threaded needles are rarely used.

Section Questions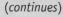

1. Describe how the diameter of sutures is identified. [Ref 78]
2. Which suture has a larger diameter: 2-0 or 4-0? [Ref 78]
3. How does tensile strength relate to the diameter of suture material? [Ref 79]
4. Which factors determine the suture that is most appropriate? [Refs 80–81]
5. In which type of tissue is absorbable suture used? [Ref 82]
6. When would nonabsorbable suture be selected? [Ref 83]
7. What is a unique application for using nonabsorbable suture with long-lasting tensile strength? [Ref 83]
8. What are common applications for nonabsorbable suture that will be removed? [Ref 84]
9. Explain the purpose of retention sutures. [Ref 85]

(continues)

Section Questions (continued)

10. Which type of information about the contents can you find on each package of suture? [Ref 87]
11. Explain the rationale for not resterilizing unused suture packages in the facility. [Ref 88]
12. What are the three basic parts of a surgical needle? [Ref 90]
13. Describe a taper needle and its application in surgery. [Ref 92]
14. What is the purpose of a cutting point on a surgical needle? [Ref 93]
15. How are blunt-tip needles used in surgical procedures? [Ref 95]
16. Describe the various shapes of surgical needles. [Ref 96]
17. Describe a swaged or atraumatic suture. [Ref 98]
18. Of what value are controlled-release sutures (pop-offs)? [Ref 99]
19. How does a French-eyed needle differ from a regular non-swaged needle? [Ref 101]
20. What are two reasons why threaded needles are rarely used? [Refs 102–103]

Other Wound Closure Devices

Stapling Devices

104. Stapling devices are available for approximation of internal tissues, for fascia, and for skin closure. Staples are made of stainless steel or titanium. Individual stapling devices are designed for stapling specific tissue and are not interchangeable. For example, skin staples are not used on fascia (Figure 10-10).

105. Staples can be applied individually, such as skin or fascia staplers with clips or staples that are delivered one at a time. Stapling devices used in intestinal and thoracic surgery deliver multiple staples simultaneously.

Skin Tapes and Skin Adhesives

106. Adhesive skin tapes (Steri Strips, Proxi-strips) are used to approximate surgical incision wound edges (Figure 10-11). When they are used in conjunction with subcuticular sutures to hold incision edges in place, skin sutures or staples are not necessary and the healed incision line has no suture tracks.

107. Skin tapes may also be used as a complement to suture or staple closures. They are often used to reinforce a wound after skin staples or sutures have been removed.

108. Skin tapes are available in widths of $^1/_8$, $^1/_4$, and $^1/_2$ inch and in lengths from $1^1/_2$ to 4 inches.

109. Skin adhesives (Dermabond, Indermil) are used to glue skin edges together. These materials are useful where cosmetic considerations are important, as they leave no suture tracks along the healed incision line.

110. Skin adhesives are also used to seal a sutured incision to prevent entry of microorganisms and are particularly useful in traumatic surgery where risk of infection is greatest.

Surgical Mesh

111. In addition to suture, knitted mesh made from polyester or polypropylene is sometimes used to reinforce tissue and provide support during and after wound healing. Mesh is particularly useful in hernia repair where a defect in the fascia exists.

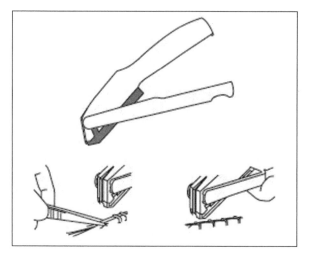

Figure 10-10 Skin staple

Source: Reprinted with permission from Ethicon, Inc. (1996), Somerville, NJ.

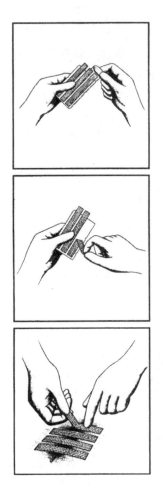

Figure 10-11 Skin tapes
Source: Reprinted with permission from Ethicon, Inc. (1996), Somerville, NJ.

Drains

112. Drains are used primarily to obliterate dead space where tissue might not have been adequately approximated, to remove foreign or harmful materials such as infected or necrotic tissue, or when hemostasis is uncertain. A drain is used when a wound is anticipated to produce fluid sufficient to place undue stress on closure.

113. The three types of drains are passive, active, and sump. Passive drains function through gravity and capillary action. Active drains employ negative pressure. Sump drains are double-lumen devices that may be attached to either continuous or intermittent low suction.

114. The most commonly used passive drain is a Penrose drain—a simple lumen drain made

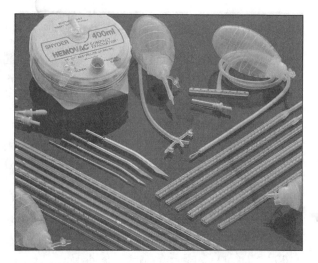

Figure 10-12 Self-contained wound drainage system
Source: Courtesy of Zimmer, Inc., Dover, OH.

from rubber or silicone. Fluid in the wound follows the path of the drain and empties because of gravity or capillary action into a surgical dressing where drainage is captured. Two important disadvantages of the Penrose drain are that it provides a pathway for microorganisms to migrate from the surrounding environment into the wound, and wound drainage cannot be accurately measured.

115. Commonly used active drains are the Hemovac and the Jackson-Pratt (Figure 10-12). Drainage flows from inside the wound through tubing that exits adjacent to the incision site and is attached to a closed reservoir. The reservoir is collapsed before being attached to the drain, creating negative pressure that directs drainage out of the wound and into the reservoir.

116. The reservoir may be emptied and negative pressure reinstated to collect additional drainage. Unlike the Penrose drain, Hemovac and Jackson-Pratt drains permit accurate measurement of drainage. They are also closed systems that provide less of a pathway for microorganisms to migrate into the wound.

117. Sump drains are double-lumened devices. One lumen provides for the passage of filtered air into the wound, and the other lumen permits passage of drainage material from the wound. In the presence of copious drainage, the sump pump may be connected to external suction.

Dressings

118. Most surgical incisions are closed primarily and covered with a sterile surgical dressing. Typically, a nonadherent dressing that will not stick to the wound and cause trauma (Telfa) is applied first, followed by a gauze dressing and tape to hold it in place. In the case of a large wound or one in which some additional absorbency is needed, the gauze layer will be covered with an absorbent pad.

119. A clean wound with minimal drainage might be covered with a nonadherent dressing (Telfa), followed a thin transparent semipermeable dressing that is oxygen permeable but serves as a barrier to bacteria and water (Tegaderm, OpSite).

120. A variety of other types of dressings are available, such as mesh nonadherent dressings, dressings impregnated with petrolatum (Vaseline gauze), and dressings impregnated with an antimicrobial.

121. In recent years, there has been an increase in development and use of dressings containing silver. Because of silver's antimicrobial properties, these dressings are particularly useful for infected wounds or wounds at risk for infection.

Nursing Responsibilities Related to Wound Management

122. The selection and use of wound-closure material and devices is primarily the surgeon's responsibility, but knowledge and understanding of suture and needle characteristics can help prevent patient injury. For example, use of a cutting needle in a vascular procedure, where a tapered point is desired and anticipated, can cause trauma to the patient and result in additional bleeding; similarly, use of an absorbable suture where permanent wound support is desired can result in wound separation. Knowledge of suture characteristics will facilitate the appropriate choice of an alternative suture when the requested suture is not available.

123. The more knowledgeable the nurse is regarding wound closure materials and devices, the less likely that inappropriate materials and devices that can compromise patient safety will be utilized. The nurse who understands sutures, drains, and dressings will be able to anticipate the surgeon's needs and assist in keeping surgery time to a minimum.

124. Prior to the procedure, the circulating nurse and the scrubbed person should review the surgeon's preference card for the intended procedure to determine the types of sutures that will be needed. Familiarity with the procedure and the surgeon's routine will assist the nurse to determine the approximate number of sutures of each type that will be needed.

125. To minimize waste, the nurse should consult with the surgeon prior to the procedure to ascertain whether any changes in suture are anticipated. Because suture cannot be resterilized, an excess of suture should not be delivered to the sterile field. An adequate supply of the suture to be used during the procedure should be available to deliver to the field when it is needed.

126. Multipack suture should be selected when a large number of the same sutures will be needed. If selected appropriately, multipack sutures can prevent waste and save time required to open individual packets.

127. On occasion, a suture packet that is not opened is returned to stock and placed into the wrong box. Before delivering suture to the sterile field, the nurse should read the label on the packet to prevent error and waste.

128. The following are additional responsibilities related to suture:

    - Both the circulating nurse and the scrubbed person should count sutures according to suture package information and verify this number upon opening the package.

    - Scrubbed person:
        - Arrange suture packets on the back table in the order in which they will be used.
        - Prepare one or two sutures for immediate use (i.e., load them on needle holders; keep the remainder in the package until needed).
        - Place loaded needle holders so as to prevent accidental exposure.
        - To prevent recoil, gently tug suture strands prior to passing them to the surgeon. Do not tug at the point of needle attachment.
        - Pass suture so as to prevent accidental exposure.
        - Place used needles on appropriate collection pad.
        - Close the needle collection pad and deposit it into a sharps container.

Section Questions www

1. What are stapling devices? [Ref 104]

2. For which purpose(s) are devices that deliver multiple staples at a time used? [Ref 105]

3. How can adhesive skin tapes be used in wound closure? [Refs 106–107]

4. What are two applications for skin adhesives? [Refs 109–110]

5. What is the value of using mesh in a surgical procedure? [Ref 111]

6. What is the primary use of a surgical drain? [Ref 112]

7. Describe how a passive drain functions. [Refs 113–114]

8. Identify two disadvantages of the passive drain. [Ref 114]

9. How does an active drain differ from a sump drain? [Refs 115, 117]

10. Explain how an active drain works. [Refs 115–116]

11. What are two advantages of active drains? [Ref 116]

12. Typically, what forms the first layer of the dressing for a surgical incision? [Ref 118]

13. Describe the benefit of transparent semipermeable dressings. [Ref 119]

14. What is the benefit of a dressing impregnated with silver? [Ref 121]

15. How can the nurse's knowledge of wound closure materials affect patient safety? [Refs 122–123]

16. What are some ways in which the nurse can minimize wasted sutures? [Refs 124–127]

17. When are multipack sutures most useful? [Ref 126]

18. How can the scrubbed person manage sutures to promote efficiency during the procedure? [Ref 128]

19. How does the scrubbed person help to prevent accidental exposure to bloodborne pathogens? [Ref 128]

20. What must the scrubbed person remember when pulling on sutures to prevent recoil? [Ref 128]

• • • References

Agency for Healthcare Research and Quality (AHRQ). Department of Health and Human Services (2010). *National healthcare quality and disparities reports*. Rockville, MD: AHRQ. Available at: www.ahrq.gov/qual/qrdr10/12_patientsafety/T12_2_9-2.htm. Accessed June 2012.

Baronoski S (2012). *Wound Care Essentials: Practice Principles* (Third Edition. Lippincott Williams & Wilkins: Philadelphia, PA.

Ethicon, Inc. (2007). *Wound closure manual*. Available at: http://surgery.uthscsa.edu/pediatric/training/wound closuremanual.pdf and http://www.orthonurse.org/portals/0/wound%20closure%20manual.pdf. Accessed June 2012.

Ortega G, Rhee D, Papandria D, et al. (2012). An evaluation of surgical site infections by wound classification system using the ACS-NSQIP. *J Surg Res*;174(1):33–38.

Phillips N (2013). *Berry & Kohn's Operating Room Technique* (12th ed.). St. Louis, MO: Mosby.

• • • Suggested Reading

Mangram A, Horan T, Pearson M, et al. (1999). Guideline for prevention of surgical site infection. *Infect Control Hosp Epidemiol*;20(4):247–278.

Post-Test

Read each question carefully. Each question may have more than one correct answer.

1. Which statement(s) is (are) true?
   a. Wound dehiscence is actual protrusion of the abdominal viscera through the incision.
   b. Abdominal and pelvic surgery patients are at greatest risk for wound dehiscence and evisceration.
   c. Inadequate wound closure accounts for most instances of dehiscence or evisceration that occur 1–3 days postoperatively.
   d. Obesity and diabetes are risk factors for wound separation.

2. Which statement(s) is (are) true?
   a. Wound healing is influenced by choice of suture and surgical technique.
   b. Dehydration and malnutrition are risk factors for delayed or complicated wound healing.
   c. A break in aseptic technique can lead to infection.
   d. Suture materials vary in their ability to prevent infection.

3. The wound classification system
   a. is an important predictor of postoperative outcomes.
   b. includes four classifications of surgical wounds.
   c. places most surgical wounds in Class I.
   d. indicates that Class I wounds are not predisposed to infection.

4. Clean contaminated wounds include
   a. wounds without inflammation.
   b. wounds involving the gastrointestinal, respiratory, and genitourinary tracts.
   c. a major break in aseptic technique.
   d. open, fresh accidental wounds.

5. Wound healing by primary intention
   a. is the preferred method of wound healing.
   b. means the wound edges are approximated at the time of surgery.
   c. involves no breaks in aseptic technique.
   d. produces a wound that heals quickly with minimal scarring.

6. Wound healing by secondary intention
   a. means the wound is sutured loosely at the time of surgery because the wound edges cannot be approximated effectively.
   b. heals from the inside or bottom upward.
   c. produces minimal scarring.
   d. is more prone to infection than healing by primary intention.

7. Wounds that heal by tertiary intention
   a. are not sutured at the time of surgery.
   b. heal by forming granulation tissue characterized by red, beefy-looking tissue.
   c. are usually wounds with extensive tissue loss.
   d. are packed with gauze for 3–5 days.

8. Which statement(s) is (are) true about wound healing?
   a. The inflammatory stage is characterized by hemostasis and phagocytosis.
   b. The proliferation stage produces granulation tissue.
   c. Platelets form a clot in the proliferation stage.
   d. Maturation can take more than a year to transform a reddish thick scar into a thin white line.

9. Which statement(s) is (are) true about sutures?
   a. As a noun, "suture" refers to a strand of material used to ligate a vessel or close a wound.
   b. Desired characteristics of sutures include sterility, pliability, consistent tensile strength, and minimal tissue reactivity.
   c. Sutures come in packages that can be delivered to the field in sterile condition.
   d. A suture is a foreign body that can create a tissue reaction.

10. Which statement(s) is (are) true about suture?
    a. Monofilament sutures drag as they are drawn through tissue.
    b. Knots tied with monofilament sutures have a tendency to loosen.
    c. Multifilament sutures provide greater tensile strength.
    d. Multifilament sutures can promote infection when fluids are carried along the strand to the wound.

11. Natural absorbable suture
    a. is purified collagen that retains its tensile strength for 90 days.
    b. is digested by body enzymes or is hydrolyzed.
    c. is used to ligate superficial blood vessels and approximate the subcutaneous tissue layer.
    d. should be soaked in water once the package is opened to prevent drying and increase tensile strength.

12. Synthetic absorbable gut suture
    a. is digested by the body's enzymes.
    b. has less tensile strength than natural absorbable suture.
    c. should be immersed in solution to increase its tensile strength.
    d. provides the longest wound support and is appropriate for patients who heal slowly.

13. Which statement(s) is (are) true about silk?
    a. Silk cannot be used for long-term support.
    b. Silk can "spit" or migrate to the wound surface.
    c. Silk is treated to resist absorption of body fluids because of its capillarity.
    d. Silk is pliable and holds a knot securely.

14. Which statement(s) is (are) true about nonabsorbable suture?
    a. Synthetic fibers cause less tissue reaction than silk.
    b. Synthetic fibers have higher tensile strength than silk.
    c. Nylon slides easily through tissue and makes knots easily and securely.
    d. Prolene is the standard nonabsorbable suture for cardiovascular surgery and other surgeries where prolonged healing is anticipated.

15. Which statement(s) is (are) true about suture?
    a. The diameter of suture decreases as the number of zeros increases.
    b. Tensile strength increases as the diameter of suture decreases.
    c. Absorbable suture is used in tissues that heal rapidly.
    d. Retention sutures are used to support a suture line in an obese patient and to support healing by secondary intention.

16. Which statement(s) is (are) true about surgical needles?

    a. The three parts of a surgical needle are the point, the shaft, and the eye.

    b. Tapered needles are used on tissue that offers little resistance.

    c. Blunt needles are used on friable tissue.

    d. Cutting needles are used on skin and tendon.

17. Which statement(s) is (are) true about surgical needles?

    a. When the suture is attached to the needle, it is called swaged or atraumatic.

    b. Controlled-release suture is threaded onto the needle by the scrubbed person.

    c. Threaded needles cause tissue trauma as two strands are pulled through the tissue instead of one.

    d. A French-eyed needle comes with suture attached.

18. Which statement(s) is (are) true?

    a. Stapling devices deliver staples one at a time.

    b. Skin staples are used on both skin and fascia.

    c. Skin tapes may be used as a complement to sutures or staples or to reinforce a wound after sutures or staples have been removed.

    d. Skin adhesives are used when cosmetic considerations are important.

19. Which statement(s) is (are) true about drains?

    a. Drains are used primarily to obliterate dead space, to removed harmful material, and when hemostasis is uncertain.

    b. A Penrose drain is passive, using gravity or capillary action to remove fluid from the wound.

    c. Active drains have a reservoir that can be collapsed to create negative pressure that draws fluid from the wound into the reservoir.

    d. Single-lumen sump drains are connected to external suction.

20. Which statement(s) is (are) true about nursing responsibilities?

    a. A nurse who is knowledgeable can prevent injury such as might result from using a cutting needle inappropriately or an absorbable suture where a permanent suture is needed.

    b. Nurses who have a good understanding of sutures, drains, and dressings can minimize surgery time and reduce waste by delivering only the supplies that are needed to the field.

    c. Knowledgeable nurses will reduce surgical time and waste by selecting multipacks of sutures that are used in large numbers.

    d. The knowledgeable nurse will handle needles and sutures in a safe and effective manner, promoting safety for both the surgical team and the patient.

• •

Competency Checklist:
Prevention of Injury—Wound Management

`www`

Under "Observer's Initials," enter initials upon successful achievement of the competency. Enter N/A if the competency is not appropriate for the institution.

Name _____

	Observer's Initials	Date
1. Sutures selected according to preference card and anticipated need	_____	_____
2. Sutures counted correctly	_____	_____
3. Package contents verified when opened	_____	_____
4. Sutures arranged on back table in order of anticipated use	_____	_____
5. Sutures loaded in anticipation of need—remaining sutures are maintained in the package	_____	_____
6. Loaded sutures placed on the Mayo/back table in a manner that avoids accidental exposure (needlestick)	_____	_____
7. Suture with memory (e.g., Prolene) pulled gently before being passed to the surgeon to prevent rebound (no pull exerted on needle attachment)	_____	_____
8. Suture passed in safe manner (e.g., sharp announced)	_____	_____
9. Needles removed from the suture in a safe manner	_____	_____
10. Needles placed carefully on a magnetic needle mat or other appropriate receptacle	_____	_____
11. Needles deposited in sharps box following procedure	_____	_____

Observer's Signature   Initials   Date

_____

Orientee's Signature

_____

Prevention of Injury: Anesthesia and Medication Safety

LEARNER OBJECTIVES

1. Identify potential patient injuries related to anesthesia.
2. Identify desired patient outcomes related to anesthesia.
3. Discuss the role of the perioperative nurse during the administration of anesthesia.
4. Describe assessment factors related to the selection of anesthetic agents and techniques.
5. Describe malignant hyperthermia and its treatment.
6. Describe four patient monitoring devices and the rationale for their use.
7. Differentiate between depolarizing and nondepolarizing neuromuscular blocking agents.
8. Describe techniques of general anesthesia, regional anesthesia, and moderate sedation/analgesia.
9. Match commonly used anesthetic agents with their actions.
10. Discuss the role of the perioperative nurse regarding medication administration and safety.

`WWW`

LESSON OUTLINE

Potential Injury: Desired Patient Outcomes

1. Little more than 100 years ago, anesthesia for surgical procedures was limited to a crude open-drop administration of ether. Depth of anesthesia and physiologic response were inconsistent and poorly controlled. The risk of complication was high.

2. In the early 1950s, the death rate associated with complications from anesthesia was approximately 1 in 10,000. The development of sophisticated anesthesia and airway management techniques, new anesthetic agents, improved preanesthesia assessment, and technologically advanced monitoring devices have combined to make delivery of anesthesia a highly refined process. The current estimate is that only 1 anesthesia death occurs per 200,000 to 300,000 procedures (Turrillazzi, 2012).

Nursing Diagnoses

3. Although the death rate associated with anesthesia is extremely low, the risk of complication persists. Anesthetic agents can compromise ventilation, perfusion, and cardiac output, and can alter hypothalamic thermoregulation.

4. Appropriate nursing diagnoses for the patient undergoing anesthesia include high risk for injury (untoward drug reaction or interaction, ineffective airway, decreased cardiac output, electrolyte or fluid imbalance, ineffective breathing pattern, alteration in thought process, and ineffective thermoregulation or hypothermia) related to anesthesia. Other diagnoses may be appropriate based on the patient's condition identified during assessment.

5. The type of anesthesia, anesthetic agents, the surgical procedure, and the patient's preanesthesia physiological condition all influence the degree of risk for complications. For example, the ambulatory patient who undergoes a minor surgical procedure with local anesthetic or moderate sedation/analgesia has less risk for hypothermia than the patient who undergoes open abdominal surgery with general anesthesia, where anesthetic agents cause dilation of blood vessels and the nature of the procedure exposes the patient's gut to room temperature.

Desired Patient Outcomes

6. The desired outcome for the patient who undergoes anesthesia is successful recovery and a return to the preanesthesia physiological state, including normothermia, unimpeded air exchange, adequate ventilation, maintenance of cardiac output and fluid volume, electrolyte and fluid balance, absence of allergic reaction, and unimpaired thought processes.

7. The time frame in which these desired outcomes will be achieved varies according to the procedure, anesthetic agents, and anesthesia technique (i.e., local, regional, or general). For example, in the immediate postoperative period, the patient should be normothermic; however, the patient may or may not be expected to breathe unassisted. Expectations for the return of independent breathing are determined by the patient's preexisting respiratory condition, the intent of the anesthesia provider, the anesthetic agents employed, and the nature of the surgery.

Outcome Criteria

8. Several postanesthesia scoring systems are used to assess the patient's recovery. The most common is the Aldrete system, which is used to assess the recovery of patients from general anesthesia. It evaluates patient activity, respiration, circulation, and oxygen saturation. Points are assigned to patient responses, and discharge from the postanesthesia care unit

Exhibit 11-1 Aldrete Score

Activity	Able to move four extremities voluntarily on command	1
	Able to move two extremities voluntarily on command	1
	Able to move no extremities voluntarily on command	0
Respiration	Able to breathe deeply and cough freely	2
	Dyspnea or limited breathing	1
	Apneic	0
Circulation	BP 1 20 of preanesthetic level	2
	BP 1 20–49 of preanesthetic level	1
	BP 1 50 of preanesthetic level	0
Consciousness	Fully awake	2
	Arousable on calling	1
	Not responding	0
O_2 Saturation	Able to maintain O_2 saturation $> 92\%$ on room air	2
	Needs O_2 inhalation to maintain O_2 saturation $> 90\%$	1
	O_2 saturation $< 90\%$ even with O_2 supplement	0

Source: From Aldrete, A.J., and Wright, A. *Anesthesiology News*, *18*(11): 17, 1992. In Litwack, K. (Ed.), *Post anesthesia care nursing*. St. Louis: Mosby Year Book, Inc., 1995.

(PACU) depends on the patient achieving an acceptable score (Exhibit 11-1).

9. The acceptable score varies with institutional policy, the anticipated recovery, and the unit to which the patient is discharged. A patient being transferred from the PACU to a step-down unit may not require as high a score as a patient who is returning to a regular unit. For obvious reasons, a patient who is discharged on the same day of surgery must achieve a high score.

Overview of Nursing Responsibilities

10. Anesthesia may be administered by the following healthcare providers:

  • An anesthesiologist: a medical doctor with at least 4 years of anesthesia training after medical school.

  • A certified registered nurse anesthetist (CRNA): a registered nurse with a bachelor's degree in nursing (or other appropriate baccalaureate degree), a minimum of 1 year of acute care experience (e.g., OR, ICU, ER), and the successful completion of both an accredited 2- to 3-year graduate-level nurse anesthesia program and the national certification examination.

    – Currently, 16 states require no supervision of CRNAs. The other states permit supervision of CRNAs by any physician, not just those specializing in anesthesia (i.e., an order for an anesthetic).

  • An anesthesiologist assistant (AA): an individual with any bachelor's degree who has completed a clinical program at the graduate level. An AA must be supervised by an anesthesiologist.

    – Anesthesia assistants are currently licensed to practice in 18 states and are physician delegated in an additional 6 states.

11. Preoperatively, the anesthesiologist, CRNA, or AA will perform a patient assessment, determine the anesthetic agents to be used, and, in collaboration with the surgeon and patient, select the anesthetic technique.

12. Intraoperative responsibility includes delivery of anesthesia with all the physiological support required throughout the procedure and through transport to the PACU.

13. The perioperative nurse circulator will assist the anesthesia provider intraoperatively, particularly during induction and extubation, and during transfer of the patient to the PACU.

14. During procedures where moderate sedation/analgesia is administered by the surgeon, and an anesthesiologist or nurse anesthetist is not present, the perioperative nurse assumes even more responsibility for patient monitoring.

15. Postoperatively, the anesthesiologist, CRNA, or AA evaluates the patient's readiness for discharge and writes a discharge order.

16. Overall responsibilities of the perioperative nurse related to anesthesia delivery include the following:

    • Preanesthesia assessment: The perioperative nurse performs a patient assessment in addition to the assessment performed by the anesthesiologist, CRNA, or AA. This assessment information serves as a safety check to ensure that all significant patient data are communicated to the surgical team. Assessment information allows the team to anticipate problems and plan appropriately for the patient's treatment and recovery.

    • Patient support: The perioperative nurse provides emotional support (answers questions, provides reassuring touch, remains close to the patient) during the preoperative period. Physiological support during the perioperative period is the responsibility of the anesthesia provider and includes applying patient monitoring devices, interpreting monitoring data, being alert to patient physiological status and changes, and providing oxygen or preparing and administering intravenous fluids as appropriate. The perioperative nurse assists the anesthesia provider by anticipating and providing needed equipment and pharmacological agents in a timely manner. Following the procedure, the perioperative nurse accompanies the patient to the PACU and continues to provide physiological and emotional support. In the postoperative period, the perioperative nurse may assist both the anesthesia provider and the PACU nurse in stabilizing the patient.

    • Communication: When the patient is transported to the operating room, a hand-off report from the last caregiver must be given to the receiving caregiver. Data communicated at this time serve as an initial step in the assessment process. Assessment data are communicated to and verified with the anesthesia provider prior to delivery of anesthesia.

    • Documentation: In addition to meeting the documentation requirements of the facility, the perioperative nurse gives a hand-off report to the PACU nurse that includes information necessary to prepare for the patient's admission to PACU and the patient's recovery from anesthesia.

    • Patient teaching: In preparation for anesthesia, the perioperative nurse provides and reinforces information regarding routines, preanesthesia preparations, instructions for the day of surgery, and procedure-specific postoperative instructions.

17. In the past, National Patient Safety Goals (2006) established by The Joint Commission (TJC) focused on improving staff communication by implementing a standardized approach to hand-off communications, including an opportunity to ask and respond to questions (TJC, 2012b). Communication should include care, treatment, services, condition, and recent or anticipated changes. In response to this mandate, healthcare facilities have developed standardized tools for hand-off communication. These tools list the type of information that should be communicated and the process for communicating it.

18. The report (hand-off) from the circulating nurse to the PACU nurse should include at least the following information:
    • Patient name, age, and sex
    • Surgical procedure
    • Surgeon and anesthesiologist/CRNA/AA
    • Anesthetic agents/technique
    • Intraoperative medications
    • Estimated blood loss
    • Fluid and blood administration
    • Urine output
    • Response to surgery/anesthesia
    • Lab results
    • Chronic and acute health history
    • Drug allergies
    • Concerns, possible problems, and desired patient outcomes not met
    • Discharge plan

19. The perioperative nurse may share responsibility for the hand-off report with anesthesia personnel, must be knowledgeable of patient status (as described in the previous list), and must be able to communicate the information to the PACU nurse.

20. In many institutions, but particularly in small rural facilities, the perioperative nurse continues to provide care through the recovery period. In many facilities, staffing variances and limited resources have made it necessary for perioperative nurses to demonstrate competence in postanesthesia care as well preoperative and intraoperative nursing.

21. The field of postanesthesia nursing is a specialty in itself and requires significant specialized training. Perioperative nurses who have responsibility for the patient's recovery phase must demonstrate skill in this specialty.

22. Even where the perioperative nurse's responsibility does not include postanesthesia care, he or she must demonstrate competence in the use of monitoring equipment and in the interpretation of the data. The perioperative nurse must also be familiar with anesthetic agents and techniques to anticipate patient events, implement nursing interventions quickly, and assist the anesthesia provider.

Preanesthesia

Assessment Data

23. In preparation for surgery and anesthesia, the patient may be required to have an assessment and preoperative testing several days prior to surgery. Diagnostic testing may include a chest X ray; electrocardiogram (ECG/EKG); blood chemistry panel, including a clotting profile; urinalysis; and other tests specific to the patient's health status. The choice of diagnostic studies is determined by the patient's medical and surgical history, the results of the physical examination, and the intended surgical procedure.

24. At the time of preoperative testing, the patient may be interviewed and examined by the anesthesia provider, who may request additional laboratory and diagnostic testing. During preoperative testing, a perioperative nurse may also interview, assess, and participate in the patient's preparation for surgery.

25. The trend today is toward minimal preoperative testing, and a healthy patient may require no laboratory or diagnostic procedures. There is a lack of evidence showing that routine laboratory testing affects patient outcomes; for this reason, most diagnostic testing today is patient and procedure specific.

26. With the continuing move from inpatient to ambulatory surgery, the patient might not be seen by the anesthesia provider or perioperative nurse until the day of surgery. Preoperative instructions may be provided by the nurse who is present at the time that the decision for surgery is made. Instructions may also be reinforced by telephone by a perioperative nurse a day or so prior to surgery.

27. Guidelines from the American Society of Anesthesiologists (ASA), coupled with institutional requirements, may require an ECG and chest X ray for patients with risk factors and/or older than a certain age who will undergo general anesthesia or moderate sedation/analgesia. Preoperative diagnostic requirements will vary according to facility policy and anesthesia provider preference.

28. During preoperative assessment, the perioperative nurse reviews the patient's chart and assessment data and assesses the patient's readiness for surgery, plans for the patient's intraoperative care, and identifies data significant to anesthesia.

29. Data collected include information about coexisting disease, history of asthma, previous surgeries, anesthetics, and complications. Family history with anesthetics can provide information suggestive of possible adverse reactions, such as malignant hyperthermia, that can be prevented.

30. Information about current medications, including herbal medications and drug allergies, is essential to prevent the use of drugs that might react unfavorably with current medications or cause an allergic reaction. Allergies to contrast dyes, iodine solutions, adhesive tape, and latex are relevant.

31. History of drug or substance abuse is important, as substance use can alter the effect of anesthesia drugs.

32. Also important is determining whether the patient has been on beta-blocker therapy. Patients on a beta-blocker should receive their beta-blocker medication prior to arrival or during the perioperative period (within 24 hours of surgery or discharge from PACU) (Centers for Medicare and Medicaid Services [CMS] Core Measure; Surgical Core Improvement Project [SCIP]).

33. Assessment for cracked lips, lacerations in or around the mouth, loose or chipped teeth, and dentures is particularly important if the patient

will have general anesthesia and intubation, both of which involve manipulation of the patient's head and mouth. The anesthesia provider will take precautions to prevent further injury to the patient. Dentures may be removed prior to general anesthesia, as they can become dislodged and interfere with intubation and anesthetic delivery.

34. Assess the patient for body piercings, studs, and other such jewelry. Mouth and tongue jewelry can interfere with or become dislodged during intubation.

35. Smoking history is important because patients who smoke perioperatively have been shown to experience more problems with local wound complications, pulmonary and cardiac complications, an increased need for postoperative intensive care, and longer periods of hospitalization than nonsmokers. Smoking has also been implicated in a need for increased anesthetic dosage as well as increased levels of postoperative pain. Benefits of smoking cessation for as few as 12 hours have been demonstrated, and patient teaching should encourage cessation for as long as possible prior to surgery.

36. Results of diagnostic testing should be checked to ensure that the tests were actually performed and that the results are present in the chart. In the event that abnormalities are noted, the perioperative nurse should confirm that all team members are aware of the test results.

37. It should be noted if female patients of childbearing age are pregnant. Confirming pregnancy status may necessitate a urine pregnancy test.

American Society of Anesthesiologists Classification

38. The anesthesia provider will classify the patient's physical status according to the ASA's classification system. Patients may be assigned a physical status (PS) from 1 to 5 as follows (ASA, 2012a):
    - PS1 patients: healthy, no organic disease
    - PS2 patients: mild systemic disease (e.g., mild obesity, controlled hypertension, smoking without chronic obstructive pulmonary disease [COPD])
    - PS3 patients: severe systemic disease (e.g., poorly controlled hypertension or history of myocardial infarction, morbid obesity, controlled congestive heart failure [CHF])

- PS4 patients: severe systemic disease that is a constant threat to life (e.g., end-stage renal hepatorenal failure, or cardiac failure, unstable angina)
- PS5 patients: moribund and not expected to survive; surgery performed as a last recourse (e.g., ruptured aneurysm, sepsis with hemodynamic instability, poorly controlled coagulopathy)
- PS6 patients: brain dead; organs harvested
- E: if the procedure is an emergency, the physical status is followed by "E" (for example, "PS2E")

39. The ASA classification system is useful in determining the anesthesia technique to be used. For example, some facility policies do not permit Class III patients to undergo surgery under general anesthesia as an ambulatory surgery patient. Class III and higher patients must have an anesthesiologist, a CRNA, or an AA present during surgery even when the anesthesia technique is limited to moderate sedation/analgesia.

Patient Teaching

40. Ideally, patient teaching will be initiated at the time the decision is made to have surgery. Instruction in preoperative routines, expected outcomes, and day-of-surgery instructions may be given in the physician's office or the clinic. Teaching and reinforcement should occur when and if the patient is instructed to report for a presurgical examination or diagnostic workup.

41. Teaching during the presurgical workup may be initiated by a nurse other than the perioperative nurse. In some facilities, a preanesthesia clinic nurse or a PACU nurse initiates preoperative teaching in preparation for anesthesia and reinforces the instructions with a phone call the night before surgery. The patient who is already hospitalized may be instructed by the nurse on the patient's unit.

42. Regardless of where the teaching was initiated or who was responsible for preanesthesia instructions, the perioperative nurse should reinforce teaching just prior to surgery and should verify that the patient is in compliance with instructions for the day of surgery.

Patient Instructions

43. Preanesthesia instructions will vary and must be individualized based on the intended surgical

procedure, patient condition, and anesthesia technique. Instructions should include the following:

- Preoperative preparation (if indicated): preoperative shower or enema.

- Preoperative medications: medications to be taken on the day of surgery, both routine and single-dose medications. (On occasion, specific medications will be ordered for a period prior to surgery and other medications that the patient routinely takes will be held.)

- Food and liquid intake: traditionally, patients receiving general anesthesia have been instructed to take nothing by mouth (NPO) for 6 to 8 hours prior to surgery. For the patient who is admitted on the day of surgery, typical instructions are "NPO after midnight."

  With the loss of a protective airway reflex under general anesthesia, a patient who vomits or regurgitates incurs a high risk of aspiration pneumonitis. Aspiration of as little as 0.4 mL of acid from the stomach with a pH of 2.5 places the patient at risk for pneumonitis.

- Postoperative routines: length of surgery, expected recovery time, postoperative anesthesia care and routines.

44. The following summary of fasting recommendations is limited to healthy patients of all ages (ASA, 2011a):

Ingested Material	Minimum Fasting Period
Clear liquids	2 hours
Breastmilk	4 hours
Infant formula	6 hours
Nonhuman milk	6 hours
Light meal	6 hours

45. These guidelines do not apply to the following patients:

- Patients who undergo procedures with no anesthesia or only local anesthesia when upper airway protective reflexes are not impaired, and when no risk factors for pulmonary aspiration are apparent

- Women in labor

46. These guidelines may not apply to, or may need to be modified for, the following patients:

- Patients with coexisting diseases or conditions that can affect gastric emptying or fluid volume (e.g., pregnancy, obesity, diabetes, hiatal hernia, gastroesophageal reflux disease, ileus or bowel obstruction, emergency care, enteral tube feeding)

- Patients in whom airway management might be difficult

- Anesthesiologists and other anesthesia providers should recognize that these conditions can increase the likelihood of regurgitation and pulmonary aspiration. Additional or alternative preventive strategies may be appropriate for such patients (ASA, 2011a).

Selection of Anesthetic Agents and Technique

47. Many factors influence the selection of anesthetic agents and technique. Each patient is unique, and the assessment will determine those drugs that best meet the surgical requirements and provide for the patient's well-being. Factors that are considered include the following:

- Age
- Medical history
- Current physical status and emotional or mental status (extreme anxiety, mental retardation, communication issues)
- Intended surgical procedure and expected length of recovery from anesthesia
- Patient preference
- Surgeon preference/requirements
- Anesthesia provider preference and expertise
- Patient's previous anesthesia/recovery experience
- Whether surgery is elective or emergent
- Considerations for postoperative pain management

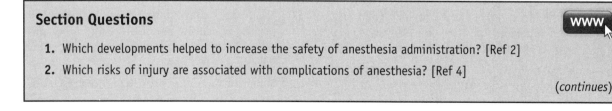

Section Questions

1. Which developments helped to increase the safety of anesthesia administration? [Ref 2]
2. Which risks of injury are associated with complications of anesthesia? [Ref 4]

(continues)

Section Questions (continued)

3. Which factors affect the patient's risk for complications of anesthesia? [Ref 5]

4. List the desired outcomes for the patient who undergoes anesthesia. [Ref 6]

5. Which factors affect the time frame for achieving desired outcomes? [Ref 7]

6. Which four parameters are assessed in the Aldrete score? [Ref 8]

7. Which factors determine the appropriate Aldrete score for discharge? [Ref 9]

8. Differentiate among the following types of anesthesia providers: anesthesiologist, CRNA, and AA. [Ref 10]

9. How is the anesthetic technique for each patient determined? [Ref 11]

10. Once in the operating room, who assists the anesthesia provider in preparing the patient for anesthesia and delivering the patient to the PACU postoperatively? [Ref 13]

11. Discuss the perioperative nurse's responsibilities related to anesthesia delivery. [Ref 16]

12. Which types of patient information should be included in hand-off communication? [Ref 18]

13. What determines the types of preoperative tests that are ordered for a patient? [Ref 23]

14. What is the current trend in preoperative testing? [Ref 25]

15. Which types of information gathered preoperatively might alert the anesthesiologist to possible adverse reactions to anesthesia? [Ref 29]

16. Which types of allergies should be documented before a surgical experience? [Ref 30]

17. Why is documentation of drug and alcohol abuse important? [Ref 31]

18. What are some important assessment details related to the mouth that might affect anesthesia delivery? [Refs 33–34]

19. How does smoking affect the response to surgery and anesthesia? [Ref 35]

20. Describe the criteria for ASA classifications PS1 though PS6. [Ref 38]

21. When should teaching begin for the surgical patient? [Ref 40]

22. Who is responsible for patient teaching? [Refs 41–42]

23. What information is included in preanesthesia instructions? [Ref 43]

24. Why are NPO orders important for patients having general anesthesia? [Ref 43]

25. Which factors are considered when selecting anesthetic agents and technique? [Ref 47]

Anesthesia Techniques: Overview

48. Anesthesia may be general, regional, local, or moderate sedation/analgesia.

49. General anesthesia depresses the central nervous system. The patient is unconscious and reflexes are obtunded. Physiologic status is controlled by the anesthesia provider. Characteristics of general anesthesia include amnesia, analgesia, and muscle relaxation.

50. Moderate sedation/analgesia is also referred to as conscious sedation, monitored anesthesia care (MAC), anesthesia standby, or local standby. The patient is given a local anesthetic at the site of surgery, and medications are administered intravenously to provide sedation and analgesia. The decision to have an anesthesia provider present is based on the patient's condition, the ASA classification, the procedure, and facility policy.

51. Moderate sedation/analgesia is also appropriate for healthy patients having minor procedures who do not require the presence of an anesthesia provider.

52. When an anesthesia provider is not present, the perioperative nurse assumes the responsibility for monitoring the patient.

53. When moderate sedation/analgesia is administered to patients too ill to tolerate general anesthesia, it is referred to as monitored anesthesia care.

54. Facility policy, in conjunction with the state's nurse practice act, determines whether the nurse, the surgeon, or both are responsible for the administration of intravenous drugs.

55. Regional anesthesia is anesthesia limited to a region of the body, such as a limb or the lower half of the body.

56. Regional anesthetic techniques can be divided into central and peripheral techniques. The central techniques include neuraxial blocks (epidural anesthesia, spinal anesthesia). Peripheral techniques can be further divided into plexus blocks (e.g., brachial plexus blocks) and single nerve blocks.

57. Regional anesthesia may be administered as a single injection or by inserting a catheter through which medication is administered over a prolonged period (e.g., continuous peripheral nerve block).

58. Regional anesthesia can be provided by injecting local anesthetics directly into the veins of an arm (provided the venous flow is impeded by a tourniquet)—a method called intravenous regional technique (Bier block). The patient is awake but does not feel pain over the anesthetized region. Regional anesthetics, such as lidocaine (Xylocaine), bupivacaine (Marcaine), chloroprocaine (Nesacaine), and tetracaine (Pontocaine), are used. Because the patient is awake, additional agents may be administered to reduce anxiety and provide sedation.

59. Local anesthesia is actually a form of regional anesthesia; however, only a small, localized area is infiltrated using an anesthetic such as lidocaine (Xylocaine) or bupivacaine (Marcaine). This infiltration is often performed by the surgeon on the field rather than by the anesthesia provider.

Premedication

Goals

60. Protocols related to preoperative medication vary among facilities and anesthesia providers. Current practices support the evaluation of each patient's needs prior to ordering and administering medications, rather than relying on standard medication protocols.

61. At one time, it was standard practice to medicate the patient in preparation for anesthesia and surgery. Today, it is not unusual for the patient to receive no preoperative medication. This is particularly true for ambulatory surgery patients, for whom preoperative medication may prolong recovery and delay discharge. In addition, residual effects of medication cannot be monitored after discharge.

62. Goals of preoperative medication may include one or more of the following:
    - Reduction of anxiety
    - Sedation
    - Analgesia
    - Amnesia
    - Prevention of nausea and vomiting
    - Reduction in gastric volume and acidity
    - Facilitation of induction
    - Reduction of risk of allergic reaction
    - Decrease of secretions
    - Prevention of infection

Medications and Protocols

63. Oral preoperative medications are usually given 60 to 90 minutes prior to surgery, and IV agents 30 to 60 minutes prior to surgery. Some agents—such as metoclopramide (Reglan), which is used to promote gastric emptying and lower stomach pH—are given 15 to 30 minutes before induction.

64. Depending on the desired outcome, a number of agents may be appropriate for use in the preoperative period.

65. Benzodiazepines, such as midazolam (Versed), diazepam (Valium), and lorazepam (Ativan), reduce anxiety and provide sedation and moderate to significant amnesia. Diazepam is given less frequently given due to its relatively long duration of action.

66. Barbiturates, such as secobarbital (Seconal) and pentobarbital (Nembutal), provide sedation with minimal cardiac or respiratory depression.

67. H_2 receptor blocking agents, such as ranitidine (Zantac, Glaxo), cimetidine (Tagamet), and famotidine (Pepcid), raise gastric pH and reduce the risk of and complications from aspiration.

68. Nonparticulate antacids, such as sodium citrate (Bicitra), raise gastric pH.

69. Dopamine antagonists, such as metoclopramide (Reglan), increase gastric emptying. Agents that raise pH or increase gastric emptying are particularly useful for patients at high risk for aspiration. Conditions that suggest high risk for aspiration include the following:

    • Morbid obesity

    • Old age

    • Pregnancy

    • History of hiatal hernia with reflux

    • Uncertain NPO status coupled with the need for emergency surgery

    • History of diabetes with gastroparesis

    • History of partial bowel obstruction

    • History of peptic ulcer disease

70. Anticholinergic agents, such as atropine, scopolamine, and glycopyrrolate (Robinul), decrease oral and tracheobronchial secretions and prevent bradycardia, which can occur during parasympathetic stimulation or with certain anesthetic agents during induction. These agents are also antiemetics and prevent postoperative nausea.

    • These drugs are particularly useful with patients who exhibit excessive salivation problems that put them at risk for aspiration.

    • They are also appropriate for toddlers and young children, who have a tendency to increase salivation up to tenfold when oral mucous membranes are stimulated (Litwack, 1995, p. 118).

    • Anticholinergics, which were once given routinely as a preoperative medication, are now ordered only for selected patients. Patients who are given anticholinergics may complain of a very dry mouth. Provide a moistened 4¾-inch gauze pad to moisten the patient's lips and tongue and provide patient comfort.

71. Antiemetic agents, such as ondansetron (Zofran), a serotonin 5-HT$_3$ receptor antagonist; diphenhydramine (Benadryl); and the scopolamine patch (TransdermScop) are given to prevent nausea and vomiting. These medications are particularly useful for patients who report a history of nausea and vomiting after anesthesia and surgery. In 2001, the FDA required droperidol (Inapsine) to carry a warning label related to "sudden cardiac death"; this change in the labeling has resulted in less frequent administration of this drug.

72. Antibiotics, such as cefazolin (Ancef, Kefzol), cefoxitin (Mefoxin), and cefotetan (Cefotan), are being used more frequently as a prophylaxis to prevent surgical-site infection (SSI). Multiple research studies have shown that the incidence of SSI can be dramatically reduced when appropriate and timely antibiotics are administered within 1 hour of surgery.

73. In an effort to reduce postoperative complications a number of organizations have developed initiatives to prevent surgical-site infection. The Surgical Care Improvement Project (SCIP) is a national quality partnership committed to improving the safety of surgical care through the reduction of postoperative complications. One of the SCIP's process and outcome measures is administration of a prophylactic antibiotic within 1 hour prior to surgical incision. To meet this criterion, most healthcare facilities have a policy that requires antibiotic administration in selected procedures within 1 hour of incision. (The exception involves administration of vancomycin, which requires an hour for infusion and must be started before the 1-hour window.)

74. The following factors determine when an antibiotic should be administered and which antibiotic is appropriate:

    • Probable risk of infection if a prophylactic agent is not administered

    • Probable contaminating flora associated with the operative site

    • Activity of the agent relative to the majority of pathogens likely to contaminate the operative site

75. Although the decision to administer an antibiotic preoperatively and the choice of antibiotic are made by the surgeon and/or anesthesia provider, institutional policy may assign responsibility for administration of the agent to the perioperative nurse.

76. Narcotics, such as meperidine (Demerol), fentanyl (Sublimaze), alfentanil (Alfenta), sufentanil (Sufenta), remifentanil (Ultiva), hydromorphine (Dilaudid), and morphine, provide relief from pain.

77. Patients who have received narcotics must be closely observed for adequate ventilation. *All* narcotics are associated with dose-related respiratory depression and can cause nausea and vomiting. In fact, narcotic analgesics such as morphine, which dramatically decrease gastrointestinal motility, can lead to constipation and GI tract obstruction or ileus.

78. It is not uncommon for patients who anticipate general anesthesia to mistakenly believe that the premedication they received should have put them to sleep for the surgery. If patients are anxious because they are still awake, provide reassurance by informing them that they will be given additional anesthetic agents for surgery, will be asleep during the procedure, and will not feel pain.

79. In the preoperative period, patients are often fearful—fear of the unknown, fear of having to relinquish control, and fear of never awakening from anesthesia are not uncommon. Perioperative nurses need to be sensitive to patients' fears, take the time to listen, remain close to the patient, and provide emotional support and reassurance. The period just prior to surgery may be the most stressful for the patient and is a time when the presence of a nurse is crucial to alleviate anxiety.

Section Questions

[www]

1. Describe the effect of general anesthesia on the patient. [Ref 49]

2. Explain moderate sedation/analgesia (conscious sedation). [Refs 50–51]

3. Differentiate between conscious sedation and monitored anesthesia care. [Ref 53]

4. Differentiate between central anesthesia and peripheral regional anesthesia. [Ref 56]

5. How is regional anesthesia administered? [Ref 57]

6. What is a Bier block? [Ref 58]

7. Explain current practice related to the premedication of surgical patients. [Refs 60–61]

8. Identify five or more goals of medications given prior to surgery. [Ref 62]

9. What differentiates Valium from other benzodiazepines? [Ref 65]

10. How do barbiturates affect cardiac and respiratory depression? [Ref 66]

11. Which drugs can be given to reduce the risk of complications from aspiration? [Ref 67]

12. List conditions that place patients at high risk for aspiration. [Ref 69]

13. Why are anticholinergic agents particularly important for toddlers and young children? [Ref 70]

14. Which types of drugs are given to prevent nausea and vomiting? [Ref 71]

15. What protocol can reduce the incidence of surgical-site infections? [Refs 72–73]

16. How does the administration of vancomycin differ from the administration of other antibiotics? [Ref 73]

17. Which factors determine when an antibiotic should be administered and which antibiotic is appropriate? [Ref 74]

18. When is responsibility for administering the antibiotic assigned to the perioperative nurse? [Ref 75]

19. What information is appropriate to share with a patient who is fearful because he or she is still awake following premedication? [Ref 78]

20. What makes the immediate preoperative period particularly stressful for patients? [Refs 78–79]

Monitoring

80. Patient monitoring is essential during anesthesia to detect physiologic changes in response to both the anesthesia and the surgical procedure. Ongoing monitoring is critical and provides the basis for appropriate and timely interventions that maintain satisfactory physiologic status.

81. The degree of monitoring required is determined by the intended procedure and the patient's history and state of health. At a minimum, monitoring for all surgical patients should include ECG, blood pressure, heart rate, and pulse oximetry. With general anesthesia, end-tidal carbon dioxide concentration, oxygen concentration, end-tidal anesthetic gas concentration, and core body temperature monitoring are also monitored.

Practice Recommendations and Standards

82. The Association of periOperative Registered Nurses (AORN) has formulated practice recommendations for the nurse who monitors the patient receiving local anesthesia and the patient receiving moderate sedation/analgesia. These recommendations state that monitoring should include the following elements (AORN, 2012, pp. 415–416):

    - Cardiac rate and rhythm
    - Level of consciousness
    - Blood pressure
    - Cardiac monitoring
    - Oxygenation using pulse oximetry with audible pulse rate and alarms
    - Ventilation monitored by direct observation and/or auscultation

83. The ASA has established standards for basic intraoperative monitoring. Qualified anesthesia personnel should be present in the room throughout the delivery of all general anesthetics, regional anesthetics, and monitored anesthesia care. During administration of all anesthetics, the patient's oxygenation, ventilation, circulation, and temperature should be continually monitored (ASA, 2012a).

    - Oxygenation: Ensure adequate oxygen concentration in the inspired gas and the blood during all anesthetics.
    - Ventilation: Ensure adequate ventilation of the patient during all anesthetics.
    - Circulation: Ensure the adequacy of the patient's circulatory function during all anesthetics.
    - Body temperature: Aid in the maintenance of appropriate body temperature during all anesthetics.
    - Carbon dioxide: Detect hypoventilation or esophageal intubation.

Monitoring Devices

84. Monitoring devices may be invasive or noninvasive. Noninvasive monitoring devices do not penetrate a body orifice.

85. Examples of noninvasive monitors include ECG electrodes, blood pressure cuffs, and pulse oximeters and capnometers. Invasive monitors are introduced beneath the skin or mucosa or enter a body cavity. Examples of invasive monitors include arterial lines and central venous catheters.

86. The choice of monitoring device is determined by the intended procedure, the patient's history and state of health, the anesthesia provider, the surgeon's judgment, and anticipated postoperative management.

87. Patients undergoing complex, critical, and extensive surgical procedures and patients with complex health problems will require extensive monitoring with a combination of invasive and noninvasive monitors. Examples where invasive monitoring is appropriate are in cardiac surgery, for procedures or patients where repeated blood samples will be required, and for patients in whom wide variations in blood pressure are anticipated. The healthy patient who undergoes a simple procedure will require only noninvasive monitoring.

88. The perioperative nurse must have knowledge of monitoring equipment and the ability to interpret data. When the entire responsibility for monitoring rests with the perioperative nurse, such as when the patient is receiving local anesthesia or moderate sedation/analgesia, monitoring is especially critical. In many facilities, supplementary monitoring competency requirements must be met before the perioperative nurse is permitted to monitor a patient independently. However, even where an anesthesiologist, a CRNA, or an AA is present, the perioperative nurse must be able to recognize normal and abnormal physiologic responses, administer oxygen

and pharmacologic therapy, and anticipate and assist in pharmacologic and emergency interventions.

Monitors for Patients Receiving General Anesthesia

Precordial or Esophageal Stethoscope

89. A stethoscope taped to the patient's chest or an esophageal stethoscope placed within the patient's esophagus facilitates continuous auscultation of the chest to monitor cardiac rate and rhythm and breath sounds. The esophageal stethoscope also has a temperature sensor attachment to continually monitor the patient's core temperature.

Electrocardiogram

90. ECG monitoring is essential to detect changes in cardiac rate and rhythm, and to detect dysrhythmia and myocardial ischemia. Myocardial ischemia in the perioperative period may lead to myocardial infarction postoperatively. Early detection and identification of cardiac irregularities permit timely and specific interventions that can prevent further complications.

91. ECG leads should be placed on clean, dry skin surfaces, and their adherence should be checked.

Pulse Oximetry

92. Pulse oximetry measures the oxygen saturation of arterial hemoglobin, which is an indicator of the oxygen transfer at the alveolar-capillary level.

93. A photodetector with one end attached to the pulse oximeter is placed on a vascular bed, such as a finger, toe, or ear lobe. The photodetector comprises a light source side and a receptor side. Two different wavelengths (red and infrared light) are transmitted through the tissue from the light source side of the photodetector. The receptor side of the photodetector measures the optical density of light that is passed through tissue. Optical density is influenced by the amount of oxygen in the hemoglobin. The absorption of light for each color indicates the ratio of saturated blood to unsaturated blood.

94. Oxygen saturation readings should be near 100%, and readings of less than 90% are generally indicative of significant hypoxemia. Hypoxemia may lead to cardiac arrest. Pulse oximetry facilitates prompt recognition of pending hypoxemia and appropriate prevention. In the event of decreased oxygen saturation, the perioperative nurse must be prepared to provide ventilatory support and to administer oxygen.

95. Satisfactory oxygen saturation readings from pulse oximetry are not a guarantee that tissues are being adequately perfused with oxygen. Other factors such as hemoglobin level must also be considered. Hemoglobin carries oxygen. Even though the hemoglobin may be saturated with oxygen, there may be insufficient hemoglobin to maintain appropriate tissues oxygen levels.

96. Pulse oximetry measures oxygenation; it does not measure ventilation. Hypoventilation for an extended period will result in an accumulation of carbon dioxide in the blood that will cause respiratory acidosis, leading to a decrease in oxygen saturation. The onset of respiratory acidosis can occur more rapidly than a decrease in oxygen saturation. It is possible for a patient on 100% oxygen to have a normal oxygen level but be suffering from respiratory acidosis. Ventilation should be assessed even when pulse oximetry readings are normal.

97. Bright lights can interfere with photodetector performance. Place the finger or toe with the probe attached under a blanket or drape.

98. Nail polish and acrylic nails do not cause clinically significant changes in pulse oximetry readings (Jakpor, 2011).

99. Intravascular dyes, such as methylene blue, interfere with the pulse oximeter's light emission, resulting in falsely depressed oxygen saturation reading (Ginimuge et al., 2010). Conditions causing vasoconstriction, such as Raynaud's disease, severe peripheral vascular disease, and hypotension, can also prevent an accurate reading (Valdez-Lowe et al., 2009).

100. Photodetectors should not be placed or secured so tightly that localized tissue ischemia results.

Blood Pressure

101. Blood pressure measures pressure in the heart during contraction and relaxation. It may be monitored manually, or an automatic monitor can take readings at preset intervals. Automatic monitors that measure blood pressure and

cardiac rate and display rhythm are standard equipment in the operating room and PACU. These monitors are also incorporated into all general anesthesia delivery machines.

102. Take care to prevent IV lines from being compressed with a blood pressure cuff. The site of cuff application should be periodically inspected to ensure that adequate deflation has taken place between readings. Extended inflation periods may lead to neurological injury.

Temperature

103. Anesthetic agents affect the patient's temperature both by dilating blood vessels and by inhibiting the temperature-regulating mechanism in the hypothalamus. Patient exposure, open surgery, and cool irrigating fluids also affect body temperature.

104. Hypothermia—defined as body temperature less than 36°C—can reduce the effectiveness of certain anesthetic agents and adversely affect pulse oximetry readings. Hypothermia has been consistently linked to shivering (which increases oxygen consumption by 400–500%), extended postoperative recovery times, and surgical-site infection (Jardeleza et al., 2011, p. 364).

105. If hypothermia develops, the patient can experience increased perioperative blood loss, longer postanesthetic recovery, postoperative shivering and thermal discomfort, increased risk of morbid cardiac events including arrhythmia, altered drug metabolism, increased risk of wound infection, reduced patient satisfaction with the surgical experience, and a longer stay in hospital (Jardeleza et al., 2011, p. 364).

106. The patients at greatest risk for unplanned hypothermia include infants, young children, the elderly, and patients with endocrine disorders. The length and type of surgical procedure also affect the risk for hypothermia.

107. There is a positive correlation between maintaining normal body temperature during the perioperative period and improved patient outcomes and increased patient satisfaction.

108. Interventions to prevent hypothermia should begin in the preoperative period and continue throughout the intraoperative and recovery periods.

109. The greatest change in patient temperature occurs during the first hour of surgery. Temperature should be monitored when the procedure is expected to last more than 30 minutes. It may be monitored with an external patch thermometer or a more accurate internal esophageal or rectal probe.

110. Keeping patients warm can also inhibit surgical-site infection. Intraoperative hypothermia can have a profound impact on SSI rates. Patient temperature less than 35°C doubles the risk for postoperative SSI (Seaman et al., 2012). Regardless of the length of the procedure, it is recommended that all patients be warmed with a forced-air warming blanket. Forced-air warming blankets are more effective in maintaining normothermia than warm blankets, warmed irrigating fluids, and head coverings such as towels.

111. For infants, a head covering made from a stockinette and use of Webril to wrap the arms and legs can help to maintain normal body temperature.

112. In addition to the application of coverings and a warming blanket, the temperature of the room may be raised to prevent hypothermia. This consideration is particularly important for burn patients, trauma patients, and babies. In some facilities, raising the room temperature may require a call to the maintenance department. If this is necessary, the request should be made as soon after assessment as possible to warm the room before the patient is brought in.

113. The stability of IV solutions can vary according to composition and container, and can be affected by temperature. Follow the fluid manufacturer's instructions to determine temperature and time limits when warming irrigating or IV solutions, and to determine whether they can be rewarmed if not used. In addition, warming cabinet temperatures should be monitored to ensure that temperatures are within the range needed to meet the manufacturer's instructions. IV solutions and especially blood products, such as packed red blood cells (PRBCs) and fresh frozen plasma (FFP), should be administered through a fluid warming device.

Capnography

114. Capnography monitors the inhaled and exhaled concentration or partial pressure of carbon dioxide in the respiratory gases. It is useful in detecting hypoventilation, esophageal intubation, and a disconnected circuit. Carbon dioxide absorbs infrared radiation. When a beam of infrared light is passed across the gas to a sensor, the carbon dioxide absorbs the light and changes the voltage in the circuit, which is then displayed on a graph. Capnography is also useful to detect acute changes in metabolic function that indicate the possibility of hypothermia or malignant hyperthermia.

115. Most capnography units provide a digital display of end-tidal CO_2 and a waveform readout of expired CO_2 partial pressure versus time.

Section Questions

1. Why is monitoring essential during the administration of anesthesia? [Ref 80]

2. What is considered minimum monitoring for all surgical patients? [Ref 81]

3. How does AORN recommend that patients receiving conscious sedation be monitored? [Ref 82]

4. Describe the American Society of Anesthesiologists' standards for monitoring patients receiving anesthesia. [Ref 83]

5. Differentiate invasive from noninvasive monitoring devices. [Ref 84]

6. Cite examples of invasive and noninvasive monitoring devices. [Ref 85]

7. What determines the choice of monitoring devices for a surgical patient? [Ref 86]

8. Cite examples of procedures where invasive monitoring is appropriate. [Ref 87]

9. Explain why a perioperative nurse must have knowledge of monitoring equipment and the ability to interpret data. [Ref 88]

10. What does an esophageal stethoscope monitor in addition to cardiac rate, rhythm, and breath sounds? [Ref 89]

11. What is the benefit of identifying myocardial ischemia in the perioperative period? [Ref 90]

12. Which criteria determine placement of ECG leads? [Ref 91]

13. Why is the oxygen saturation of arterial hemoglobin measured? [Ref 92]

14. How does a pulse oximeter work? [Ref 93]

15. What is the implication of oxygen saturations less than 90%? [Ref 94]

16. Which other factors must be measured to ensure that tissues are adequately perfused with oxygen? [Ref 95]

17. Why is it necessary to assess ventilation even when pulse oximetry readings are normal? [Ref 96]

18. How do bright lights, nail polish, and methylene blue affect pulse oximetry readings? [Refs 97–99]

19. What are some responsibilities associated with blood pressure monitoring? [Ref 102]

20. How do anesthetic agents affect the patient's temperature? [Ref 103]

21. How does hypothermia affect anesthesia and patient monitoring? [Refs 104–105]

22. Which patient populations are at greatest risk for unplanned hypothermia? [[Ref 106]

23. Describe some interventions for preventing hypothermia in surgical patients. [Refs 109–112]

24. What is monitored by capnography? [Ref 114]

25. Which patient conditions can be detected via capnography? [Ref 114]

General Anesthesia

116. Effects of general anesthesia include amnesia (loss of memory), hypnosis (loss of consciousness), analgesia, and skeletal muscle relaxation. Because different anesthetic agents produce different degrees of response, it is customary to administer more than one agent.

117. Inhalation and intravenous injection are methods used to deliver general anesthetic agents.

Inhalation Agents

118. Nitrous oxide (N_2O), isofloranene), desflurane (Suprane), and sevoflurane (Ultane) are the most commonly used inhalation anesthetic agents. They enter the system by inhalation and are removed by lung ventilation (Table 11-1).

119. Nitrous oxide is a sweet-smelling gas that acts rapidly but lacks potency. It is nonirritating and produces few aftereffects, and recovery is rapid. Because it is a relatively weak anesthetic agent, it is sometimes used as a supplement to other inhalation agents and narcotics.

120. In combination with oxygen alone, nitrous oxide is sufficient only for minor procedures that do not produce intense pain.

121. Nitrous oxide diffuses readily into gas-filled spaces such as the stomach, colon, and lungs. Its use should be avoided in cases where expansion in these areas would be a problem (e.g., bowel

Table 11-1	Inhalation Agents		
Agent	**Use**	**Advantages**	**Disadvantages**
Oxygen	Sustain life	Rapid induction and recovery; few aftereffects; nonirritating to respiratory tract	Poor relaxation, insufficient potency for general surgery, hypoxia a potential hazard
Isoflurane (Forane)	Maintenance of anesthesia; may be used for induction	Inexpensive rapid induction and recovery; minimal aftereffects, obtunds laryngeal and pharyngeal reflexes; good relaxation, potentiates all muscle relaxants; protects heart against catecholamine-induced arrhythmias; cardiovascular system remains stable	Profound respiratory depressant
Sevoflurane	Maintenance of anesthesia; may be used for induction	Most rapid induction and emergence; no ether smell; easy to breathe; protects heart against myocardial irritability	Metabolizes to inorganic fluoride; raises fluoride level in patients with renal disease—unknown consequences; mild and transient chills, fever, nausea; contraindicated in patients susceptible to malignant hyperthermia
Desflurane (Suprane)	Maintenance for short period	Rapid emergence, good relaxation	Irritating to respiratory tract; can cause transient increase in heart rate and blood pressure

obstruction, pneumothorax). Also, because it causes expansion in the stomach, this agent is associated with postoperative nausea and vomiting.

122. For major procedures, nitrous oxide can be used with other agents to potentiate the anesthetic state.

123. A major precaution with the administration of nitrous oxide is to prevent too high a concentration, which can lead to hypoxia.

124. Isoflurane, desflurane, and sevoflurane are volatile anesthetic agents that share the property of being liquid at room temperature, but evaporating easily for administration by inhalation. These anesthetics pass through a vaporizer on the anesthesia machine and are inhaled by the patient.

125. Isoflurane provides excellent relaxation and potentiates muscle relaxants. Induction and emergence are the most prolonged of the commonly used agents. The cardiovascular system remains stable when this agent is administered, and electrocardiographic abnormalities are not associated with isoflurane inhalation.

126. Isoflurane does not sensitize the myocardium to catecholamines; therefore, epinephrine may be used for local vasoconstriction.

127. Isoflurane causes peripheral vasodilation. Hypotension is common at induction; however, blood pressure rapidly returns to normal. Use of isoflurane has declined, and this anesthetic is generally being replaced by desflurane and sevoflurane.

128. Desflurane provides excellent relaxation and offers the most rapid onset and emergence. A transient increase in cardiac rate and blood pressure may occur on induction.

129. Due to desflurane's rapid induction and emergence, it is especially tailored for ambulatory surgery procedures. It is also the agent of choice for obese patients because of its low fat solubility. Because this medication is not taken up into the fat tissue as rapidly as the other agents, using it allows for faster emergence from anesthesia.

130. Because of its pungent odor, which can cause gagging and laryngospasm, desflurane is not recommended for an inhalation induction.

131. Inhalation induction—a technique often used for children—delivers only anesthetic agents by mask. Intravenous induction uses IV medications to induce a loss of consciousness.

132. Sevoflurane has a moderate rate of induction and emergence. It acts more slowly than desflurane and much more rapidly than isoflurane.

133. Sevoflurane is not irritating to the respiratory tract and does not irritate the myocardium; therefore, it is the induction inhalation agent of choice for children. It is also appropriate for ambulatory procedures.

Anesthesia Machine

134. Inhalation agents are administered to the patient through an anesthesia machine.

135. Oxygen, nitrous oxide, and air are supplied through hoses from a central source within the healthcare facility or from cylinders attached to the machine. For safety purposes, the hoses and cylinders are color coded and their fittings are not interchangeable. Oxygen cylinders and hoses are color coded green; nitrous oxide is blue; air is yellow.

136. Flow meters attached to the machine are also color coded and indicate the amount of flow of nitrous oxide, air, and oxygen being delivered to the patient. The anesthesia provider selects the ratio of these gases.

137. Another safety feature is a shutoff device, which prevents nitrous oxide from being delivered if oxygen is not also delivered at a concentration of at least 21%.

138. The anesthesia machine is equipped with an oxygen flush button that delivers 100% oxygen to the patient.

139. The anesthesia machine includes a mechanical ventilator and monitoring devices for blood pressure, ECG, inspired oxygen, and end-tidal carbon dioxide. An end-tidal measurement of the inhalational agents and gases is also commonly available. The machine also has an alarm system that indicates when the patient is experiencing apnea or the breathing circuit has become detached from the machine.

140. The anesthesia machine includes a vaporizer for vaporizing and delivering liquid anesthetic agents (isoflurane, sevoflurane, and desflurane).

141. Oxygen and other anesthetic inhalation agents are mixed and directed to and from the patient through corrugated rubber or plastic tubes. These tubes are joined with a built-in Y connector that may be attached to a face mask or an endotracheal tube. Anesthetic gases are directed to the patient through a one-way valve

in one tube, and expired gases are returned through the other tube.

142. A reservoir bag, similar to a balloon, is part of the delivery system. When the reservoir bag is manually compressed, oxygen and inhalation agents can be forced into the lungs, much like an Ambu bag.

143. As the expired gases are returned from the patient, the carbon dioxide passes through a carbon dioxide absorber and is removed. Oxygen is added to the remaining exhaled gases, and these are returned to the patient for rebreathing.

144. The presence of nitrous oxide, as well as other anesthetic gases in the atmosphere, presents a serious health hazard to operating-room staff. Nausea, dizziness, headaches, fatigue, irritability, drowsiness, decreased mental performance, reduced fertility, and miscarriages, as well as neurological, renal, and liver disease, have been associated with exposure to these gases (OSHA, 2011a, 2012).

145. The National Institute for Occupational Safety and Health (NIOSH) has set limits of exposure for anesthetic gases. Every effort must be made to prevent their escape into the atmosphere. The NIOSH guidelines limit worker exposure to 25 parts per million (ppm) nitrous oxide over an 8-hour time-weighted average (NIOSH, 2012; OSHA, 2011a, 2012).

146. The level of anesthetic waste gases is periodically tested to determine an institution's compliance with NIOSH recommendations. The perioperative nurse should be aware of limits and of testing results.

147. Anesthesia machines are equipped with a scavenger system that controls the collection of excess expired gases that are eliminated through a suction line.

148. In addition to required periodic testing to monitor the amount of waste gas in the operating room, anesthetic gases should be shut off except during delivery to the patient. Routine testing of anesthesia equipment for leaks and reviews of anesthesia technique can help prevent overexposure.

Intravenous Agents

149. Intravenous agents are introduced directly into the circulatory system, usually through a peripheral vein in the arm or hand.

150. Intravenous agents are most often used as a supplement to inhalation agents.

151. Unlike inhalation agents, which can be easily removed from the system by ventilating the lungs, most intravenous agents must be metabolized by the liver or kidneys to be eliminated from the body (excreted).

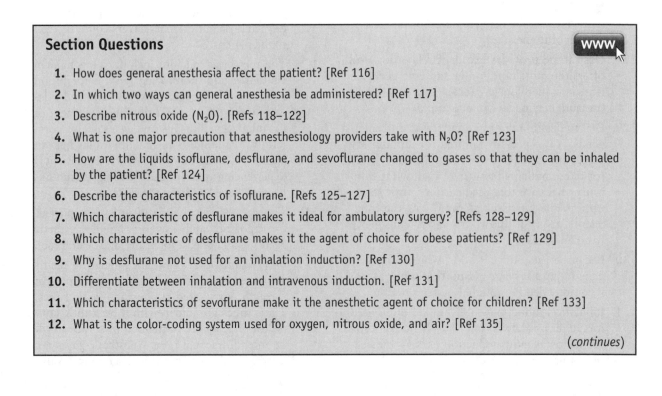

Section Questions   www

1. How does general anesthesia affect the patient? [Ref 116]

2. In which two ways can general anesthesia be administered? [Ref 117]

3. Describe nitrous oxide (N_2O). [Refs 118–122]

4. What is one major precaution that anesthesiology providers take with N_2O? [Ref 123]

5. How are the liquids isoflurane, desflurane, and sevoflurane changed to gases so that they can be inhaled by the patient? [Ref 124]

6. Describe the characteristics of isoflurane. [Refs 125–127]

7. Which characteristic of desflurane makes it ideal for ambulatory surgery? [Refs 128–129]

8. Which characteristic of desflurane makes it the agent of choice for obese patients? [Ref 129]

9. Why is desflurane not used for an inhalation induction? [Ref 130]

10. Differentiate between inhalation and intravenous induction. [Ref 131]

11. Which characteristics of sevoflurane make it the anesthetic agent of choice for children? [Ref 133]

12. What is the color-coding system used for oxygen, nitrous oxide, and air? [Ref 135]

(continues)

Section Questions (continued)

13. Which precaution is built into an anesthesia machine related to nitrous oxide and oxygen? [Ref 137]

14. What is the purpose of the oxygen flush button on an anesthesia machine? [Ref 138]

15. Which other monitoring devices are commonly built into the anesthesia machine? [Ref 139]

16. What is the purpose of the reservoir bag on the anesthesia machine? [Ref 142]

17. How might operating-room staff be adversely affected by exposure to nitrous oxide and other anesthetic gases in the air? [Ref 144]

18. Why do anesthesia machines have a scavenger system? [Ref 147]

19. How are inhalation agents removed from the patient's system? [Ref 151]

20. How are intravenous anesthetic agents removed from the patient's system? [Ref 151]

Barbiturate Induction Agents

152. Barbiturates are occasionally used for induction of anesthesia.

153. The most commonly used barbiturates are thiopental sodium (sodium pentothal), sodium thiamylal (Surital), and methohexital sodium (Brevital). These short-acting agents result in a rapid progression from sedation to loss of consciousness; however, they do not provide analgesia.

154. Barbiturates are potent respiratory depressants, and initial transient apnea is expected. For this reason, before barbiturates are administered, preparations must be made to provide oxygen and to assist or control the patient's ventilation.

155. Barbiturates also depress the cardiovascular system, and a degree of hypotension can be expected.

Nonbarbiturate Induction Agents

156. The nonbarbiturate drug propofol (Diprivan) is the most popular induction and maintenance agent. It is a hypnotic-sedative agent that produces rapid induction.

157. Propofol is delivered in a milky white intralipid emulsion. This medium supports microbial growth, and outbreaks of infection have been associated with its use (Muller et al., 2010). Propofol must be used within 6 hours of preparation, and its handling requires strict aseptic technique.

158. The patient may experience pain upon injection of propofol.

159. Recovery from propofol is more rapid than with barbiturates. This drug produces minimal aftereffects and fewer incidences of postoperative nausea and vomiting. It is often used in ambulatory surgery settings.

160. Etomidate (Amidate) is a nonbarbiturate induction agent that has minimal effects on myocardial metabolism, cardiac output, and peripheral or pulmonary circulation. It is a short-acting agent and is generally utilized for patients with a positive cardiac history and patients who cannot tolerate dramatic changes in blood pressure.

161. Etomidate does not provide analgesia.

Dissociative Induction Agents

162. Ketamine hydrochloride (Ketalar) is a dissociative agent that produces a catatonic state and provides amnesia and analgesia. The patient will breathe unassisted, may move, and may appear to be awake even after the anesthetized state has been achieved; surgery can be performed without patient response. Ketamine is rapidly metabolized, and patients emerge quickly from its effects.

163. Ketamine may be given either intravenously (IV) or intramuscularly (IM).

164. Ketamine is useful for diagnostic procedures and procedures where it is desirable to have the patient breathe unassisted. It is sometimes used for children who undergo short procedures that do not require muscle relaxation.

165. Because ketamine often produces a dramatic increase in oral secretions, an antisaligogue is often used in conjunction with it.

166. Because ketamine is a dissociative agent, patients may experience hallucinations postoperatively.

This aftereffect is more common in adults and may be minimized when diazepam or midazolam is given. The patient should recover in a quiet, darkened area.

Narcotics

167. Narcotics may be used preoperatively as a premedication or intraoperatively during anesthesia induction and maintenance.

168. Narcotics used intraoperatively include fentanyl (Sublimaze), sufentanil (Sufenta), alfentanil (Alfenta), morphine, hydromorphone (Dilaudid), and remifentenil (Ultiva). Fentanyl is 100 times more potent than morphine, and sufentanil is 5–10 times more potent than fentanyl.

169. Small doses of narcotics are used intraoperatively as adjuncts to other drugs and to provide pain relief in the early postoperative period.

170. Narcotics provide profound analgesia and can be particularly valuable in cardiac surgery because sternotomy is especially painful/stimulating.

171. Narcotics are respiratory depressants, and patients who have received high doses of narcotics intraoperatively must be monitored closely to ensure that they are breathing adequately. A patient who has received a high dose of narcotic intraoperatively may appear to be awake and alert postoperatively but may suddenly begin to hypoventilate and lose consciousness.

172. The narcotic meperidine hydrochloride (Demerol) is used in the PACU to control shivering. This drug requires caution when used with patients taking monoamine oxidase (MAO) inhibitor drugs (phenelzine, selegiline, and tranylcypromine), because it may result in hypertensive crisis, hyperpyrexia, and cardiovascular system collapse, which could be fatal. It is used infrequently for purposes other than for shivering unless the patient has unmanageable adverse reactions to other first-line opioids.

173. Naloxone (Narcan) is an opiate antagonist that competitively binds to the opioid receptors. If the patient is apneic, it is recommended that 0.4 mg or 1 ampule of naloxone be administered IV or IM with careful monitoring. If the patient is not apneic but has a falling O2 saturation, it is recommended that naloxone be titrated into effect. In the apneic patient, it is important to support the airway, and the first drug of choice to administer is oxygen. It is also important to realize that the patient may re-narcotize because the half-life of naloxone is only approximately 20 minutes—the half-life of most narcotics is longer.

174. Complications of naloxone administration include pulmonary edema and hypertension. Additionally, the patient is essentially forced into a rapid "withdrawal" and will experience pain, diaphoresis, nausea, and vomiting, similar to what an opioid addict would experience with withdrawal.

Tranquilizers: Benzodiazepines

175. Tranquilizers commonly used intraoperatively include diazepam (Valium) and midazolam (Versed).

176. Tranquilizers are used for induction and as adjuncts to other anesthetic agents. Their use permits lower doses of other agents to be administered.

177. Diazepam produces amnesia and reduces anxiety. Midazolam is an excellent amnestic and also provides significant anxiolysis.

178. Flumazenil (Romazicon) is an important drug that is used to reverse the effects of benzodiazepines. It reverses sedation and respiratory depression without producing cardiovascular effects. Patients whose anesthesia is reversed in this manner must be closely monitored because flumazenil may lose its effect sooner than the underlying benzodiazepine, and hypoventilation can recur.

Neuromuscular Blockers (Muscle Relaxants)

179. Muscle relaxants commonly used intraoperatively include succinylcholine (Anectine), cisatracurium besylate (Nimbex), rocuronium bromide (Zemuron), and vecuronium bromide (Norcuron) (Table 11-2).

180. Two primary indications for neuromuscular blockers are as follows:

- To relax the jaw and larynx to facilitate controlled breathing and tracheal intubation
- To increase muscle relaxation to permit ease of tissue handling during surgery

Table 11-2	Muscle Relaxants		
Agent	**Use**	**Advantages**	**Disadvantages**
Depolarizing Muscle Relaxant—Rapid Onset, Short Duration			
Succinylcholine (Anectine, Quelicin)	Intubation Short procedures	Rapid onset; brief duration	Can cause muscle fasciculation, postoperative myalgia; requires refrigeration, contraindicated in patients with recent burn, muscle trauma, or recurrent neuromuscular disorder; can trigger malignant hyperthermia; prolonged effect in patients with serum cholinesterase deficiency
Nondepolarizing Muscle Relaxants—Intermediate Onset, Intermediate Duration			
Atracurium (Tracrium)	Intubation Maintenance of paralysis	Transient and generally minimal cardiovascular effects	Not currently available in the US; requires refrigeration; histamine release; facial flushing; transient hypotension and reflex tachycardia
Vecuronium (Norcuron)	Intubation Maintenance of paralysis	No significant cardiovascular effects; no release of histamine	Must be mixed
Rocuronium (Zemuron)	Intubation Maintenance of paralysis	Provides excellent intubating conditions; rapid onset	May increase heart rate; eliminated via liver, contraindicated in patients with hepatic disease, contraindicated for rapid intubation for cesarean sections
Cisatracurium (Nimbex)	Intubation Maintenance of paralysis	Does not require renal or hepatic elimination (uses Hoffman/enzymatic elimination) so can use in kidney or liver failure. No histamine release so cardiovascularly stable	Requires refrigeration
Nondepolarizing Muscle Relaxants—Delayed Onset, Longer Duration			
Tubocurarine (curare)	Maintenance of paralysis		Strong histamine release; automatic blockade can cause hypotension
Pancuronium (Pavulon)	Maintenance of paralysis	Long duration	Can cause hypertension and increased heart rate

181. Muscle relaxants vary in their onset and duration. Any of the agents can be used for intubation, but the length of time to achieve prime "intubating conditions" depends on the onset of the particular drug.

182. Neuromuscular blockers paralyze the neuromuscular junction and block impulses from motor nerves to skeletal muscle. The patient becomes paralyzed. Neuromuscular blockers may be either depolarizing or nondepolarizing.

183. Succinylcholine is a depolarizing muscle relaxant. When it reaches the neuromuscular junction, it acts like acetylcholine, producing a depolarization of the membrane at the motor end plate. The depolarization causes a muscle contraction that is followed by a neuromuscular block. The drug prevents repolarization, and the muscle remains relaxed and paralyzed. The muscle contractions are sometimes obvious and appear similar to twitching. This twitching, referred to as fasciculation, progresses in cephalocaudal sequence as the drug circulates through the patient's body.

184. Succinylcholine produces paralysis within seconds and is used for intubation. Because of its rapid onset of action, it is valuable in emergency situations where rapid intubation is required.

185. Succinylcholine will cause an increase in plasma potassium levels because the acetylcholine receptor is propped open, allowing ongoing flow of potassium ions into the extracellular fluid. This increase is transient in normal patients.

186. Conditions that make patients susceptible to succinylcholine-induced hyperkalemia include burns, closed head injury, acidosis, Guillain-Barré syndrome, cerebral stroke, drowning, severe intraabdominal sepsis, massive trauma, myopathy, and tetanus.

187. Succinylcholine is a known triggering agent for malignant hyperthermia.

188. Nondepolarizing muscle relaxants block the action of acetylcholine at the neuromuscular junction but do not cause depolarization at the motor end plate, so fasciculation does not occur.

189. Nondepolarizing agents have a slower onset than depolarizing agents and their effect or duration of action is dose dependent.

   - Vecuronium, rocuronium, and cisatracurium are considered "intermediate-acting" neuromuscular blocking agents (NMBs), whose standard weight-based dose lasts approximately 45 minutes.

   - Pavulon is considered a long-acting agent and is mainly used in cardiac surgery or when the patient is not expected to be extubated at the end of the case.

190. The anesthesia provider continually monitors the patient to determine the amount of paralysis present. Applying a nerve stimulator to a peripheral nerve, such as the ulnar nerve or a branch of the facial nerve, and observing for the presence of contractions is helpful in determining the degree of paralysis present.

191. The anticholinergic or "reversal" agents spyridostigmine (Regonol) and neostigmine (Prostigmin) reverse the action of nondepolarizing agents. These two drugs are always used in combination with atropine sulfate or glycopyrrolate (Robinul) to counteract the potentially profound muscarinic effects (bradycardia and salivation) of the anticholinesterases.

192. Even if the patient has been "reversed" and demonstrates a normal twitch response on the nerve stimulator, 75–85% of the receptors at the neuromuscular junction could still be occupied (inducing paralysis).

193. Administration of the reversal agent does not make the muscle paralysis magically disappear—patients may still be weak and require extra time to breathe on their own.

Section Questions

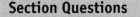

1. Which characteristics of barbiturates make them appropriate for induction? [Ref 153]

2. Which precaution is taken before administering barbiturates? [Ref 154]

3. Besides respiratory depression, which other system is affected by barbiturates? [Ref 155]

4. Describe propofol (Diprivan). [Ref 156]

(continues)

Section Questions (continued)

5. Why must propofol be used within 6 hours of preparation using strict aseptic technique? [Ref 157]

6. Which characteristics of propofol make it appropriate for ambulatory surgery? [Ref 159]

7. Which characteristics of etomidate (Amidate) make it appropriate for patients with a cardiac history? [Ref 160]

8. What is the effect of ketamine on patients? [Ref 162]

9. Under which circumstances would ketamine be chosen as an anesthetic agent? [Ref 164]

10. What is an antisaligogue? [Ref 165]

11. Which interventions address the potential for hallucinations sometimes experienced with ketamine? [Ref 166]

12. For what purpose are narcotics used intraoperatively? [Refs 169–170]

13. What must be monitored closely in postoperative patients who have received high doses of narcotics? [Ref 171]

14. What effect can meperedine (Demerol), which is used in the PACU to control shivering, have on patients who take MAO inhibitor drugs? [Ref 172]

15. How does nalaxone (Narcan) counter the adverse effects of opiates, such as apnea? [Ref 173]

16. How can a patient re-narcotize following administration of Narcan? [Ref 173]

17. Describe complications possible with use of Narcan. [Ref 174]

18. How do tranquilizers affect other anesthetic agents? [Ref 176]

19. When flumazenil (Romazicon) is used to reverse sedation and respiratory depression, why must patients be closely monitored? [Ref 178]

20. What are two primary indications for neuromuscular blockers? [Ref 180]

21. Explain the fasciculation ("twitching") that sometimes accompanies the use of a depolarizing muscle relaxant such as succinylcholine. [Ref 183]

22. Which characteristics of succinylcholine make it valuable in emergency situations? [Ref 184]

23. Succinylcholine is a triggering agent for which specific adverse outcome associated with anesthesia? [Ref 187]

24. How does the anesthesia provider use a nerve stimulator to assess the amount of paralysis present? [Ref 190]

25. Explain the need for careful monitoring after an anticholinergic has been used to reverse the action of nondepolarizing agents? [Refs 191–193]

Stages of Anesthesia

194. In 1720, Arthur Guedel integrated the four stages of anesthesia with their signs and symptoms into a system that, until recently, was used to estimate the depth of anesthesia. Depth of anesthesia was determined by observing the patient's physiological changes and reflex responses. The system applied to patients who were not premedicated, breathed spontaneously, and were anesthetized with ether.

195. The stages are as follows:

- Stage I: Relaxation—from administration of anesthesia to loss of consciousness. Patient response: dizziness, drowsiness, exaggerated hearing, and a decreased sense of pain.

- Stage II: Excitement—from loss of consciousness to onset of regular breathing. Patient response: irregular breathing, increased muscle tone and involuntary motor activity, thrashing and struggling activity (susceptible to auditory and tactile stimulation).

- Stage III: Surgical anesthesia—from onset of regular breathing to cessation of respiration. Patient response: regular thoracoabdominal breathing, a relaxed jaw, a loss of pain and auditory sensation, and loss of eyelid reflex.

- Stage IV: Danger—from cessation of respiration to circulatory failure and death. Patient response: fixed and dilated pupils, rapid and thready pulse, and paralyzed respiratory muscles. The patient should never be at this depth of anesthesia.

196. Perioperative nurses should have an appreciation of the depth of anesthesia. The excitement phase in Stage II may still be seen during induction and emergence in both children and adults, especially during a mask induction of anesthesia. Awareness of the patient's level of anesthesia allows the nurse to plan for and provide safety measures.

197. Recovery from anesthesia occurs in reverse order (moving from Stage IV to Stage I). During emergence, which often takes place at the same time as the dressing is being applied, it is important not to stimulate patients by touching them near the head or neck, pressing on the abdomen, or moving an extremity. Any of these stimulations during Stage II could trigger laryngospasm. The nurse should maintain good communication with the anesthesia provider to determine the right time to move the patient.

Preparation for Anesthesia: Nursing Responsibilities

198. As much as possible, the room should be ready and preparations for surgery completed before the patient is brought into the operating-room suite. Once the patient is in the room, it is important that the circulating nurse focus attention on providing emotional support, ensuring patient dignity, instituting safety measures, and assisting the anesthesia provider.

199. Prior to anesthesia induction, the perioperative nurse should check the suction to ensure that it is turned on and working properly. The suction catheter should be placed within easy reach of the anesthesia provider.

200. In preparation for induction, nursing responsibilities may include transfer of the patient from the stretcher to the operating-room table, placement of electrocardiographic leads, application of the blood pressure cuff, placement of the intravenous line, and application of the safety strap. Because these preparatory activities have the potential for exposing the patient's body, nursing interventions at this time should focus on maintaining patient dignity by adjusting the patient's gown and covers to ensure privacy, closing the operating-room doors, and keeping unnecessary personnel from the room.

201. As preparations are made for anesthesia induction, patients often experience feelings ranging from mild anxiety to acute fear. The perioperative nurse can help allay these feelings by being at the patient's side, speaking calmly, answering questions, and explaining activities. Nonverbal support, such as making eye contact and holding the patient's hand, can be the most supportive intervention.

202. Efforts should be made not to stimulate the patient or interrupt the calming effect of the preoperative medication. Avoid unnecessary noise. It is the perioperative nurse's responsibility to ensure a quiet atmosphere in the operating room; however, all team members must participate in the effort. All unnecessary conversation should be curtailed.

203. The scrubbed person should arrange instruments and supplies quietly. The operating room's door should remain closed. Instrument counting should not be done within range of the patient's hearing. Overhearing "blades," "needles," "mosquitoes," and so forth can be frightening to the patient. It is essential to remember that hearing is the most difficult sense to anesthetize, and it is the last sensation lost before unconsciousness.

204. In rare instances, an anesthetized patient experiences unintended awareness and has direct recall of events. The incidence of this type of event is estimated to be between 0.1% and 0.2% of all patients undergoing general anesthesia (20,000–40,000 cases per year). Forty-eight percent of these patients reported hearing during their surgery (TJC, 2004, p. 1). Conversation during the intraoperative period should always be respectful of the patient's dignity.

205. Induction is the period from when an anesthetic is first administered until the patient loses consciousness and is then stabilized at the desired level of anesthesia.

206. Induction is a critical time during the administration of anesthesia, and it is essential for patient safety that the perioperative nurse be present and available to assist the anesthesia provider with suctioning and intubation and, if necessary, to restrain the patient (particularly children).

207. The circulating nurse also assists the anesthesia provider in positioning the patient properly for

intubation. Some patients' anatomy makes them a "difficult intubation," in which case blankets or a positioning device may be necessary to achieve the "sniffing" position (a position that maximizes laryngoscopy). The nurse might also need to call for additional airway equipment (e.g., a fiber-optic scope or airway cart).

208. In young children who may not tolerate the placement of an intravenous line, and in patients with a tracheostomy tube, induction is usually begun with an inhalation agent.

Sequence for General Anesthesia: Nursing Responsibilities

209. The typical sequence for general anesthesia in patients who have an intravenous line is outlined here:

    • If the patient can tolerate it, a mask is placed over the nose and mouth while the patient breathes 100% oxygen for a few minutes. The oxygenation serves as a safety margin in the event of an airway obstruction or brief period of apnea during insertion of the endotracheal tube.

    • A narcotic and/or a benzodiazepine is injected and ventilation is monitored.

    • A barbiturate (thiopental sodium or thiamylal sodium) or a nonbarbiturate (propofol or etomidate) is injected to produce sleep. Sleep may be judged by the lack of eyelid movement when the eyelid is stroked. Sleep will usually occur within 1 or 2 minutes.

    • With the mask over the patient's nose and mouth, the anesthesia provider ventilates the patient and observes the chest rise. If the chest does not rise, the head and mandible are repositioned until a patent airway is maintained.

    • When it is established that the airway is clear, a paralyzing dose of muscle relaxant is administered to facilitate intubation. (Muscle relaxants with a longer onset may be injected before the patient is asleep, as the effect will not occur until after sleep is achieved.)

    • A laryngoscope is used to visualize the vocal cords, and the patient is intubated. (An endotracheal tube is inserted into the trachea.) The perioperative nurse can assist the anesthesia provider by pulling outwardly on the corner of the patient's mouth to permit better visualization of the vocal cords and placement of the endotracheal tube. The perioperative nurse can also assist by passing the endotracheal tube to the anesthesia provider so he or she does not have to interrupt visualization to pick up the tube, and by providing a 10-mL syringe to inflate the endotracheal tube cuff.

    • Correct endotracheal tube placement is confirmed as follows:
        1. Observe fog in the clear endotracheal tube.
        2. Observe the patient for bilateral chest excursion without epigastric enlargement.
        3. Listen for bilateral breath sounds.
        4. Identify carbon dioxide expiration through end-tidal monitoring. CO_2 waveform capnography is the gold standard for the confirmation of tube placement within the trachea.

210. If the patient is intubated, the endotracheal tube is inserted directly through the larynx into the trachea. The cuff is inflated to prevent secretions from entering the trachea and lungs. An endotracheal tube is considered a "secured" airway, as it prevents gastric contents from entering the trachea.

211. After appropriate positioning to ensure the tube is not past the carina or the bifurcation into the right and left main stem bronchi, the tube is secured in place with tape. The endotracheal tube is connected to the anesthesia machine via tubing, and inhalation agents are delivered automatically according to parameters set by the anesthesia provider. Depending on the procedure and the necessity for paralysis, the patient will either be ventilated or will breathe spontaneously.

212. For short procedures and procedures where paralysis is not necessary, the patient is usually not intubated. A combination of inhalation agents will be administered via a mask or laryngeal mask airway (LMA).

    • The mask is strapped or held over the patient's nose and mouth and connected via anesthesia tubing to the anesthesia machine. The patient may breathe spontaneously, or breathing and delivery of anesthetic agents may be accomplished manually by compressing a reservoir bag on the anesthesia machine. This is also referred to as "bagging" the patient.

- The LMA is a device that provides good airway management without intubation. It is inserted into the patient's mouth, positioned securely over the larynx, and inflated to keep it securely in place. The patient is connected to the anesthesia machine via an anesthesia circuit. The patient may breathe spontaneously or be mechanically ventilated. An LMA is not a "secured airway," as it does not have a cuff that prevents gastric contents from entering the trachea (Figure 11-1 and Figure 11-2).

213. When a barbiturate or hypnotic is given at the start of induction, it will quickly reach the patient's brain, causing apnea. The patient's pharyngeal muscles and tongue relax, and airway obstruction can occur. If a clear airway is not maintained, the patient will attempt to breathe as the drug washes out of the brain. The abdominal muscles may strain and pull the diaphragm down, compressing the stomach and causing the patient to regurgitate. If the patient regurgitates and attempts to breathe, he or she can aspirate gastric contents into the lungs, resulting in aspiration pneumonia. The perioperative nurse must be prepared to provide suction immediately, turn the patient's head to one side, adjust the table to the Trendelenburg position, and assist the anesthesia provider as needed.

214. Patients who have not been NPO for the required period of time are not given general anesthesia except in emergency situations when regional anesthesia is not appropriate.

- The patient who ate before becoming ill, the trauma victim with blood in the stomach, and the patient with a hiatal hernia are at risk for aspiration.

- Aspiration of stomach contents can be fatal.

- The perioperative nurse's first priority is to remain at the patient's side at the head of the table, prepared to assist the anesthesia provider until intubation is complete and assistance is no longer needed.

- A suction catheter or tip, a nasogastric tube, an emesis basin, and a towel should be immediately available.

215. During intubation, cricoid pressure may be necessary.

- The perioperative nurse may be asked to assist by firmly pressing the cricoid cartilage posteriorly with the index finger or thumb and forefinger.

- This maneuver (called the Sellick maneuver) compresses the esophagus between the cricoid cartilage and the vertebral column.

- The Sellick maneuver aids in visualization of the tracheal lumen for intubation

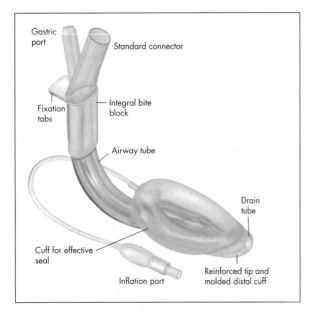

Figure 11-1 Laryngeal mask airway (LMA)

Source: Image courtesy of LMA North America, Inc., San Diego, CA.

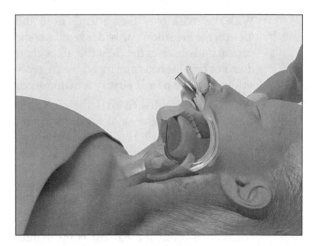

Figure 11-2 Laryngeal mask airway in place

Source: Image courtesy of LMA North America, Inc., San Diego, CA.

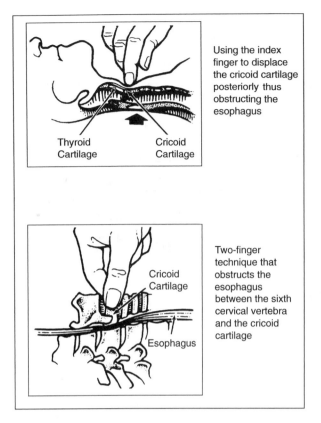

Using the index finger to displace the cricoid cartilage posteriorly thus obstructing the esophagus

Thyroid Cartilage

Cricoid Cartilage

Cricoid Cartilage

Two-finger technique that obstructs the esophagus between the sixth cervical vertebra and the cricoid cartilage

Esophagus

Figure 11-3 Sellick Maneuver

Source: Courtesy of Gensia Pharmaceuticals, Inc., San Diego, CA.

and occludes the esophagus to prevent regurgitation.

- Pressure must be maintained until the endotracheal tube is in place, inflated, and placement verified by an anesthesia provider (Figure 11-3).
- The nurse should not release the pressure until advised to do so by the anesthesia provider.

216. Once the cuff is inflated, the endotracheal (ET) tube is connected to the anesthesia machine, from which the inhalation agents are delivered and by which ventilation is controlled.

217. General anesthesia depresses the hypothalamus, preventing the patient from compensating for the temperature in the room. If the operating room is cold, the anesthetized patient can become hypothermic. Nursing interventions should be directed toward maintaining the patient's body temperature within normal limits.

218. Automated forced-air warming devices should be used strictly in accordance with the manufacturer's instructions. The air hose should never be used without being connected to the warming blanket provided with the device. The hose end has a dangerously high air temperature and the blanket serves to disperse this heat. Using the air unit without a blanket has resulted in serious burns (AORN, 2012, p. 372).

219. Following the induction of anesthesia and positioning for the surgical procedure, the perioperative nurse should scan the patient from head to foot and, if necessary, take corrective action to ensure that the body alignment is maintained and padding is adequate to prevent pressure damage. This is a critical review—once the patient is draped, positioning cannot be visualized.

220. If the patient is moved or repositioned during the procedure, another check is required to ensure a safe and proper position.

221. Before repositioning the patient, the perioperative nurse should confer with the anesthesia provider to determine that the patient can be moved without compromise to the airway and to ventilation, and that he or she is ready to assist in repositioning by guiding and securing the patient's head to prevent accidental extubation or disconnection from the ventilator.

222. During the surgical procedure, the perioperative nurse monitors fluid output and replacement, blood loss, blood and blood product replacement, and the amount of irrigating solution used.

223. Emergence from anesthesia, particularly from extubation, is a critical period when the perioperative nurse must be at the patient's side and immediately available to assist the anesthesia provider.

224. Extubation can initiate bronchospasm or laryngospasm reflex. The airway may become obstructed, and vomiting can occur. Airway management and adequate ventilation are priorities. Prior to extubation, the perioperative nurse should confirm that a suction catheter is within reach of the anesthesia provider and that suction is turned on and working.

Section Questions

www

1. Describe the patient response in each of the four stages of anesthesia. [Ref 195]

2. Why is it important for the perioperative nurse to recognize all of the stages of anesthesia, even though today's anesthesia techniques take the patient rapidly to Stage III? [Refs 195–196]

3. What is the importance of avoiding stimulation of patients during Stage II, when they are emerging from anesthesia? [Ref 197]

4. Once the patient enters the operating room, what is the circulating nurse's primary focus? [Ref 198]

5. In which ways does the circulating nurse support the patient and assist the anesthesia provider with the induction of anesthesia? [Refs 199–202]

6. What is the scrubbed person's responsibility to the patient during the induction of anesthesia? [Ref 203]

7. Why is it important to monitor the quality of conversation in the operating room, even after the patient is anesthetized? [Ref 204]

8. Define "induction of anesthesia." [Ref 205]

9. Describe some nursing responsibilities during the induction period. [Refs 206–207]

10. Describe the typical sequence of administering general anesthesia. [Ref 209]

11. How can the perioperative nurse assist the anesthesia provider during intubation? [Ref 209]

12. Why is an endotracheal tube considered a "secured airway"? [Ref 210]

13. Under which circumstances might the patient not be intubated? [Ref 212]

14. What must the perioperative nurse be prepared to do for a patient at risk for aspiration during induction? [Ref 213]

15. Describe the Sellick maneuver and the purpose in using it. [Ref 215]

16. How does anesthesia place the patient at risk for hypothermia? [Ref 217]

17. When using forced-air heating devices, what is one very important precaution? [Ref 218]

18. Why should the nurse confer with the anesthesia provider in preparation for positioning the patient? [Ref 221]

19. Which challenging situations can occur during extubation? [Refs 223–224]

20. What are the perioperative nurse's responsibilities during extubation? [Refs 223–224]

Malignant Hyperthermia

Overview

225. Malignant hyperthermia (MH) is an inherited muscle disorder triggered by certain types of anesthesia that may cause a fast-acting, life-threatening crisis. The incidence of MH is low; however, if left untreated, it can result in cardiac arrest, kidney failure, blood coagulation problems, internal hemorrhage, brain injury and can be fatal. (Malignant Hyperthermia Association [MHAUS], 2012).

226. MH is characterized by a rapid rise in temperature, with body temperatures rising as high as 109.4°F (43°C). Other signs and symptoms associated with an MH crisis that may present in any particular sequence include masseter muscle rigidity, unexplained tachycardia, hypercarbia, metabolic acidosis, rhabdomyolysis (AORN, 2012, pp. 625–627).

227. The exact incidence of MH is unknown. The rate of occurrence has been estimated to be as frequent as one in 5000 or as rare as one in 65,000 administrations of general anesthesia with triggering agents. The incidence varies depending on the concentration of MH-carrier families in a given geographic area. High-incidence areas in the United States include

Wisconsin, Nebraska, West Virginia, and Michigan (MHAUS, 2012).

228. The MH mortality rate has been reduced from as high as 70% to less than 5% with better screening, the establishment of a pharmacologic basis for MH, sophisticated monitoring techniques, and the use of dantrolene sodium (AORN, 2012, pp. 622–623).

229. In patients who experience malignant hyperthermia, the sarcoplasmic reticulum (the calcium-storing membrane of the muscle cell) is unable to regulate calcium within the muscle cell in the presence of certain anesthetic agents.

230. When malignant hyperthermia occurs, intracellular calcium increases, and the result is sustained contracture of skeletal muscle. These contractions cause muscles to consume higher than normal amounts of oxygen, in a process that produces lactic acid and heat. The patient's temperature rises rapidly and dramatically. Electrolytes, enzymes, and myoglobin leak from the cells. Hyperkalemia may result and lead to cardiac arrhythmias. The loss of myoglobin can result in renal failure.

231. Symptoms may be multifocal and include sudden inappropriate tachycardia with tachypnea, unstable blood pressure, generalized rigidity, masseter muscle spasm, metabolic and respiratory acidosis, increased end-tidal CO_2, fever, profuse sweating, cyanotic mottling of the skin, and dark unoxygenated blood in the field. Temperature can rise as much as 1.8°F (1°C) every 5 minutes.

232. Tachycardia and increased end-tidal CO_2 are often the first symptoms to appear and may be attributed to causes other than malignant hyperthermia. The classic symptom of fever may occur after the appearance of other symptoms.

233. Certain inhalation agents and depolarizing muscle relaxants are known to be malignant hyperthermia triggers. The following anesthetic agents are known triggers of MH and are not safe for use in MH-susceptible patients (MHAUS, 2012):
    - Desflurane
    - Enflurane
    - Isoflurane
    - Methoxyflurane
    - Sevoflurane
    - Halothane
    - Ether
    - Succinylcholine

234. When succinylcholine is the triggering agent, a sudden severe rigidity of the jaw may be seen following administration of the drug.

235. Depending on the patient and the triggering agent, malignant hyperthermia can occur immediately or as late as 24 hours following the administration of anesthesia.

236. MH is considered a genetic disorder with an autosomal mode of inheritance; however, multiple risk factors such as Duchene's muscular dystrophy and other myopathies have also been identified (AORN, 2012, p. 623).

237. The following risk factors can sometimes be identified through preoperative assessment:
    - Personal or family history of malignant hyperthermia or complications arising from anesthesia
    - A family history of suspicious anesthesia experience
    - Unexplained death during surgery
    - History of unexplained muscle cramps with fever
    - Inherited skeletal muscle disorders

238. If it is suspected that the patient is susceptible to malignant hyperthermia, the surgery may need to be postponed until a skeletal muscle biopsy test is performed to confirm the diagnosis.

239. Alternatively, the surgery may proceed if none of the possible triggering agents is utilized. A total intravenous anesthesia (TIVA) is performed. The patient may be intubated using a nondepolarizing muscle relaxant, and amnesia and analgesia are maintained using a propofol infusion and narcotic. No inhalation agents other than oxygen are delivered to the patient.

240. Molecular diagnostic testing is also available for diagnosing patients suspected to be susceptible to MH. Genetic testing will not detect all patients at risk, whereas a muscle biopsy test is considered definitive.

Treatment

241. If a patient experiences a malignant hyperthermia episode during surgery, *get help and get dantrolene sodium!* Every operating room where general anesthesia is administered should have immediate access to dantrolene sodium and a written, readily accessible protocol for the

management of MH. A cart containing supplies needed to manage an MH occurrence should be readily available, and staff should be familiar with the contents and the treatment protocol. (Exhibits 11-2 and 11-3).

242. In addition to a posted policy and a cart with necessary supplies, many operating-room departments have an anesthesia machine reserved for use in the event of an MH episode. Should an episode occur, the reserved anesthesia machine is brought to the room to replace the one in use. This saves time by eliminating the necessity to change the anesthesia circuit and replace the CO_2 absorbent on the existing machine.

243. Initial treatment is to immediately discontinue all triggering anesthetic agents, hyperventilate with 100% oxygen, administer dantrolene sodium (Dantrium), and rapidly terminate surgery. Dantrolene sodium is a skeletal muscle relaxant that blocks the release of calcium from the sarcoplasmic reticulum, which in turn decreases muscle contractions.

244. Each operating-room pharmacy where general anesthesia might be performed is required to stock 36 vials for a potential case of MH. Dantrolene sodium is supplied in a 20-mg vial and requires 60 mL of preservative-free sterile water for reconstitution.

245. A major task is reconstituting the dantrolene sodium. Each vial is reconstituted with 60 mL of preservative-free sterile water. It can take from two to four licensed individuals to reconstitute the amount required to accomplish rapid administration (AORN, 2012, p. 624).

246. The anesthesia circuit and CO_2 absorbent should be changed to reduce risk from residual triggering agents.

247. Glucose, insulin, and calcium should be available to treat hyperkalemia, bicarbonate to treat metabolic acidosis, and a diuretic to maintain urinary output.

248. Tests frequently performed during an MH crisis include creatinine phosphokinase (CPK), lactic dehydrogenase (LDH), and blood-clotting analysis.

249. Cooling of the patient is achieved by wound irrigation with cold saline, administration of cold intravenous solutions, surface cooling with ice or a cooling blanket, and cold gastric and rectal lavage.

250. If it is impossible to terminate surgery, anesthesia is continued with nontriggering agents.

251. Following an episode of malignant hyperthermia, the patient must be closely monitored for a possible recurrent episode. Dantrolene sodium is continued for 48 hours or more.

Nursing Responsibilities

252. During the preoperative interview, the perioperative nurse should assess the patient for risk factors associated with malignant hyperthermia.

253. The perioperative nurse should be familiar with the malignant hyperthermia protocol and be able to institute prompt and appropriate treatment. Competencies include the ability to perform the following tasks:

- Assess the patient preoperatively for MH risk factors.
- Prepare the room with appropriate supplies for a patient known to be susceptible to MH.
- Recognize signs and symptoms of MH.
- Rapidly supply and reconstitute dantrolene sodium.
- Provide the necessary supplies without hesitation.
- Assist the anesthesia provider with intravenous line setup and placement, drug preparation and administration, implementation of laboratory testing, and as otherwise directed.
- Cool the patient—surface, intravenous, and lavage.

254. If the patient is known or considered to be susceptible to malignant hyperthermia, regional anesthesia or only nontriggering anesthetics are administered, and fresh anesthesia circuitry and CO_2 absorbent are used.

255. Perioperative nursing interventions include preparation of the operating-room table with a cooling blanket, and transfer of the malignant hyperthermia cart and supplies into the room.

256. Depending on institutional policy, prophylactic administration of dantrolene sodium may be ordered.

Exhibit 11-2 Sample Malignant Hyperthermia Policy and Procedure

SPIVEY STATION SURGERY CENTER   ENVIRONMENT OF CARE

Malignant Hyperthermia

Policy

Professional staff will be prepared to respond to a malignant hyperthermia (MH) medical emergency.

Purpose

Establish a calm and effective response to a malignant hyperthermia medical emergency.

Procedure

Responsibility

Clinical staff is responsible for providing emergency response to a MH occurrence.

Process

Clinical Educator will conduct a simulation of a MH response drill annually.

Treatment of MH will be according to the guidelines published by the Malignant Hyperthermia Association of the United States and AORN.

Assess preoperative patients for family history of anesthetic deaths and/or complications. Family history of any muscle weakness, condition, or disease will be assessed and documented. Deaths have occurred even though a patient has undergone prior surgeries without complication.

Stock a minimum of 36 vials of dantrolene sodium and all other medications and devices needed to treat an MH reaction.

Assessment

Any unexpected tachypnea, hypercarbia, tachycardia, or arrhythmia should be evaluated. The unanticipated doubling or tripling of end-tidal carbon dioxide is the most sensitive indicator of MH in the operating room. Avoid suppressing tachycardia with beta-blockers until MH is ruled out. Most arrhythmias respond to correction of hyperkalemia and acidosis. Calcium channel blockers, when used with dantrolene, may produce life-threatening hyperkalemia and myocardial depression.

The most specific sign of MH is total body rigidity (i.e., limbs, abdomen, and chest). If MH is suspected, the staff should determine whether peripheral muscle rigidity is present. Consider MH with sustained masseter muscle rigidity (MMR) during general anesthesia. Dantrolene is not recommended for MMR only.

Consider MH with any temperature rise during general anesthesia. Monitor core temperature. Skin temperature may not adequately reflect core temperature during a MH episode. Temperature increase is often a late sign in a MH episode.

Cardiac arrest that occurs suddenly in a male child with normal oxygen levels may be secondary to hyperkalemia. Treatment should be directed to correction of hyperkalemia with calcium chloride, bicarbonate, insulin, glucose, and hyperventilation.

Treatment of Acute MH Medical Emergency

Anesthesia Provider

- Stop inhalation anesthetic if muscle rigidity occurs and do not administer additional succinylcholine. If surgery must continue, switch to nontriggering anesthetic agents.
- Hyperventilate with 100% oxygen at high gas flow, at least 10 L/min.
- The circle system and carbon dioxide absorbent need not be changed when MH is diagnosed during a procedure.

(continues)

Exhibit 11-2 Malignant Hyperthermia Policy and Procedure (continued)

Circulating Nurse
- Assist anesthesia provider and act as recorder.
- Call for additional staff members stat to assist with MH:
  - dantrolene nurse (preop nurse) brings MH cart;
  - medication nurse (PACU nurse) brings crash cart;
  - cooling nurse (clinical coordonator) brings ice and cold saline; and
  - other staff available for additional assistance as needed.
- Follow MALIGNANT HYPERTHERMIA EMERGENCY RESPONSE chart for duties of each nurse.
- Transfer patient to nearby hospital as soon as medically stable.

Cool hyperthermic patient.
- Use IV cold saline, not Ringer's lactate.
- Lavage stomach, bladder, rectum, and open cavities with cold saline as appropriate. Surface cool, but avoid hypothermia.

Arrhythmias will usually respond to treatment of acidosis and hyperkalemia. If they persist or are life-threatening, standard anti-arrhythmic agents may be used, with the exception of calcium channel blockers, which may cause life-threatening hyperkalemia and cardiovascular collapse. Verapamil also is contraindicated.

Treat hyperkalemia in adults with hyperventilation, bicarbonate, IV glucose, and insulin per physician order. Life-threatening hyperkalemia may also be treated with calcium administration.

Ensure urine output of greater than 2 mL/kg/hr by hydration; administration of mannitol or furosemide may be needed. To prevent renal failure, urinary output greater than 2 mL/kg/hr must be maintained. Consider cardiovascular or PA monitoring because of fluid shifts and hemodynamic instability that may occur.

Patient Follow-Up
Counsel patient and family regarding MH and refer to MHAUS.

Fill out an adverse metabolic reaction to anesthesia (AMRA) report, available through the MHAUS registry at (717) 531-6936. Information about the malignant hyperthermia registry is available online at *http://naregistry.mhaus.org.*

MH Resources
- MH Hotline: (209) 634-4917 or (800) MH-HYPER (644-9737).
- Information on MH is available online at *https://www.mhaus.org/index.cfm/fuseaction /Hotline.Home.cfm.*
- For general MH Information, call (607) 674-7901.
- Emergency therapy wall charts can be ordered from MHAUS by calling the nonemergency telephone number (800) 986-4287 or online at *http://www.mhaus.org.*

  Related form following this policy and procedure:
- Malignant Hyperthermia Emergency Response (SA-5.7-1)

Complies with Joint Commission Standard:
EC.1.10   EC.1.20   EC.4.10   EC.4.20   EC.6.20
PC.5.10   PC.5.60PC.9.10PC.9.20

Source: Spivey Station Surgery Center, Jonesboro, GA.

Exhibit 11-3 Malignant Hyperthermia Emergency Response Protocol

CIRCULATING NURSE (OR)	DANTROLENE NURSE (PRE OP)	MEDICATION NURSE (PACU)	COOLING NURSE TECHS
1. Call for three additional nurses. 2. Assist anesthesia and record.	1. Bring MH cart. 2. Mix and administer dantrolene. **Inject directly thru INT or central line port without fluids infusing.**	1. Bring crash cart. 2. Mix and administer medications as highlighted. 3. Bring insulin from medication fridge.	1. Bring cold IVFs and irrigation saline from medication fridge and ice. 2. Cool and monitor patient temperature.

Supplies needed:
  (*Possible*) New anesthesia machine and/or new circuit filter and soda absorber
CVP and A line x 2
Lab study supplies
Blood tubes (red, blue and purple tops) repeat x 6 of CK, LDH, Na, K, Cl, Ca, Mg, myoglobin
Heparinized 5 mL blood gas syringes x 6
Tubes for coagulation studies (eg, PT, PTT, platelet count, fibrinogen, and fibrin split product)
Urine specimen container for myoglobin
Urine dipstick for hemoglobin
Record medications, dosages, time of administration, and response.
	Supplies needed:
	  Dantrolene sodium IV, 36 amps
	2,000 mL sterile H_2O for injection (without a bacteriostatic agent)
	Multi-ad fluid transfer set or mini-spike IV additive pins
	
	Mix:
	  Dantrolene 20 mg vial with 50 cc of sterile water.
	
	Administer:
	  Dantrolene 2.5 mg/kg IV for initial bolus
	Kg _____ x 2.5 mg.
	= _____
	This dose may be repeated up to 4 times per continued MH signs and anesthesia order.
		Supplies needed:
		  Medications/syringes on MH cart and, if necessary, on crash cart
		Draw, prepare, and label medications.
		Administer per anesthesia orders.
		Prepare bicarbonate 1–2 mEq/kg
		Kg _____ x 1 mEq = _____ bicarb and repeat as directed
		Prepare 0.15 units/kg regular insulin in 1 cc/kg 50% glucose:
		Kg _____ x 0.15 units = _____ insulin
		Mix in:
		Kg _____ x 1 cc = _____ volume of 50% glucose
		Prepare $CaCl_2$, 2 mg/kg
		Kg_____ x 2 mg = _____ $CaCl_2$
		Prepare furosemide (40 mg/amp) 4 mL x 2.
		Prepare antiarrythemic drugs as directed (e.g., lidocaine, procainamide).
		Have mannitol 50 ml available.
			Supplies needed:
			  Nasogastric tube
			Foley (urimeter)
			Rectal tube (large RR cath)
			Cold IV saline 1,000 x 3 or 4 for IV administration and several for lavage cooling
			Bags and bucket of ice
			Core temp probe
			Prepare and administer:
			15 mL/kg IV cold saline x 3
			Kg _____ x 15 mL = _____ volume
			NaCl x 3
			Nasogastric tube and core temp probe to anesthesia
			Place Foley catheter and rectal tube.
			Lavage stomach, bladder, rectum, and open cavities as appropriate with cold normal saline.
			Monitor and record patient temperature.

NOTE: Medications cannot be administered without a physician's order. Dosages must be calculated individually for each patient.

Section Questions

1. Which factors have helped to reduce the mortality rate of malignant hyperthermia? [Ref 228]
2. Describe the pathophysiology of MH. [Refs 229–230]
3. What are some of the symptoms triggered by MH? [Ref 231]
4. Which symptoms of MH are often the first to appear? [Ref 232]
5. Which types of anesthetic agents are known to be triggers for MH? [Ref 233]
6. How long does it take MH to manifest following administration of the triggering agent? [Ref 235]
7. Which questions might be asked during patient assessment that might identify a patient at risk for MH? [Ref 237]
8. Which decisions might be made about the surgical procedure when assessment identifies a patient at risk for MH? [Refs 238–239]
9. Which kind of testing is available for patients suspected of having MH? [Refs 238, 240]
10. What is the drug of choice (the only drug) for treating MH? [Ref 241]
11. Which precautions for managing an MH emergency should every facility have in place? [Ref 242]
12. What is the initial treatment when MH occurs? [Ref 243]
13. Which challenge is associated with the administration of dantrolene sodium? [Ref 245]
14. In addition to administering dantrolene sodium, which other steps are taken during an MH episode? [Refs 246–247]
15. Which lab tests provide important information during an MH crisis? [Ref 248]
16. Which interventions can be used to bring down the patient's temperature? [Ref 249]
17. How is the patient managed following an MH crisis? [Ref 251]
18. If surgery is to proceed on a patient at risk for MH, which precautions will the anesthesia provider take? [Ref 254]
19. How will the perioperative nurse prepare for a patient at risk for MH? [Ref 255]
20. What determines whether dantrolene sodium will be administered prophylactically? [Ref 256]

Moderate Sedation/Analgesia

Overview

257. Moderate sedation/analgesia, also known as conscious sedation or IV conscious sedation, is a drug-induced depression of consciousness. The patient is able to respond purposefully to verbal commands, either alone or accompanied by light tactile stimulation. No interventions are required to maintain a patent airway. Spontaneous ventilation is adequate.

258. Moderate sedation/analgesia is frequently employed for diagnostic procedures or minor surgery where the presence of an anesthesiologist is not routinely necessary. Examples of such procedures include colonoscopy, incision and drainage of an abscess, excision of small mass, vascular access, vasectomy, and the reduction of a dislocation with a cast application.

259. Goals of moderate sedation/analgesia:
   - Allay fear and anxiety.
   - Enhance cooperation.
   - Maintain consciousness and the ability to respond to verbal stimulation.
   - Maintain respirations unassisted.
   - Provide adequate analgesia.
   - Maintain stable vital signs.
   - Achieve partial amnesia.
   - Facilitate prompt return to activities of daily living.

260. Desired outcomes of moderate sedation/analgesia:

    - The patient demonstrates or reports adequate pain control throughout the perioperative period.
    - The patient's cardiac status is consistent with or improved from baseline levels established preoperatively.
    - The patient breathes unassisted and is easily aroused, and respiratory status is consistent with or improved from baseline levels established preoperatively.
    - The patient is relaxed, comfortable, and cooperative.
    - The patient's protective reflexes are intact.

261. Each institution should develop criteria to identify patients who are suitable candidates for moderate sedation/analgesia. Patients classified as PS2 and medically stable PS3 are normally considered appropriate for registered nurse–administered moderate sedation (AORN, 2012, p. 412).

262. Assessment should include physiological status, psychological maturity, and the patient's ability to tolerate and maintain the desired position for the duration of the procedure.

263. An airway assessment will determine if the patient would be difficult to intubate if necessary. Factors that could make intubation difficult include significant obesity, especially of the face, neck, and tongue; significantly recessed or protruding jaw; limited range of neck motion; protruding or missing teeth, edentulous; history of sleep apnea; and presence of stridor (AORN, 2012, p. 413).

264. Sedatives and analgesic agents are delivered intravenously. Commonly used agents include diazepam (Valium), midazolam (Versed), morphine sulfate (Duramorph), meperidine (Demerol), and fentanyl (Sublimaze).

265. Reversal agents include naloxone hydrochloride (Narcan) for narcotics and flumazenil (Romazicon) for benzodiazepines.

Nursing Responsibilities

266. The registered nurse who monitors the patient receiving moderate sedation/analgesia should have no other responsibilities during the procedure that would require leaving the patient unattended and might compromise continuous monitoring (AORN, 2012, p. 413). An additional nurse should be present to function in the circulating role.

267. At a minimum, the following knowledge and skills are necessary:

    - Patient selection and assessment criteria
    - Selection, function, and proficiency in use of physiologic monitoring equipment
    - Pharmacology of the medications used
    - Airway management
    - Continuous positive airway pressure (CPAP) use
    - Basic dysrhythmia recognition and management
    - Emergency response and management
    - Advanced cardiac life support (ACLS) and pediatric advanced life support (PALS) according to the type of patients served
    - Recognition of complications associated with sedation/analgesia
    - Knowledge of anatomy and physiology (AORN, 2012, pp. 416–417)

268. Some facilities require ACLS certification for nurses who monitor patients receiving moderate sedation/analgesia.

269. In addition to the ability to perform a thorough preoperative assessment, the nurse who is monitoring the patient should have a working knowledge of resuscitation equipment and the function and use of monitoring equipment, and the ability to interpret any data that are obtained.

270. Monitoring equipment should include airway management devices (e.g., oral, nasal airways, mask ventilation devices, pulse oximeter, noninvasive blood pressure monitor, and electrocardiograph). Suction should be immediately available, turned on, and functioning. The patient should have an established intravenous line, and sedative and analgesic antagonists should be in the room and immediately available. The crash cart should be immediately available (AORN, 2012, pp. 412–416).

271. The patient who receives moderate sedation/analgesia must be continuously monitored for any reaction to drugs and for physiological and psychological changes that might cause the patient to progress to a state of deep sedation. Because of the rapid patient response to

pharmacologic agents, it is possible for the patient to lapse into unconsciousness. Deep sedation may be characterized by extremely slurred speech, not easily being aroused, inability to independently maintain a patent airway, and nonresponsiveness to verbal commands. In the event that a patient progresses to a state of deep sedation and cannot be easily aroused and cannot maintain independent ventilatory function, the nurse must be competent to provide rescue measures.

272. Patients who are discharged to another unit should be monitored for several hours to ensure the maintenance of a satisfactory level of consciousness, a patent airway, and stable vital signs.

273. Criteria for discharge may include, but are not limited to, the following:

- Return to preoperative, baseline level of consciousness
- Stable vital signs
- Sufficient time interval since the last administration of an antagonist to prevent resedation of the patient
- Use of an objective patient assessment scoring system (e.g., Aldrete score)
- Absence of protracted nausea
- Adequate pain control
- Return of motor/sensory control (AORN, 2012, pp. 416–417)

274. Patients should be given written postoperative instructions because medications used in moderate sedation/analgesia can diminish the ability to recall information that has been given verbally.

Section Questions   www

1. Describe moderate sedation/analgesia. [Ref 257]

2. For which types of procedures is moderate sedation frequently used? [Ref 258]

3. What are the goals of moderate sedation? [Ref 259]

4. Identify four desired outcomes of moderate sedation. [Ref 260]

5. Which patients are considered appropriate candidates for moderate sedation? [Ref 261]

6. Describe the assessment of a patient for moderate sedation. [Ref 262]

7. What are the components of an airway assessment for moderate sedation? [Ref 263]

8. Which reversal agents are available for narcotics and benzodiazepines? [Ref 265]

9. What is important about circulating duties and monitoring the patient receiving moderate sedation? [Ref 266]

10. Which knowledge and skills are important for the perioperative nurse who will monitor patients receiving moderate sedation? [Refs 267–269]

11. Which equipment should be available to monitor the patient receiving moderate sedation? [Ref 270]

12. What are the characteristics of deep sedation? [Ref 271]

13. What is the implication of deep sedation for the perioperative nurse monitoring the patient? [Ref 271]

14. List criteria for discharge for patients who have received moderate sedation. [Ref 273]

15. Why are written instructions important for patients who have received moderate sedation? [Ref 274]

Regional Anesthesia

Overview

275. The decision to use regional anesthesia involves many factors. Generally, the respiratory and cardiac systems remain relatively stable with regional anesthesia.

276. Regional anesthesia is preferable for patients who require emergency surgery, have a full stomach, and do not need to be unconscious for the procedure. It is important to avoid providing too much sedation in addition to the regional anesthetic because of the potential for aspiration.

277. Regional anesthesia is also used when general anesthetic agents are contraindicated, such as with patients who have severe metabolic, renal, cardiac, pulmonary, or hepatic disease.

278. Regional anesthetic may be utilized in conjunction with a general anesthetic, especially in orthopedic or major abdominal procedures to assist with postoperative pain management.

279. Regional anesthesia techniques include spinal, epidural, and caudal block; intravenous block; nerve block; local infiltration; and topical administration.

Spinal

280. Spinal anesthesia involves injecting the anesthetic agent into the cerebrospinal fluid in the subarachnoid space. Injection is made through a lumbar interspace usually between L2 and L3 or lower, so that the needle is not inserted into the spinal cord, which normally ends at L1 to L2.

281. As the anesthetic is absorbed by the nerve fibers, nerve transmission is blocked. Spread of the anesthetic agent and the subsequent level of anesthesia are determined by cerebrospinal pressure; the injection site; the amount, concentration, and specific gravity of the anesthetic solution; the speed of injection; and the position of the patient during and immediately following the injection.

282. Spinal anesthetic solutions are generally a mixture of local anesthetic and dextrose. These solutions settle by gravity. The block can be directed upward, downward, or to one side of the spinal cord by adjusting the patient's position. After 10 or 15 minutes, the block is set and does not extend farther.

283. Agents frequently used for spinal anesthesia include lidocaine (Xylocaine), pontocaine (Tetracaine), and bupivacaine (Marcaine). A narcotic may also be added to the injection.

284. Spinal anesthesia is used for lower abdominal, pelvic, lower extremity, and urologic procedures, and for cesarean sections.

285. The administration of spinal anesthesia requires patient cooperation. Proper positioning is the key to successful placement of the anesthetic injection. Nursing interventions should be directed toward positioning the patient and providing support during administration of the spinal.

286. During preparation for spinal anesthesia, the perioperative nurse should help to position the patient, assist the anesthesia provider as needed, and reassure the patient. The patient in the lateral decubitus position is very close to the edge of the table, and safety measures to prevent falling are necessary. The perioperative nurse should remain with the patient, institute measures to prevent falling, and help the patient feel secure.

287. Injection of the anesthetic is done with the patient in a sitting or lateral decubitus position. In the sitting position, the patient sits on the operating table with the legs over the side and feet on a stool high enough to raise the patient's knees above the level of the waist. The patient should be encouraged to arch the back outward and lower the chin to the chest (Figure 11-4).

288. In the lateral decubitus position, the patient's hips, back, and shoulders are aligned parallel with the edge of the table. The patient brings the knees up toward the chest and flexes the head and neck. These maneuvers assist in spreading the vertebrae and exposing the desired interspaces to facilitate correct needle insertion.

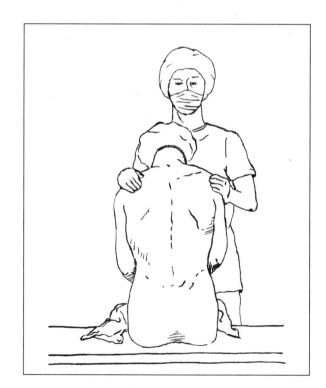

Figure 11-4 Position for spinal anesthesia
Source: Courtesy of Andrew Maillard.

289. When administering spinal anesthesia, strict attention to asepsis is important to prevent entry of pathogens that can cause meningitis into the subarachnoid space.

290. Complications of spinal anesthesia include a rapid drop in blood pressure, nausea and vomiting, total spinal anesthesia, postdural headache, and neurological or integumentary positioning injury.

291. Sudden hypotension is caused by vasodilation when sympathetic nerves that control vasomotor tone are blocked. Peripheral pooling, decreased venous return, and decreased cardiac output can also result. Ephedrine may be administered to restore normotension.

292. Nausea and vomiting can occur as a result of hypotension or as a reaction to sedation medication. Suction should be immediately available, as well as an emesis basin and wet towel.

293. Total spinal anesthesia occurs when the level of anesthesia becomes high enough to paralyze the respiratory muscles and respiratory distress occurs. This is an emergency situation. Ventilation must be supported, and intubation may be required.

294. Patients may experience headache 24 to 48 hours following spinal anesthesia if the dura at the site of injection does not seal itself off and cerebrospinal fluid leaks into the epidural space. The loss of cerebrospinal fluid decreases cerebrospinal pressure, leaves less fluid to cushion the brain, and can cause headache.

295. In most cases, treatment consists of hydration, intravenous or oral caffeine, sedation, and bed rest. If symptoms persist longer than 24 hours, a blood patch of the patient's blood may be administered at the puncture site to seal the epidural leak.

296. Neurological or integumentary injuries can occur because the patient's sensory pathways are blocked and the patient cannot respond to improper positioning.

Epidural and Caudal

297. Epidural anesthesia is achieved by injection of the anesthetic agent into the epidural space (Figure 11-5). The agent is usually injected through the interspaces of the lumbar vertebrae; however, depending on the surgical site, thoracic or cervical vertebrae may be used.

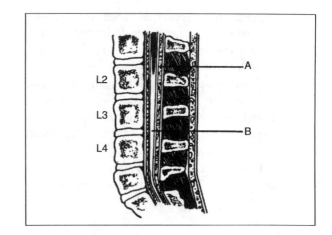

Figure 11-5 Regional anesthesia sites
Source: Courtesy of Jeanne Spry.

298. Lumbar epidural anesthesia is useful in anorectal, vaginal, and perineal procedures and is often used in obstetric surgery. It is also combined with a general anesthetic for orthopedic procedures and urologic procedures.

299. Thoracic epidural anesthesia will cover the surgical site for abdominal and thoracic surgeries.

300. For caudal anesthesia, the anesthetic is injected into the epidural space through the caudal canal in the sacrum. Caudal anesthesia used in obstetrics and in small children for circumcisions.

301. Commonly used epidural and caudal anesthetic agents include lidocaine hydrochloride (Xylocaine), bupivacaine (Marcaine), ropivacaine, and chloroprocaine (Nesacaine). A narcotic agent is very often added to the local anesthetic to enhance the analgesic effects.

302. Epidural anesthesia can be delivered as a single dose, or a small catheter can be left in place for continuous infusion. Continuous infusion is useful for pain management in the postoperative period.

303. Anesthetic agents that are injected into the epidural space are not as affected by positioning as in spinal anesthesia.

304. The following complications of epidural anesthesia are possible:

- Dural puncture—postdural headache
- Inadvertent subarachnoid injection—total spinal anesthesia
- Inadvertent intravascular injection—extreme hypotension and cardiac arrest

Section Questions

1. For which patients is regional anesthesia preferable? [Refs 275–278]

2. List the variety of available regional anesthesia techniques. [Ref 279]

3. For spinal anesthesia, where is the anesthetic injected? [Ref 280]

4. How is the level of anesthesia determined? [Ref 282]

5. For which procedures is spinal anesthesia used? [Ref 284]

6. What is the perioperative nurse's responsibility in assisting with spinal anesthesia? [Refs 285–286]

7. Describe the positions that are appropriate for administering spinal anesthesia. [Refs 287–288]

8. Why is strict aseptic technique important during the administration of spinal anesthesia? [Ref 289]

9. Describe the potential complications of spinal anesthesia. [Refs 290–292]

10. What is "total spinal anesthesia" and what are the implications of its use? [Ref 293]

11. Explain the etiology of headaches that might occur following spinal anesthesia. [Ref 294]

12. How can post–spinal anesthesia headaches be managed? [Ref 295]

13. Which patient injuries can result when spinal anesthesia is used? [Ref 296]

14. Contrast epidural anesthesia with spinal anesthesia. [Refs 297, 302–303]

15. Which complications can be associated with epidural anesthesia? [Ref 304]

Intravenous Block (Bier Block)

305. A Bier block involves the injection of a local anesthetic agent into the vein of a tourniquet-occluded extremity. In this procedure, an intravenous catheter is inserted into the operative extremity. Two side-by-side tourniquets or one double-cuffed tourniquet is applied, but not inflated, on the extremity. The extremity is elevated and drained of blood with an Esmarch or elastic bandage. The proximal tourniquet or cuff is then inflated, and a fixed amount of anesthetic agent—lidocaine (Xylocaine)—is injected. The anesthetic agent infiltrates the extremity and is confined to the tissues that are distal to the tourniquet. To alleviate tourniquet pain, the second distal cuff is inflated after the anesthetic agent has taken effect. The proximal cuff is then deflated.

306. This technique is used most often for surgeries of the upper extremities that last an hour or less.

307. After the procedure, the tourniquet is released slowly to control the release of the remaining anesthetic into the general circulation. Rapid release can result in cardiovascular collapse or central nervous system toxicity.

Nerve Block

308. In nerve block, the anesthetic agent—usually lidocaine (Xylocaine)—is injected into and around a nerve or nerve group that supplies sensation to a small area of the body.

309. Nerve blocks can be used for purposes of surgical intervention but are more commonly used for sustained relief in patients with chronic pain and to increase circulation in some vascular diseases.

310. Nerve blocks can be minor or major. Major blocks involve multiple nerves or a plexus. Minor blocks block a single nerve.

311. Major nerve blocks used in operative procedures include the brachial plexus block for procedures of the arm (intrascalene, supraclavicular, infraclavicular, and axillary), orbital blocks for eye procedures, and cervical blocks for procedures involving the neck.

312. Common minor blocks are radial and ulnar nerve blocks for procedures of the elbow, wrist, or digits.

313. The perioperative nurse may assist during nerve block by aspirating the needle during placement to check for inadvertent vascular

injection. The nurse may also be asked to inject the local anesthetic while the anesthesia provider secures the placement of the needle. Whether it is appropriate for the nurse to inject the anesthetic will depend on facility policy, state board of nursing regulations, and demonstrated competency.

Local Infiltration

314. Local infiltration involves the injection of the anesthetic agent into subcutaneous tissue at, or close to, the anticipated incision site.

315. Local infiltration is useful for minor, superficial procedures.

316. The most frequently used local anesthetic is lidocaine (Xylocaine). Epinephrine may be added to the lidocaine to cause vasoconstriction, reduce bleeding, and slow absorption of the drug.

317. During local anesthesia, the perioperative nurse should monitor the patient's blood pressure, cardiac rate and rhythm, respiratory rate, oxygen saturation, level of consciousness, pain level, skin temperature and color, amount and local anesthetic administered, and response to medications (AORN, 2012, pp. 414–415).

318. Toxic reactions from local anesthetics can occur if too rapid an absorption from a vascular site occurs or if there is an inadvertent intravascular injection. Toxic reactions include central nervous system and cardiovascular depression. The nurse must be alert to the possibility of a toxic reaction.

319. Initial signs of central nervous system toxicity include restlessness, lightheadedness, visual and auditory disturbances, dizziness, tremors, and convulsions, sometimes followed by unconsciousness, apnea, and cardiac arrest.

320. Patients who say that they hear unusual sounds or express a feeling of uneasiness may be experiencing a toxic reaction. Initial treatment consists of establishing and maintaining an airway, assisting or controlling ventilation with oxygen, and administering sedation.

321. It is the perioperative nurse's responsibility to ensure that resuscitation equipment is available when local anesthetics are administered.

Topical

322. In topical anesthesia, the anesthetic is applied directly to a mucous membrane or an open wound. Topical anesthetics are readily absorbed by mucous membranes and, therefore, act rapidly.

323. Topical anesthesia is often used for nasal surgery, cystoscopy, and procedures of the respiratory tract in which it is advantageous to eliminate cough and laryngeal reflex (gag reflex).

324. Sudden cardiovascular collapse is possible following the application of topical anesthetic in the respiratory tract. Resuscitation equipment should be immediately available.

325. Commonly used topical anesthetics include pontocaine (Tetracaine), cocaine, and lidocaine (Xylocaine). Lidocaine may be supplied as a liquid, liquid spray, or jelly.

326. Cocaine is used in nasal passages; pontocaine in the eye; and lidocaine in the throat, nose, esophagus, and genitourinary tract.

Regional Anesthesia: Nursing Responsibilities

327. Responsibilities of the perioperative nurse will vary according to the type of regional anesthesia being administered.

328. Patients who are scheduled to receive regional anesthesia may be apprehensive about being awake during surgery. They may mistakenly believe that they will experience pain or they will be unable to avoid observing the surgery. Providing assurance, answering questions, and remaining close to the patient will, in most instances, significantly reduce anxiety. Even patients who are sedated should be aware that the nurse is close by and is available to provide support.

329. For some surgeries, it is important that the patient be alert and cooperate with the surgeon to facilitate the procedure. In these circumstances, the perioperative nurse can provide encouragement, support, and information that the patient needs.

330. Patients who receive regional anesthesia are awake, and conversation in the operating suite should be respectful. These patients are usually given supplemental tranquilizers and may sleep. However, they are arousable and may be startled by noise or made anxious by inappropriate conversation. It is appropriate to place a sign on the door of the operating suite stating that the patient is awake. This will serve as a reminder to persons who enter.

331. During placement of the needle for spinal, epidural, caudal, and nerve block, the patient should be protected from unnecessary exposure to prevent embarrassment and cooling. Pillows and blankets should be provided to increase patient comfort.

332. Preparation of the incision site with an antiseptic scrub may necessitate exposing the patient and may cause the awake patient to become embarrassed or anxious. It is important to maintain the patient's dignity and minimize exposure.

333. Every patient receiving some type of regional anesthesia should be monitored. The extent of monitoring and the person responsible for monitoring are determined by the anesthesia technique, the results of preoperative assessment, the surgical procedure, recognized anesthesia standards and practices, and the facility's policy.

334. Administration of topical and local infiltration anesthetics is the surgeon's responsibility. During spinal, epidural, and caudal anesthesia; intravenous block; and nerve block, an anesthesia provider is present. However, during local anesthesia, it is unusual for an anesthesia provider to be present; in this situation, monitoring the patient's physiological and psychological status is the responsibility of the perioperative nurse.

335. The nurse who monitors the patient receiving local anesthesia must be able to establish a normal baseline and recognize any changes that occur. Baseline data must include blood pressure, cardiac rate and rhythm, respirations, oxygen saturation, skin condition, and mental status. In addition, knowledge of the drugs used as well as possible reactions to them is necessary for the perioperative nurse to be able to respond appropriately.

336. During local anesthesia, the perioperative nurse should track and monitor the amount of anesthetic agent given. The maximum recommended dose of 1% lidocaine without epinephrine should not exceed 4.5 mg/kg, and the maximum total dose should not exceed 300 mg. The maximum recommended dose of lidocaine with epinephrine should not exceed 7 mg/kg and the maximum total dose is 500 mg (Kapitanyan, 2012).

337. Lidocaine with epinephrine should not be used on fingers or toes (Murhammer et al., 2004);

vasoconstriction can cause vascular compromise. The amount that is administered should be reported to the surgeon.

338. Nursing interventions for all patients who receive regional anesthesia should include preparation for toxic systemic reactions of the central nervous system and cardiovascular collapse.

339. Resuscitation equipment must be immediately available, and the perioperative nurse monitoring the patient must be competent in the use of such equipment. Competency in preparation of related medications and knowledge of their actions is also imperative. Current cardiopulmonary resuscitation (CPR) certification is an essential requirement for the perioperative nurse.

Medication Safety

Overview

340. In response to the significant risk of patient injury related to medication errors, two of The Joint Commission's patient safety goals relate to medication use. Goal 3 is "Improve the safety of using medications." Goal 8 is "Accurately and completely reconcile medications across the continuum of care" (TJC, 2012a).

Responsibilities of Team Members

341. The perioperative nurse who functions in either the scrubbed person or the circulating nurse role shares responsibility for achieving the desired patient outcome: "The correct patient receives the correct medication(s) in accurate doses, at the correct time, and via the correct route through the perioperative experience" (AORN, 2011, p. 203).

342. The Joint Commission requires that all medications/solutions on and off the sterile field be labeled. Many operating rooms have purchased sterile labeling kits for this purpose. Some kits contain printed labels. If a kit is not available, the scrubbed person can prepare a label using a sterile marking pen and sterile label. Items that must be labeled include the following:

- Syringes
- Basins
- Medicine cups

- Bowls
- Other containers

343. Before dispensing a medication, the circulating nurse should confirm that the medication is not contraindicated because of patient allergy or interaction with other substance(s) the patient may be taking. The healthcare facility pharmacist should be consulted if any question arises regarding the appropriateness of the medication.

344. Whenever a medication is delivered to the sterile field, the scrubbed person and the circulating nurse should visually, verbally, and concurrently confirm the medication name, strength, dose, concentration, and expiration date.

345. If the scrubbed person or circulating nurse is relieved, the hand-off report given to the relieving personnel should include verification of all medications. Any unlabeled medications or solutions should be discarded.

346. It is not uncommon for verbal medication orders to be given to the circulating nurse during surgery. It is critical that the circulating nurse confirm the order. The operating room can be a busy place with multiple distractions. Background noise from activity, talking, telephone and beeper rings, equipment alarms, monitoring equipment sounds, and music can interfere with communication and result in a misunderstood verbal medication order. When a verbal order is given by someone wearing a surgical mask that covers the nose and mouth, it is essential to take steps to ensure clear communication and prevent misunderstanding.

347. At a minimum, the verbal order should be repeated and confirmed by the person to whom it is directed. Ideally, the verbal order should be written on a dry-erase board and read back to the person who issued the order. Verbal confirmation, coupled with visual confirmation, can decrease the risk of error and prevent injury to the patient.

348. The Joint Commission requirement on medication reconciliation states that "A complete list of the patient's medications is communicated to the next provider of service when a patient is referred or transferred to another setting, service, practitioner, or level of care within or outside the organization" (TJC, 2012a).

349. The perioperative nurse should ensure that the patient's medication list is readily available and visible. This list should be checked for completeness—medication history, medication, dose, and schedule. Responsibility for medication reconciliation may vary according to facility and department. It is the responsibility of the perioperative nurse to know the policy for medication reconciliation and his or her related responsibilities.

Section Questions

1. Describe the process of creating a Bier block. [Ref 305]
2. For which type of procedure is the Bier block commonly used? [Ref 306]
3. What is the purpose of deflating the tourniquet slowly? [Ref 307]
4. Differentiate between major and minor nerve blocks. [Refs 310–312]
5. How are nerve blocks most commonly used? [Ref 311]
6. How does the perioperative nurse assist the anesthesia provider during nerve blocks? [Ref 313]
7. Describe local infiltration of an anesthetic agent. [Ref 314]
8. What is the purpose of epinephrine when added to lidocaine for a local infiltration? [Ref 316]
9. What does the perioperative nurse monitor during local infiltration of anesthetic? [Ref 317]
10. How can toxic reactions to local infiltration occur? [Ref 318]
11. What are the symptoms of toxic infiltration? [Ref 319–320]
12. What is the perioperative nurse's responsibility in case of a toxic reaction? [Ref 321]
13. When is topical anesthesia most frequently used? [Ref 323]

(continues)

Section Questions (continued)

14. Why is topical anesthesia especially helpful in procedures involving the respiratory tract? [Ref 323]

15. What must be present when topical anesthesia is used in the respiratory tract? [Ref 324]

16. How can the perioperative nurse allay the fear of a patient who worries about being awake during a procedure being performed with regional anesthesia? [Refs 328–329]

17. Which nursing interventions are appropriate during the administration of regional anesthesia? [Refs 331–332]

18. During the administration of topical and local anesthesia, who is primarily responsible for monitoring the patient? [Ref 334]

19. When the patient is receiving a local infiltration, what will the perioperative nurse monitor? [Refs 335–336]

20. For what reason does TJC require that all medications on and off the sterile field be labeled? [Refs 341–342]

21. Which precautions does the perioperative nurse take before dispensing any medication? [Ref 343]

22. How do the circulating nurse and the scrubbed person handle medications delivered to the sterile field? [Ref 344]

23. When personnel relieve one another, how should unlabeled medications be managed? [Ref 345]

24. What is a safe approach to verifying verbal orders? [Refs 346–347]

25. How does TJC expect that a patient's medication information will be communicated from one provider to another? [Refs 348–349]

● ● ● **References**

American Society of Anesthesiologists (ASA) (2012a). *ASA physical status classification system.* Park Ridge, IL: ASA. Available at: www.asahq.org/clinical/physicalstatus.htm. Accessed June 2012.

American Society of Anesthesiologists (ASA) (2012b). Practice Advisory for Preanesthesia Evaluation An Updated Report by the American Society of Anesthesiologists Task Force on Preanesthesia Evaluation. *Anesthesiology*;116(3); 1–17.

American Society of Anesthesiologists (ASA), Committee on Standards and Practice Parameters (ASA) (2011a). Practice guidelines for preoperative fasting and the use of pharmacologic agents to reduce the risk of pulmonary aspiration: application to healthy patients undergoing elective procedures. *Anesthesiology*;114(3):495–511.

American Society of Anesthesiologists (ASA) (2011b). *Practice guidelines for sedation and analgesia by non-anesthesiologists.* Park Ridge, IL: ASA. Available at: www.asahq.org/for-healthcare-professionals/education-and-events/guidelines-for-sedation-and-analgesia-by-non-anesthesiologists.aspx. Accessed June 2012.

American Society of Anesthesiologists (ASA) (2010). *Standards for basic anesthetic monitoring.* Available at: https://ecommerce.asahq.org/p-365-asa-standards-guidelines-and-statements.aspx. Accessed June 2012.

Association of periOperative Registered Nurses (AORN) (2012). *Standards, Recommended Practices and Guidelines.* Denver, CO: AORN.

Association of periOperative Registered Nurses (AORN) (2011). *Perioperative Nursing Data Set* (3rd ed.). Denver, CO: AORN.

Ginimuge P, Jyothi S (2010). Methylene blue: revisited. *Clin Pharmacol*;26(4): 517–520. Available at: http://www.ncbi.nlm.nih.gov/pmc/articles/PMC3087269/. Accessed June 2012.

Jakpor O (2011). Do artificial nails and nail polish interfere with accurate measurement of oxygen saturation by pulse oximetry? *Young Scientists J*;4(9):33–37. Available at: www.butrousfoundation.com/ysjournal/sites/default/files/YoungScientistsJ4933-3568108_095441.pdf. Accessed June 2012.

Jardeleza A, Fleig D, Davis N, Spreen-Parker R (2011). The effectiveness and cost of passive warming in adult ambulatory surgery patients. *AORN J*;94(4):363–369.

Kapitanyan R (2012). Local anesthetic toxicity. In: *Medscape Reference: Drugs, Disease, and Procedures.* Available at: http://emedicine.medscape.com/article/1844551-overview. Accessed June 2012.

Litwack K (1995). *Post Anesthesia Nursing Care.* St. Louis, MO: Mosby Year Book.

Malignant Hyperthermia Association of the United States (MHAUS) (2012). *What is MH?* Sherburne, NY: MHAUS. Available at http://mhaus.org/mhaus-faqs-healthcare-professionals/what-is-malignant-hyperthermia. Accessed October 2012.

Muller A, Huisman I, Roos P, et al. (2010). Outbreak of severe sepsis due to contaminated propofol: lessons to learn. *J Hosp Infect*;76(3):225–230. Available at: www.ncbi.nlm.nih.gov/pubmed/20692067. Accessed June 2012.

Murhammer J, Ross M, Bebout K (2004). Lidocaine: maximum dosing requirements. *University of Iowa Rx Update.* Available at: www.healthcare.uiowa.edu/pharmacy/RxUpdate/2004/12rxu.html. Accessed June 14, 2008.

National Institutes of Occupational Safety and Health (NIOSH) (2012). *Criteria for a Recommended Standard: Occupational Exposure to Waste Anesthetic Gases and Vapors.* Publication No. 77-140. Washington, DC: NIOSH. Available at: www.cdc.gov/niosh/docs/1970/77-140.html. Accessed June 2012.

Occupational Safety and Health Administration (OSHA) (2012a). *Occupational safety and health guideline for nitrous oxide.* Available at: www.osha.gov/SLTC/health guidelines/nitrousoxide/recognition.html. Accessed June 2012.

Occupational Safety and Health Administration (OSHA) (2012b). Surgical Suite module. Washington, DC: OSHA. Available at: www.osha.gov/SLTC/etools/hospital/surgical/surgical.html. Accessed June 2012.

Seaman M, Wobb J, Gaughan J, et al. (2012). The effects of intraoperative hypothermia on surgical site infection. *Ann Surg*;224(4):789–795.

Surgical Care Improvement Project (SCIP) (2011). Core Measures. Available at: www.jointcommission.org/assets/1/6/Surgical%20Care%20Improvement%20Project.pdf

The Joint Commission (TJC) (2012a). *Comprehensive Accreditation Manual for Hospitals.* Oakbrook Terrace, IL: TJC.

The Joint Commission (TJC) (2012b). *2011–2012 National Patient Safety Goals.* Available at: www.joint commission.org/assets/1/18/2011-2012_npsg_presentation_final_8-4-11.pdf. Accessed June 2012.

The Joint Commision (TJC) (2010b). *Specifications Manual for Joint Commission National Quality Core Measures.* Available at: http://manual.jointcommission.org/releases/archive/TJC2010B/DataElem0023.html

The Joint Commission (TJC) (2004). Sentinel Event Alert: *Preventing and managing the impact of anesthesia awareness, 32;* 1–3. www.jointcommission.org/sentinel_event_alert_issue_32_preventing_and_managing_the_impact_of_anesthesia_awareness/. Accessed October 2012.

Turillazzi E, Bellow S, Bonsignore A, et al. (2012). Retrospective analysis of anaesthesia-related deaths during a 12-year period: looking at the data from a forensic point of view. *Med Sci Law*;52(2):112–115. Available at: http://msl.rsmjournals.com/content/52/2/112.full. Accessed June 2012.

Valdez-Lowe C, Ghareeb S, Artinian N (2009). Pulse oximetry in adults. *Am J Nursing*;109(6):52–59. Available at: http://journals.lww.com/ajnonline/Fulltext/2009/06000Pulse_Oximetry_in_Adults.37.aspx. Accessed June 2012.

Post-Test

Read each question carefully. Each question may have more than one correct answer.

1. Which statement(s) is (are) true about risk factors?

    a. Anesthetic agents can compromise ventilation, perfusion, cardiac output, electrolyte and fluid balance, and thought processes.

    b. The risk of complications is determined by the type of anesthesia, anesthetic agents, the surgical procedure, and the patient's condition.

    c. Desired outcomes include normothermia, effective air exchange, adequate ventilation, and unimpaired thought processes.

    d. Patients should achieve desired outcomes within 45 minutes after extubation.

2. The Aldrete scoring system evaluates all of the following *except*

    a. activity.

    b. respiration.

    c. circulation.

    d. CO_2 saturation.

3. Anesthesia providers include all of the following *except*

    a. an anesthesiologist.

    b. a CRNFA.

    c. an AA.

    d. a CRNA.

4. Which of the following are the perioperative nurse's responsibilities related to anesthesia delivery?

    a. Preanesthesia assessment

    b. Patient support and patient teaching

    c. Communication

    d. Documentation

5. The hand-off report from the circulator to the PACU nurse should include

    a. drug allergies.

    b. a surgical safety checklist.

    c. estimated blood loss.

    d. intraoperative medications.

6. Which statement(s) is (are) true about preanesthesia data?

    a. The perioperative nurse is responsible for gathering all preoperative data and communicating this information to other health professionals.

    b. In healthy patients, there is no evidence that routine preoperative testing affects patient outcomes.

    c. It is important to know if a patient is taking beta-blocker medication.

    d. Guidelines may require certain preoperative tests based on the age of the patient.

7. Smoking history is important because smokers can experience

    a. more problems with wound complications.

    b. pulmonary and cardiac complications.

    c. a need for increased anesthetic dosage

    d. increased postoperative pain.

8. Benefits of smoking cessation can be evident in as few as _____ hours.
   a. 72
   b. 48
   c. 24
   d. 12

9. Anesthesia uses the following classes for communicating physical status (PS):
   a. PS1—healthy, no organic disease
   b. PS2—mild systemic disease (e.g., controlled hypertension)
   c. PS3—severe systemic disease (e.g., morbid obesity)
   d. PS4—severe systemic disease that is a threat to life (e.g., unstable angina, symptomatic CHF, hepatorenal failure)

10. The following are fasting recommendations for patients of all ages:
    a. Clear liquids—2 hours before surgery
    b. Light meal—6 hours before surgery
    c. Heavy meal—surgery should be canceled
    d. Infant formula—6 hours before surgery

11. Factors that are considered when selecting anesthetic agents and technique include
    a. age.
    b. patient preference.
    c. surgeon preference.
    d. anesthesia provider preference.

12. When conscious sedation is administered by an anesthesia provider, it is called
    a. AAS—anesthesia-assisted sedation.
    b. MAC—monitored anesthesia care.
    c. CSA—conscious sedation by anesthesia.
    d. ADS—anesthesia-delivered sedation.

13. Regional anesthesia is anesthesia delivered
    a. to a section of the body, such as a limb or the lower half of the body.
    b. as a single injection or over a long period of time.
    c. via mask induction.
    d. by both central and peripheral techniques.

14. Which statement(s) is (are) true about preoperative medications/protocols?
    a. IV agents are administered 60–90 minutes prior to surgery.
    b. Midazolam (Versed) and diazepam (Valium) reduce anxiety and provide some amnesia.
    c. Valium is used infrequently because of its short duration of action.
    d. Metoclopramide (Reglan) is given to patients with conditions that place them at high risk for aspiration.

15. Anticholinergics are
    a. given routinely to all patients.
    b. useful in preventing postoperative nausea.
    c. useful with patients who salivate excessively.
    d. appropriate for toddlers and children.

16. One SCIP measure is the delivery of an antibiotic for certain procedures within
   a. 120 minutes prior to surgery.
   b. 90 minutes prior to surgery.
   c. 60 minutes prior to surgery.
   d. 30 minutes prior to surgery.

17. Patients who receive narcotics must be observed closely because
   a. narcotics provide relief from pain.
   b. narcotics can be abused.
   c. it is not uncommon for patients to have adverse reactions to narcotics.
   d. all narcotics are associated with a dose-related respiratory depression and can cause nausea and vomiting.

18. Minimum monitoring for all surgical patients should include
   a. ECG.
   b. blood pressure.
   c. heart rate.
   d. pulse oximetry.

19. The choice of monitoring device is determined by
   a. the procedure.
   b. the anesthesia provider's and surgeon's preference.
   c. the patient's history and state of health.
   d. anticipated postoperative management.

20. Which statement(s) is (are) true about pulse oximetry?
   a. Pulse oximetry measures the oxygen saturation of arterial hemoglobin.
   b. O_2 saturation readings should be near 100%.
   c. O_2 saturation readings less than 95% are usually indicative of hypoxemia.
   d. Dark nail polish and acrylic nails can affect pulse oximetry readings.

21. Which statement(s) is (are) true about hypothermia?
   a. Hypothermia is defined as body temperature less than 34°C.
   b. Hypothermia is linked to shivering, which increases O_2 consumption.
   c. Hypothermia is linked to extended recovery and surgical-site infection.
   d. Hypothermia can result in increased perioperative blood loss.

22. The greatest change in patient temperature during anesthesia administration occurs within the first
   a. 30 minutes.
   b. 60 minutes.
   c. 90 minutes.
   d. 120 minutes.

23. The best approach to warming the patient who has received anesthesia is
   a. warm blankets.
   b. warmed irrigating fluids.
   c. raising the room temperature.
   d. a forced-air warming blanket.

24. Capnography is useful in detecting
    a. hypoventilation.
    b. respiratory insufficiency.
    c. esophageal intubation.
    d. a disconnected circuit.

25. The effects of general anesthesia include
    a. amnesia.
    b. hypnosis.
    c. analgesia.
    d. skeletal muscle relaxation.

26. Which statement(s) is (are) true about nitrous oxide?
    a. Nitrous oxide acts rapidly but lacks potency.
    b. Nitrous oxide is nonirritating and produces few aftereffects.
    c. Nitrous oxide diffuses readily into gas-filled spaces (e.g., stomach, lungs, colon).
    d. A high concentration of nitrous oxide can lead to hypoxia.

27. Which statement(s) is (are) true about isoflurane?
    a. Isoflurane is a volatile anesthetic.
    b. Isoflurane provides excellent relaxation and potentiates muscle relaxants.
    c. Induction and emergence are the shortest with isoflurane among commonly used agents.
    d. Isoflurane potentiates myocardial irritability and cannot be used with epinephrine.

28. Which statement(s) is (are) true about desflurane?
    a. Desflurane's rapid induction and emergency make it especially useful in ambulatory surgery.
    b. Desflurane has high fat solubility and cannot be used with obese patients.
    c. Desflurane's pungent odor can cause laryngospasm.
    d. Desflurane is highly recommended for inhalation anesthesia.

29. What are the color codes for tanks and fittings of O_2, N_2O, and air?
    a. Oxygen tanks and fittings are green.
    b. Nitrous tanks and fittings are blue.
    c. Nitrous tanks and fittings are white.
    d. Air tanks and fittings are white.

30. Which statement(s) is (are) true about anesthesia machines?
    a. The machine has a reservoir bag that can be compressed like an Ambu bag.
    b. Anesthesia gases that escape into the air can cause a variety of symptoms in operating-room personnel.
    c. A scavenger system on the machine collects expired gases and eliminates them through a suction line.
    d. The perioperative nurse should be aware of limits for exposure to anesthetic gases and confirm that test results are within normal limits.

31. Which statement(s) is (are) true about induction agents?
    a. Sodium pentothal results in a rapid progression from sedation to loss of consciousness.
    b. A degree of hypotension can be expected with barbiturates.
    c. Diprivan is the most popular nonbarbiturate induction and maintenance agent.
    d. Propofol hurts when injected, but is associated with rapid recovery and minimal aftereffects, including nausea and vomiting.

32. Which statement(s) is (are) true about ketamine?
    a. Ketamine produces a catatonic state; the patient may appear to be awake.
    b. Ketamine is used only for children.
    c. An antisaligogue is often used in conjunction with ketamine.
    d. It is a myth that patients hallucinate postoperatively when ketamine is used.

33. Which statement(s) is (are) true about narcotics?
    a. Fentanyl is more potent than morphine; sufentanil is more potent than fentanyl.
    b. Narcotics provide profound analgesia; they can also provide pain relief in the early postoperative period.
    c. Narcotics are respiratory stimulants.
    d. Potential complications of the opioid antagonist Narcan include pulmonary edema and hypertension.

34. Which statement(s) is (are) true about tranquilizers?
    a. Valium and Versed are used intraoperatively
    b. Using a tranquilizer intraoperatively permits the use of lower doses of other anesthetic agents.
    c. Tranquilizers produce amnesia and reduce anxiety.
    d. Respiratory depression from tranquilizers can be reversed with flumazenil (Romazicon).

35. Which statement(s) is (are) true about the perioperative nurse's responsibilities related to preparation for anesthesia?
    a. The room should be ready when the patient arrives so the perioperative nurse can focus on the patient throughout induction.
    b. Suction should be working and available to the anesthesia provider.
    c. Talking should be kept to a minimum.
    d. The scrubbed person should work quietly at the back table.

36. Induction is the period from when
    a. the patient enters the room until he or she is asleep.
    b. the patient is moved onto the operating-room table into the anesthesia provider's care until he or she is asleep.
    c. the anesthesia provider injects the first anesthetic medication to when the patient loses consciousness and is stabilized at the desired level of anesthesia.
    d. the anesthesia provider places the mask over the patient's face until the patient is intubated.

37. Induction is a critical time when the perioperative nurse should be present to
    a. position the patient.
    b. assist with suctioning and intubation.
    c. collect routine supplies for the anesthesia provider.
    d. restrain or calm the patient if necessary.

38. Place the following activities in order of the typical sequence of inducing a patient having general anesthesia:
    a. The patient breathes 100% O_2 by mask.
    b. The endotracheal tube is inserted and secured.
    c. A paralyzing dose of muscle relaxant is administered.
    d. Sodium pentothal or propofol is injected.

39. Which statement(s) is (are) true about the perioperative nurse's role when the patient is given a barbiturate or hypnotic at the start of induction?
    a. Suction if the patient regurgitates to prevent aspiration.
    b. Turn the patient's head to one side to prevent aspiration.

    c. Adjust the table to the reverse Trendelenburg position.

    d. Provide an emesis basin if the patient begins to regurgitate.

40. The Sellick maneuver

    a. involves firmly pressing the cricoid cartilage posteriorly with the thumb and forefinger.

    b. compresses the esophagus between the cricoid cartilage and the vertebral column.

    c. aids in visualization of the esophagus for intubation.

    d. is done until the endotracheal tube is in place and the anesthesia provider indicates it can be released.

41. Malignant hyperthermia (MH) might present with which of the following symptoms?

    a. Unexplained rise in temperature

    b. Masseter muscle rigidity

    c. Unexplained tachycardia

    d. Metabolic alkalosis

42. MH can be triggered by which of the following anesthetic agents?

    a. Valium

    b. Halothane

    c. Isoflurane

    d. Succinylcholine

43. Risk factors for MH include

    a. family history of MH or unexplained death from anesthesia experience.

    b. unexplained death during surgery.

    c. history of unexplained muscle cramps with fever.

    d. inherited skeletal muscle disorders.

44. In the event of an MH diagnosis during surgery,

    a. get help.

    b. get dantrolene sodium.

    c. get the MH cart.

    d. get a replacement anesthesia machine, if available.

45. The most significant challenge in addressing an MH event is

    a. finding the needed supplies.

    b. getting assistance in the room.

    c. reconstituting the dantrolene sodium.

    d. finding the MH policy.

46. Following an episode of MH,

    a. the patient must be monitored closely for a recurrent episode.

    b. the prognosis for recovery is poor.

    c. dantrolene sodium is continued for 48 hours or more.

    d. the patient should not undergo surgery in the future.

47. Monitoring the patient receiving conscious/moderate sedation

    a. should be done by an anesthesia provider.

    b. can be done by the surgeon.

    c. can be done by the circulating nurse if he or she can spend most of the time with the patient.

    d. can be done by a perioperative nurse who has no other responsibilities during the procedure.

48. At a minimum, which equipment should be available when the patient is receiving conscious sedation?

    a. Pulse oximeter

    b. Blood pressure monitor

    c. Temperature monitor

    d. ECG

49. Which of the following are criteria for discharge following conscious sedation?

    a. Return to baseline level of consciousness

    b. Absence of nausea and vomiting

    c. Adequate pain control

    d. Return of motor/sensory control

50. Which statement(s) is (are) true about regional anesthesia?

    a. Regional anesthesia is preferable for emergency surgery when the patient has a full stomach.

    b. With regional anesthesia, the respiratory system remains relatively stable.

    c. Regional anesthesia can cause cardiac instability.

    d. Regional anesthesia can be used with patients in whom general anesthesia is contraindicated (e.g., patients with metabolic, hepatic, or renal disease).

51. Which statement(s) is (are) true about spinal anesthesia?

    a. Administration of spinal anesthesia requires cooperation from the patient.

    b. Aseptic technique is essential to prevent meningitis.

    c. Anesthetic agents settle by gravity and the block is sensitive to the patient's position.

    d. Potential complications of spinal anesthesia include rapid drop in blood pressure, nausea and vomiting, postprocedure headache, and total spinal anesthesia when the level of anesthesia paralyzes respiratory muscles.

52. Which statement(s) is (are) true about a Bier block?

    a. A Bier block involves the use of a double tourniquet.

    b. Anesthetic is injected into the artery after the proximal tourniquet is inflated.

    c. The second cuff inflated and the first cuff deflated to alleviate tourniquet pain.

    d. The tourniquet is released rapidly to release of the remaining anesthetic from the extremity.

53. Major nerve blocks used in operative procedures include

    a. brachial plexus block.

    b. orbital block.

    c. spinal block.

    d. cervical block.

54. Which statement(s) is (are) true about toxic reactions to local infiltration?

    a. Toxic reaction can occur if absorption from a vascular site is too rapid.

    b. Toxic reaction can occur following inadvertent intravascular injection.

    c. Cardiovascular depression can be a toxic reaction.

    d. Restlessness and visual and auditory disturbances are symptoms of central nervous system toxicity.

55. Which statement(s) is (are) true about nursing responsibilities related to regional anesthesia?

    a. Every patient receiving some type of regional anesthesia should be monitored.

    b. During local anesthesia, the perioperative nurse should monitor the amount of anesthetic agent given.

    c. Resuscitation equipment should be immediately available.

    d. All medications should be labeled.

• •

Competency Checklist: Anesthesia

Under "Observer's Initials," enter initials upon successful achievement of the competency. Enter N/A if the competency is not appropriate for the institution.

Name _____

	Observer's Initials	Date

Preoperative Assessment

1. Assesses the patient/chart for anesthetic considerations (as applicable):
   a. Coexisting disease
   b. NPO status
   c. Allergies to medications, contrast dyes, tape, or latex
   d. Current medications, including herbal and nutritional supplements
   e. Previous surgeries
   f. Patient/family history of anesthesia complications
   g. Substance abuse
   h. Pregnancy
   i. Diagnostic testing
   j. Response to preoperative medications
   k. Anxiety level
   l. Knowledge level
   m. Previous anesthesia—complications
   n. Other
2. Verifies that patient is in compliance with preoperative instructions.
3. Communicates assessment data to the surgical team as appropriate.
4. Provides emotional support (e.g., answers patient concerns, provides reassuring touch) to the patient/family.
5. Provides information as needed to the patient/family.
6. Reinforces preoperative teaching with the patient/family.

General Anesthesia

7. In preparation for induction:
   a. Checks suction and places it for easy access to the patient's mouth
   b. Applies monitoring equipment (ECG leads, blood pressure cuff, pulse oximeter)
   c. Places IV line
   d. Applies safety strap
   e. Limits patient exposure
   f. Maintains a quiet atmosphere
   g. Remains at the patient's side at the head of the table, provides reassurance
8. At induction, assists in intubation as needed (e.g., provides endotracheal tube, applies cricoid pressure, suctions, inflates cuff).

9. Following induction:

    a. Checks position and pressure points and provides protective
devices as needed   _____ _____

    b. Applies warming devices as appropriate (e.g., with a lengthy
procedure, large/deep incision)   _____ _____

10. Monitors fluid output and replacement and irrigating fluid.   _____ _____

11. During emergence and extubation:

    a. Checks suction and places for it easy access to the patient's mouth _____ _____

    b. Remains at the head of the OR table by the patient   _____ _____

    c. Assists the anesthesia care provider as needed (e.g., suction,
Ambu bag, O_2)   _____ _____

12. Provides hand-off report to postanesthesia care unit (e.g., patient name
and age, surgical procedure, surgeon and anesthesiologist, anesthesia
technique, estimated blood loss, fluid and blood administration, urine
output, response to surgery/anesthesia, lab results, chronic and acute
health history, drug allergies, expected problems/suggested interventions,
discharge plan, other).   _____ _____

Regional Anesthesia

13. Implements procedures to alert others that the patient is awake. _____ _____

14. Assists in positioning the patient for administration of regional anesthetic
(e.g., provides stool for feet, instructs patient). _____ _____

15. Provides a safe environment for the patient during positioning for
administration of regional anesthetic (e.g., remains with patient). _____ _____

16. Limits patient exposure during preparation for and administration
of anesthesia. _____ _____

17. Monitors and reports the amount of local anesthetic agent administered. _____ _____

Monitoring

18. Demonstrates ability to apply and use monitoring devices and interpret
data for:

    a. Blood pressure   _____ _____

    b. Cardiac rate and rhythm   _____ _____

    c. Respiratory rate   _____ _____

    d. Oxygen saturation   _____ _____

    e. Mental status/level of consciousness   _____ _____

19. Demonstrates airway management, including use of oxygen delivery
devices and equipment. _____ _____

20. Demonstrates ability to use resuscitative equipment. _____ _____

Emergency Preparations

21. Retrieves malignant hyperthermia supplies without hesitation. _____ _____

22. Explains the protocol for malignant hyperthermia crisis. _____ _____

	Observer's Initials	Date

23. Ensures immediate availability of resuscitative equipment (IV, conscious sedation, and local procedures).   _____ _____

24. Reports changes in patient condition and implements appropriate interventions.   _____ _____

Documentation

25. Documents data as required by institutional policy.   _____ _____

Anesthesia Machine

26. Identifies the anesthesia machine components—oxygen flush button, monitors for ECG, blood pressure, pulse, respirations, breathing bag, carbon dioxide absorber canister, ventilator, flow meters, scavenging system.   _____ _____

27. Repeats/confirms verbal medication orders.   _____ _____

28. Labels all medications.   _____ _____

Additional Safety Measures

29. Verifies that the surgical site is marked (if appropriate to the surgery).   _____ _____

30. Participates in "time-out."   _____ _____

31. Verifies the presence and application of a forced-air warming blanket as appropriate.   _____ _____

32. Raises the room temperature as appropriate.   _____ _____

33. Verifies preoperative antibiotic orders and administration when appropriate.   _____ _____

34. Applies sequential compression devices when appropriate.   _____ _____

Observer's Signature   Initials   Date

_____

Orientee's Signature

_____

12

Workplace Safety

LEARNER OBJECTIVES

1. List elements of a safety officer's responsibilities.
2. Identify chemical and physical hazards present in the operating room environment.
3. List the government organizations that publish regulations for healthcare worker safety.
4. List accrediting organizations' safety standards.
5. Define a sentinel event.
6. Define failure mode effects analysis (FMEA).
7. Discuss the most common causes of operating-room fires.
8. Identify the ECRI recommendations to decrease the chance of a fire in the operating room.
9. Define the acronyms RACE and PASS.
10. Describe the components of a fire safety plan.
11. Discuss elements of a fire drill report card.
12. Define the purpose of the line isolation monitoring (LIM) system.
13. Discuss elements of sharps safety.
14. State the guidelines for healthcare workers to follow when working in a room where radiation is present.
15. State the guidelines for healthcare workers to follow when working with lasers.
16. Discuss possible causes of low back pain in healthcare workers and the recommendations for preventing injury.
17. Describe the precautions for working with methyl methacrylate.
18. Discuss the difference between localized and systemic latex allergy reactions.
19. Discuss hazards of surgical smoke.
20. Discuss the personal protective equipment required in a perioperative setting.
21. Discuss the requirements of eye wash stations.

www

LESSON OUTLINE

This chapter addresses those aspects of workplace safety that perioperative nurses most often cite as cause for concern. It does not cover all aspects of workplace safety or patient safety. Exposure to bloodborne pathogens is covered in the Prevention of Infection: Aseptic Practices chapter, and patient safety is addressed throughout the text.

Regulations

1. Trained safety personnel can be a valuable resource when designing and developing a safety program for the operating room. All staff should master the basic safety requirements for the perioperative environment.

2. Building, electrical, and fire codes developed for each state and city are part of creating a safe environment for patients and healthcare workers.

3. In addition to state and city regulations, the following organizations create regulations and recommendations for healthcare facilities that affect the workplace environment and perioperative nursing practice:

   - Centers for Disease Control and Prevention (CDC)
   - National Institute of Occupational Safety and Health (NIOSH)
   - Occupational Safety and Health Administration (OSHA)
   - The Joint Commission (TJC)
   - Accreditation Association for Ambulatory Health Care (AAAHC)
   - American Association for Accreditation of Ambulatory Surgery Facilities (AAAASF)
   - Healthcare Facilities Accreditation Program (HFAP)
   - Center for Medicare and Medicaid Services (CMS)
   - National Fire Protection Association (NFPA)
   - Environmental Protection Agency (EPA)

4. Healthcare organizations define safe practices for the perioperative environment and guide clinical staff to achieving a culture of safety. The following organizations influence the safe practice and standards of care for the perioperative team:

   - American Association of Nurse Anesthetists (AANA)
   - American Association of Surgical Physician Assistants (AASPA)
   - American College of Surgeons (ACS)
   - American Society of Anesthesiologists (ASA)
   - American Society of PeriAnesthesia Nurses (ASPAN)
   - Association of periOperative Registered Nurses (AORN)
   - Association of Surgical Technologists (AST)

Standards and Recommendations

Occupational Safety and Health Administration (www.osha.gov)

5. OSHA has the primary responsibility for publishing and enforcing workplace safety and health standards. Established in 1970, this federal agency creates legal standards that must be economically feasible. OSHA can also assess the workplace for hazards and mandate changes to correct unsafe conditions. OSHA regulations carry the weight of law, and health-care facilities are generally vigilant in ensuring compliance.

6. Under OSHA's General Duty Clause, each employer must furnish each employee with a place of employment free from recognized hazards that are capable of causing or likely to cause death or serious physical harm. Employers must create and implement an effective process that provides management support, involves employees in the plan, identifies problems, implements corrective actions, addresses employee and patient injury reports, provides periodic employee training, and evaluates ergonomics efforts.

National Institute for Occupational Safety and Health (www.cdc.gov/niosh)

7. NIOSH, which was also created in 1970, recommends standards based on public health considerations. Categories of standards include biological hazards such as bloodborne pathogens and tuberculosis; chemical hazards including ethylene oxide, glutaraldehyde, latex, and laser smoke control; physical hazards of ergonomics and musculoskeletal disorders; and violence in the workplace.

8. NIOSH focuses on safety and health, quality, and human resources development. A facility must promote safety and health as part of the facility's culture, which includes the participation of management as well as staff. Quality is the driver of a safe work environment; thus NIOSH promotes continuous quality improvement activity that is understood by all staff members of the facility. Training and assessing knowledge and competence of all staff members are ongoing in an organization that supports and promotes safety.

9. Voluntary organizations, such as The Joint Commission and the National Fire Protection Association, have also developed important standards and recommendations.

Environmental Protection Agency (www.epa.gov /lawsregs)

10. Under the EPA, the environment is protected from dumping of medical waste, medications, and emissions of pollutants into the air that would be harmful to the public. Proper medical waste disposal is the responsibility of every employee, and each facility is held accountable for abiding by the laws and regulations. Employees should be educated on the proper disposal of all types of medical waste. OSHA requires that all employees be provided with personal protection equipment (PPE) to ensure they are protected from harm while disposing of medical waste.

The Joint Commission (www.jointcommission.org)

11. The Environment of Care (EC) chapter of The Joint Commission's standards focuses on the promotion of safety. TJC expects both facility and staff to embrace the goal of fostering an environment that supports and promotes a culture of safety.

12. There are three basic elements of a safe environment:
    - A building design that protects patients, visitors, and employees
    - Equipment that is maintained and deemed safe to use on a regular basis
    - People who enter the environment and understand the roles they play in minimizing risks in the environment (TJC, 2012, pp. EC1–EC3)

13. The healthcare organization addresses the elements of an environment of safety by creating a plan addressing a variety of environmental risks:
    - Safety and security of the building
    - Security-sensitive areas such as the emergency room, children's ward, and nursery
    - Product failures or recalls
    - Smoking
    - Biohazardous materials

- Hazardous wastes or materials such as radiation, radioactive materials, medications, gases and vapors that are dangerous to people and the environment

14. Fire safety is addressed in the environmental safety plan. Fire safety includes the following issues:

   - A response plan
   - Fire drills
   - Alarm testing
   - Equipment maintenance and testing
   - Employee competence through fire drills
   - Report cards addressing the response of staff and others during the drill

15. A medical equipment maintenance and replacement policy is included in the environmental safety plan. Utilities are inspected and tested on a regular basis. The disaster plan should describe the type of equipment or supplies needed for each type of disaster the facility might experience (TJC, 2012, pp. EC5–EC24).

Accreditation Association for Ambulatory Health Care (www.aaahc.org)

16. Chapter 7, Infection Prevention and Control and Safety, and Chapter 8, Facilities and Environment, in the AAAHC's manual describe the standards for and expectations of a healthcare facility to meet national, state, and local standards and to provide a safe environment for patients, visitors, and staff members.

17. The AAAHC safety plan provides a safe environment by embracing practices that promote an infection-free facility:

   - Hand washing
   - Proper environmental cleaning
   - Proper use of cleaning agents
   - Proper decontamination and reprocessing of equipment and instruments

18. The AAAHC promotes an active safety program that identifies the following:

   - Environmental hazards
   - Medical waste hazards
   - Potential threats
   - Near misses
   - Equipment failure

   - Building security
   - Medication safety
   - Internal and external disasters (AAAHC, 2012, pp. 64–65, 68–70)

19. The facility's governing body assumes ultimate responsibility for overseeing the safety plan. Its members are responsible for ensuring that staff have been properly trained in safety processes and are competent all safety processes, such as responding to fire, internal and external disasters, cardiac arrest, and malignant hyperthermia. In addition, they are responsible for ensuring that all biohazardous materials and hazardous materials are disposed of properly.

Healthcare Facilities Accreditation Program (www.hfap.org)

20. Chapter 11, Physical Environment, of the HFAP describes the standards, elements, and expectations of a healthcare facility's safety program. The basic elements include the following:

   - Fire drills and the equipment required in each department
   - Disaster response plans for internal and external disasters, including annual drills
   - Staff education on safety of the environment
   - Facilities maintenance program for building and equipment
   - Monitoring for compliance with safety plan
   - Actual overall safety of the building and equipment (HFAP, 2009, pp. 11-8 to 11-38)

21. The facility leadership team is responsible for environmental safety, to include the safety plan; standards of performance; competency of staff; security of the building and protection of the patients, visitors, and staff; and monitoring for compliance.

22. The safety team and safety officer are responsible for educating the staff at least annually; reviewing and updating safety policies and procedures; emergency call system monitoring; life safety monitoring; equipment safety inspections; utility safety inspections; environmental safety such as fire walls, fire doors, safety equipment, and storage and disposal of hazardous materials and wastes; OSHA compliance; and Safe Medical Device Act compliance.

American National Standards Institute (www.ansi.org/)

23. The American National Standards Institute (ANSI) was created in 1918 as a not-for-profit organization to be the voice of the United States marketplace for standards, and to assess compliance with the standards. The organization has prepared standards that govern medical devices safety and integrity, as well as standards for aseptic processing of medical devices and supplies. ANSI works with other agencies such as CDC, OSHA, and the Association for the Advancement of Medical Instrumentation (AAMI) to set and govern safety standards.

Association for the Advancement of Medical Instrumentation (www.aami.org)

24. AAMI was founded in 1967. A not-for-profit organization, it has become the primary resource for national and international standards for the use of safe and effective medical technology. ANSI/AAMI publication ST79, *Comprehensive Guide to Steam Sterilization and Sterility Assurance in Health Care Facilities,* provides the perioperative staff and the sterile processing department with standards for properly cleaning and reprocessing of equipment and instrumentation.

Section Questions

1. Which resources are available in each state that should be considered when developing a facility safety plan? [Refs 2–3]

2. In addition to state and city resources, identify at least eight organizations that create regulations and recommendations for workplace safety. [Ref 3]

3. List at least six healthcare organizations that influence safe practice and standards for the perioperative team. [Ref 4]

4. What is OSHA's primary responsibility? [Ref 5]

5. What are some of the requirements that OSHA places on each employer? [Ref 6]

6. What type of standards does NIOSH recommend? [Ref 7]

7. What does NIOSH consider the driver of a safe work environment? [Ref 8]

8. Which voluntary agencies participate in workplace safety? [Ref 9]

9. How does the EPA affect the healthcare industry? [Ref 10]

10. The TJC chapter on Environment of Care identifies three basic elements of a safe environment. What are they? [Ref 12]

11. What components should be included in a facility's safety plan? [Ref 13]

12. What should a facility include in its fire safety plan? [Ref 14]

13. How is medical equipment addressed in an environmental safety plan? [Ref 15]

14. How does the environment safety plan address disaster planning? [Ref 15]

15. What is the AAAHC and how does it promote workplace safety? [Refs 16–18]

16. Who is ultimately responsible for overseeing the safety plan in an ambulatory surgery facility? [Ref 19]

17. What is included in the chapter on physical environment in the HFAP? [Ref 20]

18. Which responsibilities do facility leadership, the safety team, and the safety officer have? [Refs 21–22]

19. Describe the purpose and function of ANSI. [Ref 23]

20. Describe the purpose and function of AAMI. [Ref 24]

Job Safety Analysis

25. Job safety analysis can be applied to many work situations, including the operating room, to analyze hazards and identify ways to overcome or eliminate them. Safety analysis methodology includes the following considerations:

    - Identification of the various tasks in the work site
    - Breakdown of each task into the steps required to accomplish the task
    - Identification of any potential hazards
    - Suggestion of ways to reduce or eliminate the hazards
    - Development of standards for accomplishing the tasks
    - Periodic review of conditions in the work area

26. Safety standards are developed by each department in conjunction with infection control and employee health personnel. All employees receive education training on appropriate protective attire and work methodology designed to avoid hazardous situations.

27. Ongoing monitoring ensures that all personnel are familiar with the standards and practice according to standard protocols. Monitoring results should be shared with personnel. Training activities should be scheduled regularly to ensure that all personnel continue to comply with the standards. Any deviations from the standards should be addressed.

28. An effective method of monitoring compliance with standard safety protocols and identifying new hazards is the implementation of periodic rounds using a checklist of workplace safety issues.

Physical Hazards

29. There should be periodic (quarterly or at least annual) training for all employees that focuses on preventing the most important physical hazards:

    - Fire
    - Electricity
    - Radiation
    - Lifting and moving
    - Slips, trips, and falls

Assessment results should be used to make changes in the environment to reduce risk, identify educational needs, and provide follow-up education for staff.

Fire

30. Reports indicate that 50 to 100 surgical fires occur every year. ECRI (formerly known as the Emergency Care Research Institute), however, estimates that 550 to 650 fires actually occur in the United States each year, but not all are reported. Of those incidents reported, ECRI states that 10% to 20% of fires result in serious patient injury and one or two events—usually tracheal tube fires—are fatal. Seventy-five percent of these fires occur in the oxygen-enriched area surrounding the patient's face. Frequent ignition sources include electrosurgery (70%), lasers (10%), light sources, sparks from burrs, and defibrillators (20%). Airway fires account for 21% of the total number of surgical fires, with 44% occurring on the face, head, neck, and chest (Bruley, 2012).

31. A small fire in an oxygen-enriched operating room can progress to a large, life-threatening fire in seconds. Flames can reach a temperature of approximately 1700°F (926°C) (ECRI, 2012, p. 21). Smoke can diminish visibility, and toxic fumes from burning synthetic materials can cause eye irritation or death if inhaled.

32. The Joint Commission requires adherence to the National Fire Protection Association's Life Safety Code for hospitals, ambulatory care centers, and other facilities. The Life Safety Code defines the requirements for facilities and procedures for safety from fire (NFPA, 2012).

33. In June 2003, The Joint Commission issued a "Sentinel Event Alert on Preventing Surgical Fires" (TJC, 2003). A sentinel event is defined as an "unexpected occurrence involving death or serious physical or psychological injury, or risk thereof." All TJC-accredited healthcare organizations are required to report any sentinel events that occur; to conduct a timely, thorough, and credible root-cause analysis; to develop an action plan to implement improvements to reduce risk; to implement the improvements; and to monitor the effectiveness of these improvements.

34. The sentinel alert on fires in the operating room requires that personnel meet the following criteria:

- Be trained in use of firefighting equipment.
- Know methods for rescue and escape.
- Know the location of alarm systems and their use.
- Know how to contact the local fire department.
- Know the location of the medical gas shutoff valves and electrical controls.

35. The fire triangle represents the three critical elements that must be present for a fire to occur:
    - An ignition source (e.g., electrosurgery, laser, and fiber-optic cords)
    - Fuel (anything that can burn)
    - Oxygen

36. Flammable anesthetics such as Halothane and ether have been eliminated from operating rooms, but the operating room remains an oxygen-enriched environment and is home to many other hazards that must be closely monitored:
    - Electrical equipment
    - Alcohol-based prepping and hand washing solutions
    - Flammable chemicals
    - Cylinders of compressed gas
    - Draping materials
    - Lasers
    - Fiber-optic light sources and cables
    - Flammable patient care supplies and trash

37. ECRI has identified electrosurgical devices as the most common cause of operating-room fires.

38. The scrubbed person should know the location of the active electrode (ESU pencil) at all times. The ESU pencil should be treated as follows:
    - Be stored away from the patient's airway
    - Be stored in a protective holder that is secured so it will not be dislodged by personnel movements during the surgical procedure
    - Not be wrapped around a metal surgical instrument to secure it to the drapes
    - Have an active electrode that is cleaned periodically to remove buildup of eschar that might trap heat (AORN, 2012b, pp. 105–106)
    - Not be activated when the environment is enriched with flammable materials

39. Whenever an electrosurgical device is in use, wet towels, normal saline, or sterile water should be readily available (AORN, 2012b, pp. 105–106).

40. It is imperative that the surgical prep be dry and all vapors evaporated before placing drapes on the patient to eliminate the risk of trapped vapors that can ignite when a device such as electrosurgical cautery devise is used.

41. Fiber-optic cords and connectors become heated during use. They should never be placed uncoupled on the drapes, because they have the potential to burn both the patient and the draping materials.

42. The fiber-optic cord for a headlight should be kept attached to the light source; it should not be allowed to hang loose on the surgeon's back, where it has a potential to ignite the gown. Headlights should be removed when not in use.

43. Oxygen supports combustion and, when used in close proximity to electrical equipment, requires constant vigilance. Surgery on or near the oxygen source—for example, surgery on the face—creates an increased risk of fire. Often, surgical drapes used in conjunction with facial surgery create a tent effect where oxygen delivered via nasal cannula or endotracheal tube can become concentrated, creating a highly enriched oxygen environment. A spark in this environment can be disastrous. Draping should be done in a manner to prevent pockets where oxygen can concentrate.

44. Materials that can contribute to the potential for combustion include patient hair, gases in the gastrointestinal (GI) tract, skin degreasers, aerosol adhesives, ointments, breathing circuits, suction tubing, endotracheal tubes, and alcohol-based products (Exhibit 12-1).

45. To reduce the risk of fires, alcohol-based hand washing products and patient prep solutions must be allowed to dry thoroughly or to evaporate following application. Prep solutions should not be allowed to saturate the drapes or soak into the patient's hair or linens or pillow.

46. The perioperative nurse may implement the following ECRI recommendations:
    - Question the need for 100% oxygen during facial surgery and replacing it with a lower concentration.
    - Ensure that all flammable preps are thoroughly dry prior to placing drapes on the patient.
    - Coat facial hair near the surgical site with a water-soluble lubricant.

Exhibit 12-1 Fire Hazards and Appropriate Responses

Department/Services	Fire Hazard(s)/Fire Response Consideration(s)
Laboratory	Flammable materials such as xylene, methanol, and other solvents with low flashpoints.
	Large volumes of formaldehyde solutions could present toxic environments for emergency responders in a fire situation.
Central supply/sterile processing	Cartridges of 100% ethylene oxide (EtO) are flammable. EtO in any mixture (e.g., 90/10) could present a toxic environment for emergency responders in a fire situation.
Surgical suites	Surgical suites are considered to have oxygen-enriched atmosphere (OEAs) due to the fact that oxygen concentration can exceed 23.5% by volume. Heat is present in overhead surgical lights, defibrillators, electrosurgical units, electrocautery units, and other sources. Fuels include prepping agents, open bottles or basins of volatile solutions, and most textiles (e.g., surgical drapes and gowns). Therefore, all the necessary ingredients are available in ample quantities to create a fire, which puts both patients and staff at risk.
Kitchens/food service	Grease fires represent a common fire hazard for those who prepare food.
Respiratory therapy	Generally responsible for the storage and maintenance of large quantities of portable oxygen cylinders. Storage areas for bulk storage of these cylinders should be approved by the authority having jurisdiction (AHJ).
Hyperbaric facilities	These areas are considered OEAs. Design and protocols should be conducted in accordance with NFPA 99 standards.
Magnetic resonance imaging (MRI)	MRI facilities represent evacuation issues for the patients being treated, and response issues for emergency responders. The magnet poses a potential risk for fire fighters responding to a room. In addition, emergency responders may have to purge the oxygen within the room to execute an emergency response, which then creates an oxygen-deficient atmosphere.
Engineering/building and grounds	Flammable materials such as gasoline and other fuels, oil-based paints, and paint thinners are all present in large quantities.
Critical care/general nursing areas	Areas such as the intensive care unit; neo-natal intensive care unit; maternity, labor, and delivery unit; and hemodialysis unit may have OEAs and also may represent significant challenges from an evacuation standpoint because these patients are connected to hospital equipment or may outnumber staff by large numbers. Evacuation plans should be developed and approved by the AHJ.
Print shops	Flammable solvents with large quantities of combustible material may be present.
Psychiatric units	Evacuation may be an issue because the unit may be secured in accordance with the facility's security management plan. Consult with the AHJ.
Linen and laundry	Dryers and other heat sources are present. Ensure combustible material such as lint is adequately controlled.

Source: Reprinted with permission from ECRI, Plymouth Meeting, PA; www.ecri.org.

- Keep sponges, gauze, and pledgets moist during surgery.
- Place the electrosurgical pencil in a properly placed holster when not in use.
- Disconnect and remove contaminated ESU pencils.
- Check the ESU alarm before use.
- Remove foot pedals that are not being used from the area around the surgeon's feet.
- Place the laser on standby when it is not being used.
- Place wet towels around the laser incision site, and use nonreflective instrumentation.
- Keep activated fiber-optic light sources from contacting surgical drapes or gowns.
- Store alcohol-based hand rubs in an area away from ignition and heat sources (ECRI, 2012).

47. ECRI Institute maintains a Medical Device Safety Reports (MDSR) database of incident and hazard information. The database is not meant to be an "alert" and is periodically updated. It is searchable at ECRI's online site (www.mdsr.ecri.org).

48. Prevention is the best way to combat operating-room fires. Prior to a procedure, the perioperative nurse should assess the risk for fire, such as materials, draping requirements, condition of equipment (integrity, function, current biomedical inspection), and chemicals, and should take steps to reduce this risk.

49. An AORN Fire Risk Assessment tool for the perioperative setting is part of the AORN Fire Tool Kit (AORN, 2012c).

50. In the event of a fire in the operating room, healthcare workers must be concerned about protecting both the patient and themselves. The acronym RACE is used to define personnel roles and responsibilities during a fire:
    - **R:** Rescue people from flaming materials.
    - **A:** Alert others by announcing "Code Red" and the location of the fire three times. (Institutional policy may dictate a specific phone number to call in the event of a fire or disaster.)
    - **C:** Confine or contain fire and smoke. Close the doors and shut off medical gas valves when leaving the room or when going from the fire area to a safe zone.
    - **E:** Extinguish the fire. Smother a small fire with a wet sponge or towel, extinguish the fire with water or saline, or, if needed, use a fire extinguisher. If the fire is immediately extinguished, call "Code Red all clear" and notify the fire department.
    Or
    - **E:** Evacuate to a safe place beyond the smoke or fire barrier doors, or outside. Activate the fire pull station when exiting the area. Remain with the patients and others in the safe area (ECRI, 2012).

51. Fire safety training should include instruction in the use of fire extinguishers. When using an extinguisher, the acronym PASS identifies the steps of the process:
    - **P:** Pull the pin.
    - **A:** Aim the nozzle.
    - **S:** Squeeze the handle.
    - **S:** Sweep at the base of the fire.

52. Fire extinguishers are classified according to the NFPA's system:
    - Class A: Suitable for wood, cloth, paper, and most plastics
    - Class B: Suitable for flammable liquids or grease
    - Class C: Suitable for electrical equipment

53. The best fire extinguisher for the operating room is a halon extinguisher. It is usually marked for Class B and C fires but is also effective against Class A fires. This device is lightweight and easy to handle.

54. A carbon dioxide extinguisher can be used for Class A, B, and C fires. It is heavier than a halon extinguisher; because of its size, it is usually wall mounted.

55. A pressurized water extinguisher, typically found in older operating room departments, is most suitable for Class A fires. However, the fire hose sprays approximately 50 gallons per minute and is difficult to operate, and the force of the hose itself can cause injury.

56. Actual training sessions in a controlled area outside the building under the supervision of the local fire department can help employees gain expertise and confidence when using fire extinguishers.

57. The education of staff begins at new-employee orientation and is reinforced annually.

Employees must demonstrate knowledge and competence in fire prevention, use of fire extinguishers, emergency response activities, and prevention of fire in the operating room.

58. Everyone on the surgical team must know the location of fire extinguishers, fire alarms, fire exits, and emergency shutoff gas valves. The locations of the alarms, extinguishers, and hoses must be posted in several sites.

59. Evacuation routes from all areas of the perioperative suite should be defined and posted in the hallways, operating-room lounge, and operating rooms. Hallways should be free of clutter that could hinder an evacuation. Every perioperative nurse should be able to describe the evacuation route.

60. Fire blankets should not be kept in the operating room; they will burn in the intense heat of a fire. They should be stored outside the operating room and may be used in an area that is not oxygen enriched.

61. Each healthcare facility must plan for fire incidents:
    - Have a fire safety plan.
    - Schedule safety education programs.
    - Conduct periodic fire drills—at least one fire drill quarterly each shift.
    - Evaluate fire drills based on expected criteria in the fire safety plan.
    - Complete education of staff on an annual basis.

62. Each facility should develop a fire safety plan with input from clinical representatives from all departments, clinical education, anesthesia, security, and the local fire and police departments. The chain of command should be clearly documented and disseminated to all departments.

63. The fire safety plan should include the following elements:
    - A clear definition of responsibilities
    - Methods for training staff members
    - Scenarios for fire drills
    - Instruction in the use of fire extinguishers
    - A plan for implementation of the code requirements
    - Documents for life safety surveillance
    - An interim life safety plan for use in the event of construction
    - The equipment, packaging materials, and supplies that must be retained for the fire investigation following any operating-room fire

64. Once the fire safety plan is finalized, education sessions should be scheduled to familiarize the entire staff with the plan and their roles in it. A safety officer should assume responsibility for surveillance, conducting the fire drills, overseeing the required documentation, and overseeing an annual review of the plan.

65. The perioperative nurse must have a clear understanding of his or her responsibilities:
    - Remove burning material from the patient and smother fire.
    - Extinguish small fires with extinguisher.
    - Turn off emergency shutoff valves.
    - Identify the evacuation route.
    - Stay with the patient during evacuation.
    - Complete appropriate documentation.

66. Conducting periodic fire drills will ensure that healthcare workers know their roles, whether they are at the location of the fire or away from the area. All employees should know the process for contacting the fire department, the location of the medical gases shutoff valves, the operation of fire alarm systems, the use of fire extinguishers, the evacuation plans, and proper methods of rescue and escape.

67. Critique sessions following fire drills using different scenarios are invaluable for identifying portions of the plan that need revision or updating and the need for further education.

68. Life safety surveillance information should be collected and evaluated in a systematic way. In addition to fire safety, other life safety topics may include facility and personnel security, hazardous substances, radiation safety, emergency preparedness, utilities, and infection control.

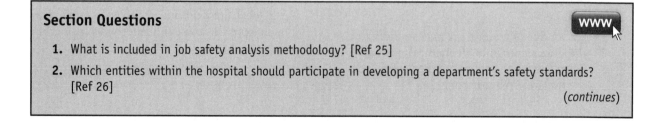

Section Questions   www

1. What is included in job safety analysis methodology? [Ref 25]
2. Which entities within the hospital should participate in developing a department's safety standards? [Ref 26]

(continues)

Section Questions (continued)

3. How does a department ensure that personnel are familiar with standards and practice accordingly? [Refs 27–28]

4. What are the five most important physical hazards in the perioperative environment? [Ref 29]

5. Where do the majority of surgical fires occur? [Ref 30]

6. Identify at least five sources of ignition of surgical fires. [Ref 30]

7. Which elements involved in fire, besides the heat, can cause injury? [Ref 31]

8. What is the purpose of the NFPA's Life Safety Code that The Joint Commission adopted? [Ref 32]

9. What is a "sentinel event" as defined by TJC? [Ref 33]

10. What does TJC require of hospitals when a sentinel event occurs? [Ref 33]

11. What does TJC's sentinel alert on fire expect of personnel? [Ref 34]

12. What are the three elements of the fire triangle? [Ref 35]

13. Which fire hazards in the operating room must be closely monitored? [Ref 36]

14. Which fire hazard in the operating room has ECRI identified as the most common source of fires? [Ref 37]

15. How should the scrubbed person manage the active electrode? [Refs 38–39]

16. How should the surgical prep be managed to avoid the potential for fire? [Ref 40]

17. How should fiber-optic light cords be managed to avoid the potential for fire? [Refs 41–42]

18. Which precautions can be taken during a procedure (e.g., on the face) that is being performed near an oxygen source to minimize the potential for fire? [Ref 43]

19. Which materials present during surgical procedures can contribute to the potential for combustion? [Ref 44]

20. How must alcohol-based products be managed to reduce the potential for combustion? [Ref 45]

21. Identify at least eight practices that the perioperative nurse can implement to reduce the potential for a surgical fire. [Ref 46]

22. What is the single most effective way to combat operating-room fires? [Ref 48]

23. What are the personnel roles and responsibilities defined by the acronym RACE? [Ref 50]

24. Which steps in using a fire extinguisher are associated with the acronym PASS? [Ref 51]

25. What is the most effective fire extinguisher for the operating room? [Ref 53]

26. What are some characteristics of the carbon dioxide fire extinguisher? [Ref 54]

27. How should personnel be trained in the use of a fire extinguisher? [Refs 56–57]

28. Who is responsible for knowing the locations of fire extinguishers, alarms, shutoff valves, and fire exits? [Refs 58–59]

29. Why should fire blankets not be stored in the operating room? [Ref 60]

30. Identify five responsibilities of a healthcare facility in relation to fire safety. [Refs 61–62]

Electricity

69. Electricity is one of the primary causes of hospital fires. Electrical hazard increases with the use of inappropriate extension cords and/or equipment with frayed or faulty electrical cords.

70. Avoid the use of extension cords; many fire safety regulations prohibit their use. Equipment manufacturers must supply cords of sufficient length to allow equipment to be placed in the area of use.

71. Any new equipment should be inspected by a biomedical engineer prior to use. Labels or stickers with the date of inspection and a department inventory number should be affixed to each piece of equipment. If the

inspection sticker is missing, or if the inspection has expired, the equipment should not be used. Biomedical engineering personnel are also responsible for documentation of regular inspections and preventive maintenance of all electrical and mechanical equipment.

72. Each piece of equipment that is used in the operating room should be checked by the facility's biomedical engineering department. Before use, the electrical outlets, switch plates, plugs, and power cords should be inspected for defects or damage. Electrical equipment that is not functioning properly can cause shock, explosion, and burns.

73. Operating rooms are also equipped with a line isolation monitoring (LIM) system that continuously monitors ungrounded power systems that may allow leaking electricity to flow from the power system to ground. An alarm will sound if leakage exceeds the threshold for safety. The LIM system reduces the potential for electrical shock, cardiac fibrillation, or burns produced by excess electrical current flowing through the patient's body to ground.

74. In the event of an alarm, the perioperative nurse should immediately unplug the piece of equipment most recently plugged in and continue this process until the alarm ceases. The equipment responsible for the alarm should be removed from service until it has been assessed and cleared by biomedical engineering.

Radiation

75. The majority of the facilities today do not have hybrid operating rooms, nor do they house diagnostic radiology equipment. However, the trend is changing and more facilities are adding diagnostic imaging to the services provided in the operating room for specialized procedures.

76. In August 2011, The Joint Commission issued a sentinel event alert (Issue 47) describing the dangers of diagnostic imaging, which have been identified as cancer, burns, and other radiation injuries (TJC, 2011). In an operating room providing diagnostic radiological procedures, staff can take the following steps to prevent potential injury to patients and employees:

    - Develop a comprehensive patient safety program, including education for patients and family members.
    - Educate staff on the types of dangers to which they and their patients are exposed when performing diagnostic radiation procedures.
    - Ensure physician education and competency to include awareness of proper dose levels for each diagnostic test.
    - Provide extensive training for physicians and staff on how to use diagnostic equipment.
    - Develop clear protocols describing the maximum limit (dose) of radiation for each type of test being performed in the facility.
    - Work closely with a medical physicist to ensure staff are competent, equipment is being used properly, and the equipment is safe.
    - Communicate.
    - Ensure the staff have a safety checklist that is being used appropriately.
    - Develop policies and procedures that are detailed and can be understood by all levels of staff education.
    - Develop a culture of radiation safety (TJC, 2011).

77. Surgical procedures performed under fluoroscopy or using intraoperative X rays are the primary sources of potential exposure to radiation for operating-room staff. Radiation safety training should be conducted as part of new-employee orientation and periodically thereafter. The safety training should include not only how each staff member should be protected, but also how to protect patients based on the area of exposure.

78. The principles of time, distance, and shielding assist perioperative personnel to minimize their exposure to X rays. When radiation is emitted at a constant rate, the dose received depends on the amount of exposure time. The amount of time spent near the patient while radiation is being emitted should be kept as short as possible.

79. During fluoroscopy or other procedures involving radiation, all personnel should remain at least 6 feet away from the X-ray tube (AORN, 2012b, p. 303).

80. Perioperative personnel who must remain with the patient while radiation is being used should wear lead aprons and thyroid shields. Additionally, leaded gloves and leaded eye protection are available for instances of lengthy exposure. A portable lead screen is another form of protection from radiation. Personnel should face the source of radiation while the radiation is

being emitted. If the staff member cannot face the source of radiation during exposure, the staff member should have on a wrap-around lead apron on to protect the back (AORN, 2012b, p. 303).

81. Lead shielding devices should be checked at regular intervals by the X-ray department, safety officer, or radiation physicist to ensure their integrity. If lead aprons are not handled properly, they can develop cracks and subsequently provide inadequate protection. Devices with cracks should be discarded and replaced. Aprons should be hung on a mobile or fixed rack designed for this purpose. They should not be folded.

82. Mobile lead shields may be placed in the room for non-scrubbed personnel to stand behind during the radiation emission time. For rooms designed for procedures requiring radiation exposure, the facility can purchase and install retracted radiation shields mounted to the ceiling. Shielding devices available for protection from radiation include the following items:

    - Lead-lined walls, lead windows, control rooms, and doors
    - Mobile shields on wheels
    - Aprons, vest, gloves, thyroid shields, and glasses with side shields (AORN, 2012b, p. 304)

83. Personnel who are frequently assigned to procedures in which radiation is used should be monitored for exposure. A radiation monitoring badge (dosimeter) consists of a strip of X-ray film encased in a plastic holder. Personnel should wear the dosimeter on the same area of their scrub attire above the lead apron. If two badges are worn, one should be worn at the neck above the lead apron and the other inside the apron (AORN, 2012b, p. 307). The amount of radiation absorbed by each badge should be measured monthly. The facility's safety officer is responsible for collecting the badges, analyzing the dosimeter readings, and passing out new badges. All reports should be kept according to federal and state regulations.

84. Any healthcare facility that uses therapeutic radionuclides for patient care should identify a radiation safety officer to supervise the operation of the radiation safety program. Radionuclides are absorbed by the body, so personnel caring for those patients receiving such therapy must take radiation safety precautions in addition to standard precautions with any bodily secretions from these patients.

85. The radiation safety officer will assist perioperative personnel in complying with government safety regulations and standards. Protective measures for perioperative personnel who are caring for a patient who has received or is receiving therapeutic radionuclides include the following:

    - Using the principles of shielding, time, and distance to limit exposure to the radionuclides
    - Instituting contamination control measures
    - Notifying personnel caring for the patient postoperatively about the type and location of the radiation
    - Observing radiation precautions when transporting the patient
    - Keeping radioactive materials in a lead-lined container
    - Handling radioactive needles and capsules with forceps
    - Posting radiation warning signs on the doors to the operating room where the patient is located
    - Documenting all protective measures on the perioperative record

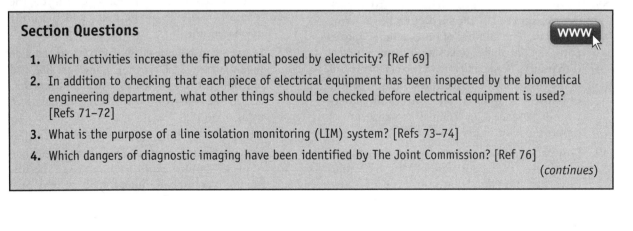

Section Questions

1. Which activities increase the fire potential posed by electricity? [Ref 69]

2. In addition to checking that each piece of electrical equipment has been inspected by the biomedical engineering department, what other things should be checked before electrical equipment is used? [Refs 71–72]

3. What is the purpose of a line isolation monitoring (LIM) system? [Refs 73–74]

4. Which dangers of diagnostic imaging have been identified by The Joint Commission? [Ref 76]

(continues)

Lifting and Moving

86. Musculoskeletal disorders (MSDs), often referred to as ergonomic injuries, account for 29% of all workplace injuries and illnesses requiring time away from work (Bureau of Labor Statistics [BLS], 2012, p. 5).

87. Back injury prevention is an important factor in keeping nurses on the job. Back injuries rate second only to the common cold as employees' reason to miss work. Researchers estimate that 80% of healthcare workers will experience a back injury and approximately 10% of those workers will experience a second injury. The U.S. Department of Labor, Bureau of Labor Statistics, reported that healthcare workers are 4.5 times more likely to sustain an overexertion injury than other types of workers.

88. It is estimated that more than one-third of back injuries suffered by nurses occur when moving a patient. The number of times a nurse moves patients contributes to sustaining an overexertion injury. Bernice Owen, a former professor at the University of Wisconsin–Madison School of Nursing, states that one-third of the nurses who experience a back injury at work do not report the back injury.

89. Low back pain occurs more frequently in nurses than in the general population. Most back injuries are of short duration, and workers are able to return to work. However, some healthcare workers sustain back injuries that result in permanent disability and the end of a career in nursing.

90. Lifting and moving heavy pieces of equipment, instrument sets, and patients who exceed the nurse's physical capacity put excess force on the spine. Most work-related back injuries are cumulative injuries. Although the injury appears to be caused by a single incident, it is often the result of repetitive trauma over a period of time. Lifting injuries include sprains and strains, acute or chronic lower back pain, and injury to the shoulder and neck.

91. Factors that influence the number of back injuries include the advancing age of the nursing workforce, staffing shortages, obesity of patients and staff, and sicker, less mobile patients. Lifting injuries are also influenced by the height from which an item is lifted, the location and size of the item, and the body mechanics the nurse uses during lifting.

92. Injuries can be caused by twisting to the side when lifting and moving heavy items, and reaching for items such as instrument sets that are stored above shoulder level, rather than using a ladder.

93. Using proper body mechanics when lifting heavy instrument sets can reduce the incidence of neck, shoulder, and back injuries. The following recommendations for lifting may prevent injury:

- Keep the back straight.
- Bend the knees.
- Hold the load close to the body.
- Use the leg muscles to lift.
- Do not turn or twist to pick up something or while carrying a heavy object.
- Avoid reaching for items above shoulder level; reach for objects no higher than chest high, and use a ladder/stool if necessary.
- When lifting, place the feet apart to create a wide base of support.

94. Facilities can promote safe lifting by implementing the following measures:
    - Engineering designs that ensure the physical conditions are safe for lifting
    - Employee training in correct body mechanics for lifting
    - A consistent review of injury reports to identify common causes of injury that might motivate work redesign or further education

95. Managing the patient in surgery can also lead to injury:
    - Pushing and pulling a stretcher, bed, or other equipment
    - Transferring a patient between a stretcher and the operating-room bed
    - Positioning a patient
    - Holding an extremity during a prep

96. An adequate number of staff members must be involved when transferring patients to and from the operating-room table. A careful assessment of the patient will determine the number of personnel needed to maintain patient alignment, support extremities, and maintain the airway during transfer. Four is often considered the minimum number of staff needed to transfer an anesthetized adult patient. Safety devices used in the perioperative setting include slides, roller devices, and mechanical lifts.

97. Bariatric patients present special challenges. As of 2010, 35.7% of the adult population and 16.9% of children and adolescents in the United States were obese (Ogden et al., 2012, p. 1). An adult who has a body mass index (BMI) of 30 or greater is considered obese (CDC, 2012). Special bariatric equipment is required for obese patients. Lateral transfer devices or mechanical lifts should be used to move obese patients. An air-driven mattress or friction-reducing sheet is useful. An assistive device should be used whenever a caregiver is required to lift more than 35 pounds of a patient's weight (AORN, 2012b, p. 694).

98. Long periods of standing in one spot, coupled with poor posture, can cause back pain. It is important for the scrubbed person to maintain good posture, stand with one foot on a standing stool, and change positions often. Standing on an antifatigue mat may also reduce risk of injury.

99. Research demonstrates that specific interventions can reduce the rate of musculoskeletal disorders for workers who perform high-risk tasks. Support from administration and management is essential for a successful program. Both OSHA and TJC have identified safety as a top priority for healthcare institutions. Reduction of injuries and lost work time saves money in worker's compensation costs and can lower the insurance premium for the facility. Promotion of a back injury prevention program requires a careful look at the extent and cost of injuries in the institution, a realistic and measurable goal, and a plan of action.

100. OSHA has identified the elements for a program to prevent back injuries (OSHA, 2012a):
    - Wheels and other devices to move heavy equipment
    - Mechanical devices for patient lifting
    - Adequate staffing to prevent staff from lifting patients alone
    - Training for new and experienced staff, addressing avoidance of back injuries
    - Supervision of newly trained employees to validate learning
    - Evaluation of workers prior to employment to identify preexisting back disorders

101. Today, a variety of equipment is available to healthcare workers to assist with lifting and moving patients safely, and protecting both healthcare workers and patients from injury. Facilities should work with staff to perform a needs assessment to determine the types of equipment necessary to serve the facility's patient population. A needs assessment should include the following at a minimum:
    - Lifting techniques being used in the facility
    - Type of lifting required in the facility
    - Patient positioning techniques especially in the perioperative setting
    - Current process and content of staff education

- Gaps between expectations and results (Premier, Inc., 2012)

102. An action plan should follow the needs assessment:
     - Define criteria for each type of lift or move identified.
     - Identify the type of equipment needed for each lift or move.
     - Update policies and procedures.
     - Update staff education content and process.
     - Develop strategies that motivate support for changes.
     - Implement the plan.
     - Review and revise as required.

103. The Washington Industrial Safety and Health Act (WISHA) provides examples of safety checklists that can be adapted to a specific facility's action plan (Washington State Department of Labor and Industries [WSDLI], 2012).

Slips, Trips, and Falls

104. Workplace occupational hazards have been identified as a major contributor to nurses leaving the profession. According to the U.S. Bureau of Labor Statistics, the incidence rate of lost-workday injuries from slips, trips, and falls (STFs) in hospitals was 38.2 per 10,000 employees—90% greater than the average rate for all other private industries combined (Bell et al., 2010, p. 3).

105. An analysis of worker's compensation injury claims from acute care hospitals showed that the lower extremities (i.e., knees, ankles, feet) were the body parts most commonly injured after STFs, resulting most often in sprains, strains, dislocations, and tears. STFs were also significantly more likely to result in fractures and multiple injuries than were other types of injuries (Bell et al., 2010, p. 4).

106. Prevention is the best action for an organization to take when addressing the risk of anyone slipping, tripping, or falling. A prevention plan should address at least the following strategies:
     - Develop a housekeeping program that addresses what all employees should know about their responsibility to provide a safe work environment, such as location of mops, signage for warnings, cleaning materials, housekeeping employee schedule, and who to call in an emergency or dangerous situation for help.
     - Encourage all employees to assist in keeping floors clean and dry.
     - Provide safety mats where spills occur frequently, such as by sinks.
     - Provide umbrella bags by entrance doors.
     - Develop a floor cleaning program. Research recommends the two-step process where the cleaning solution is applied to a small section of the floor with a dripping mop. Follow the manufacturer's direction on proper use of the solution. Mop the area to dry it using a wrung mop.
     - Encourage staff to wear slip-resistant shoes.
     - Use barriers when possible for wet floors so no one enters the area. If barriers cannot be placed in an area, be sure there are plenty of warning signs identifying wet floors.
     - Check drains frequently to ensure they are working properly.
     - Observe the condition of all floors and replace or repair any areas identified as buckled, torn, or loose.
     - Repair cracks in foundations, sidewalks, and parking lots.
     - Create visual clues to warn people of changes in elevation so they do not trip.
     - Floors in areas that are subject to water spillage and other spills such as grease or particulate matter should have a rough surface.
     - Make sure all elevators line up with floors properly when the doors open.
     - Make sure there is adequate lighting throughout the building.
     - Stairwells should be kept clean and free of any hazards such as uneven floors, cracks, trash, and spills.
     - All stairwells should have handrails. Test handrails to make sure they are secure. Make sure handrails are mounted at 34 to 36 inches from the stepping surface. Stairwells that are greater than 44 inches wide must have two sets of handrails.
     - Eliminate clutter.
     - Provide safety devices to control electrical cords.

107. Investigate all falls, trips, and slips to determine their cause. Eliminate these causes as soon as possible.

108. Each person in the operating room can take action to decrease the incidence of slips, trips, and falls:

- Placement of equipment, operating-room furniture, and supplies should allow for safe passage between them while carrying out patient care tasks.

- The multiple cords and hoses of electrical and mechanical equipment used in surgery present a tripping hazard and should be positioned out of the traffic pattern or safeguarded.

- Wet floors in the scrub sink area and in the operating rooms can cause slips and falls. Solutions spilled on the floor should be wiped up promptly. The use of brush-free, gel solutions for hand hygiene can minimize wet floors. Although an absorptive mat may reduce the incidence of a wet floor, it can also become a trip hazard, and if oversaturated, can lose its slip-resistant properties.

- Nonskid protective footwear and support hosiery should be worn to safeguard the employee.

For additional information contact NIOSH: 800-232-4636 or www.cdc.gov/niosh.

Head Injury

109. Overhead operating-room lights that are positioned low pose a risk for head injury. It is not uncommon for operating-room personnel to inadvertently walk into a light that is positioned lower than their head. To prevent this kind of injury, position the light up high and out of the way when not in use.

110. In preparation for surgery, the nurse or surgeon may position the light before the patient is transferred to the operating room bed. Once positioned, the light may remain raised until the start of surgery, at which time it may be lowered. Once the procedure is complete, the light should be moved up and out of the way.

Section Questions

1. Musculoskeletal disorders are also known as what kind of injury? [Ref 86]
2. Healthcare workers are more likely than other workers to sustain what type of injury? [Ref 87]
3. What is the most common cause of back injuries for nurses? [Ref 88]
4. Which activities that nurses perform put excess force on the spine? [Ref 90]
5. Explain why back injuries sustained by nurses are thought to be cumulative injuries. [Ref 90]
6. Which factors influence the number of back injuries sustained by nurses? [Ref 91]
7. Which types of activities can cause musculoskeletal injuries? [Ref 92]
8. Identify seven components of good body mechanics. [Ref 93]
9. How can facilities promote safe lifting? [Ref 94]
10. Which patient care activities have the potential to cause musculoskeletal injuries? [Ref 95]
11. Which considerations in preparing for transferring a patient can prevent musculoskeletal injuries? [Ref 96]
12. How can bariatric patients be managed to prevent injury? [Ref 97]
13. How can the scrubbed person maintain good posture? [Ref 98]
14. Which elements of a program to prevent back injuries has OSHA identified? [Ref 100]
15. Which items should be included in a needs assessment to determine the type of equipment necessary to serve the facility's patient population? [Ref 101]
16. Identify some of the major components of an action plan to prevent lifting injuries. [Ref 102]
17. What is the best approach to addressing the potential for slips, trips, and falls? [Ref 106]
18. Identify at least 15 activities within a healthcare facility that help to prevent slips, trips, and falls. [Ref 106]
19. Identify activities within the operating room that help to prevent slips, trips, and falls. [Ref 108]
20. How are head injuries most often sustained in the operating room setting? [Ref 109]

Chemical Hazards

111. Each employee must be informed of the potential hazards of all chemicals used in the work setting, including information about disinfectants, skin prep agents, tissue preservatives, bone cement, chemotherapy agents, and any other chemicals used in the department. The material safety data sheet (MSDS) for each chemical must be readily available.

112. Manufacturers of chemical products must provide an MSDS for each chemical contained in the product. The MSDS describes hazards associated with the chemicals and describes first-aid measures in the event of exposure. Staff should know the location of MSDSs and be familiar with hazards and first-aid measures for the chemicals with which they work.

113. The employer is responsible for providing appropriate PPE, and all employees must follow label instructions and use the appropriate PPE and/or precautions when working with chemicals.

114. Employers should train staff on the safe and effective use of all potentially hazardous materials used in the workplace.

115. Eye wash stations and body drenching stations must be located where there is potential for exposure to corrosive materials.

Formaldehyde

116. A 37% aqueous solution of formaldehyde is used in the operating room for preservation of surgical specimens. Formaldehyde can also be combined with water and methanol to make formalin.

117. Formaldehyde is a carcinogen that affects the nose and upper respiratory tract. It has a strong, pungent odor that can cause watery eyes and respiratory irritation. When using formaldehyde, healthcare workers should wear gloves and ensure that the work area is adequately ventilated.

Glutaraldehyde

118. Glutaraldehyde is a toxic chemical used as a cold sterilant to disinfect heat-sensitive instruments and equipment. This chemical is also used as a fixative in pathology and histology as well as a fixative for developing X rays.

119. Potential side effects that healthcare workers exposed to glutaraldehyde can experience include eye irritation (mild to severe) and burns to the skin if exposed to high concentrations of the chemical. Breathing in glutaraldehyde can cause a number of respiratory issues, such as irritation of the nose, throat, and respiratory tract. Other side effects include coughing, wheezing, nausea, headaches, nosebleeds, dizziness, and drowsiness.

120. Long-term exposure to glutaraldehyde can cause the employee to be sensitized. Once sensitized, if the employee is exposed to glutaraldehyde again, he or she may experience the following side effects: sudden asthma attacks, difficulty breathing, wheezing, coughing, and tightness in the chest. Some employees have developed skin irritation such as eczema.

121. Protect the healthcare worker by using glutaraldehyde in a room that has at least 10 air exchanges per hour. Best practice is to provide a room that has an exhaust ventilation system such as a fume hood.

122. Post signs in areas where glutaraldehyde is stored and used, warning staff of the hazards as well as how to safely work with this chemical.

123. Use appropriate PPE when working with glutaraldehyde. Appropriate practice includes, but is not limited to, the following items:
    - Wear gloves impervious to glutaraldehyde. Gloves made of butyl rubber, nitrile, and vitorn are preferred.
    - Wear protective covering such as an apron or gown made of polypropylene.
    - Protect your eyes by using splash-proof goggles or a face shield.
    - Provide eye wash stations in area where glutaraldehyde is stored or used.
    - Use respirators for employees who tend to have respiratory reactions to glutaraldehyde.

Methyl Methacrylate

124. Methyl methacrylate (MMA) is an acrylic cement-type compound that polymerizes to form a strong plastic. Its uses include securing orthopedic prostheses and neurosurgical reconstruction of cranial bone (EPA, 2012).

125. Precautions must be taken when using methyl methacrylate, as this chemical can cause skin rashes, itching and watering of the eyes,

headache, and respiratory tract irritation. Prolonged exposure can result in respiratory issues as well as damage to the liver, brain, and kidney. Other major issues may occur with the eyes and nasal cavity. EPA does not consider methyl methacrylate carcinogenic.

126. Breathing methyl methacrylate for short periods of time irritates the nose and throat. The ability to erode olfactory function is considered to be the most sensitive effect of methyl methacrylate and perhaps its most serious potential human hazard following inhalation exposure (EPA, 1998, p. 48).

127. Methyl methacrylate also causes headaches and fatigue, and is a potent skin sensitizer in laboratory animals (EPA, 1994, p. 1).

128. Other effects (e.g., cardiovascular and neurologic effects) that have been noted are generally nonspecific, occur at higher exposures, and are often not clearly attributable to MMA exposure.

129. Methyl methacrylate is supplied in separate containers of a liquid and a powder that are mixed just prior to being used. The combination forms polymethyl methacrylate (PMMA). The liquid should always be poured into the powder to decrease the chance of aerosolization. The liquid component of PMMA is flammable. The MSDS for methyl methacrylate must be readily available in the operating room.

130. A face shield should always be worn while mixing cement. Sterile suction evacuation mixing devices are available for mixing methyl methacrylate on the sterile field. When mixing in an unsterile environment, PPE and an exhaust hood will protect the healthcare worker.

131. Contact lenses should not be worn when working with methyl methacrylate because the vapors can penetrate permeable lenses, causing damage to the lens of the eye.

132. Double gloving is recommended when mixing the liquid and the powder. The outside pair of gloves should be discarded once the cement has been mixed. Double gloving should be used by any staff who will be handling the cement to avoid penetration of the surgical gloves by the cement fumes (AORN, 2012b, pp. 228–229).

133. NIOSH recommends limited exposure to methyl methacrylate. OSHA sets a time limit for exposure at 8 hours per day and no more than 40 hours per week. OSHA also states that exposure limits should be set for the employee. Limits suggested are 100 ppm or a time-weighted average of 410 mg/m^3 (OSHA, 2012a).

134. Follow the manufacturer's recommendation when storing methyl methacrylate (AORN, 2012b, pp. 228–229).

135. If a spill occurs, the area should be secured and isolated until all fumes have been exhausted and the material is cleaned up. Activated charcoal absorbent should be placed over the material. Dispose of the methyl methacrylate according to state and federal requirements, as this material is hazardous to the environment (AORN, 2012b, pp. 228–229).

Surgical Smoke

136. During surgical procedures using a laser or electrosurgical unit, the thermal destruction of tissue creates a smoke by-product referred to as surgical smoke or plume.

137. Research studies have confirmed that this smoke plume can contain toxic gases and vapors such as benzene, hydrogen cyanide, and formaldehyde; bioaerosols; dead and live cellular material (including blood fragments); and viruses (NIOSH, 1996).

138. At high concentrations, surgical smoke causes ocular and upper respiratory tract irritation in healthcare personnel, and creates visual problems for the surgeon. The smoke has unpleasant odors and has been shown to have mutagenic potential (NIOSH, 1996).

139. Health symptoms that the perioperative team may suffer if smoke is not properly evacuated include, but are not limited to, the following:

   • Eye irritation
   • Headache
   • Nausea
   • Respiratory changes
   • Nasopharyngeal changes
   • Neurologic issues such as weakness, fatigue, and lightheadedness

140. OSHA estimates that 500,000 healthcare workers are exposed to surgical smoke each year. Smoke evacuation recommendations for the perioperative environment are available,

and perioperative nurses should be aware of these recommendations and take steps to be compliant to protect themselves and other members of the perioperative team (AORN, 2012c).

141. Smoke evacuation recommendations (AORN, 2012c):

    • Use the central or portable smoke evacuation system for large amounts of plume.

    • Use of wall suction with an inline filter for small amounts of plume is acceptable practice.

    • Use of a laparoscopic filtration system for laparoscopic cases is acceptable.

    • Wear protective equipment such as a high-filtration mask, protective eye wear, long sleeves to protect arms, and gloves to protect hands.

    • Develop competencies for surgical smoke evacuation.

    • Educate staff.

    • Document education of staff.

    • Comply with all federal and state laws concerning safety in the healthcare environment.

142. The leaders in the organization should provide education and tools for the perioperative team members to be compliant with smoke evacuation recommendations that are designed to protect those personnel. The perioperative team members are responsible for complying with the organization's policy and procedure on smoke evacuation and demonstrating competency with the process.

Latex Considerations

143. Localized allergic reactions and skin irritation following contact with natural rubber latex have been recognized for many years, with the first reported case of hypersensitivity appearing in 1979. Irritant skin reactions range from acute, with an immediate burning sensation and redness, to cumulative, with symptoms occurring after several weeks of exposure.

144. Localized allergic reactions can occur 1 to 2 days following contact with latex. Symptoms include redness followed by a rash and vesicles, with the skin becoming darker in color over time. Patch testing can assist with identification of the chemical causing the reaction. Once the

chemical is identified, alternatives can be pursued. In severe cases, a temporary or permanent change of work area may be necessary.

145. Latex allergy is different from irritant contact dermatitis. A true latex allergy may either be a type IV sensitivity or a type I hypersensitivity. Exhibit 12-2 illustrates the difference.

146. Systemic allergic reactions to latex are less common but are the most hazardous types of reactions. Such a reaction may occur immediately on exposure of the skin and mucous membranes to the allergen or after several instances of contact with rubber latex. Usually caused by the proteins in latex, systemic reactions can occur on any contact with products made of rubber. Symptoms range from mild urticaria to anaphylaxis, and must be treated immediately.

147. Staff members diagnosed with a type I hypersensitivity to latex must avoid latex altogether and cannot work in an operating room environment. Many healthcare facilities have created latex-free protocols and often reserve specific operating rooms for patients who are allergic to latex. Staff members are provided with alternative latex-free products. The Safe Medical Devices Act requires all incidents of serious injury or death related to use of a medical device to be reported, including events involving latex allergy.

148. Alternatives for operating-room personnel include selection of nonlatex gloves, wearing glove liners, or changing brands of gloves, and monitoring for continuation of the allergic symptoms.

Exposure Control Plan and Personal Protective Equipment

149. The identification of the personal protective equipment worn today was the result of OSHA's Bloodborne Pathogen Standard, which was designed to protect healthcare workers from biological hazards. This standard benefits not only the healthcare worker but also the patient.

150. PPE must be provided by the organization. It must be available in sizes that fit each healthcare worker and must be present in a quantity that allows the healthcare worker to wear and replace it appropriately.

Exhibit 12-2 Reactions to Latex

Irritation	Delayed Hypersensitivity (also known as Type IV allergic reaction)	Immediate Type I Hypersensitivity

Non allergic condition
 	
Dry skin
Crusted skin lesions
Papules
Localized to contact area
	Chemical allergy that activates the cellular immune system
	
	Symptoms appear 6 to 48 hours following contact.
	  Dry crusted skin
	  Eczema
	  Hives
	  Itching
	  Redness
	  Possible blisters
	Symptoms are localized but with repeated exposure may spread.
		Allergic reaction mediated by lgE antibodies. It is a systemic reaction.
		Immediate onset
		  Itchy eyes
		  Rhinitis
		  Hives
		  Eczema
		  Wheezing
		  Swollen lips and tongue
		  Asthma
		In rare instances may lead to shock and death.

Caused by friction or chemicals used in glove manufacturing.	Caused by reaction to chemicals used during the manufacturing process or by a manufacturing deficiency.	Caused by the proteins in latex.
Symptoms resolve when contact discontinued.	Symptoms resolve when contact discontinued. May not have reaction with change to another glove product.	Must avoid contact with all items containing latex.

151. The organization must develop and perform a biohazard risk analysis covering the following issues:

    - Type of risk facing the healthcare worker

    - Type of PPE needed to protect the healthcare worker from the risk

    - The frequency with which the healthcare worker will be at risk in the area identified as high risk

152. Wearing PPE is not optional; OSHA mandates that all healthcare workers wear PPE in the areas of risk identified in the risk analysis. The healthcare worker cannot waive the right to wear PPE.

153. PPE worn in the perioperative setting includes goggles or glasses with shields, mask, gloves, gowns, hats, and shoe covers.

154. All PPE must be discarded immediately after being used in a patient care or hazardous setting, either before leaving the setting or as the healthcare worker is leaving the setting. No PPE can be taken out of the setting or laundered at home.

155. The organization must provide annual training for all healthcare workers at risk for exposure to bloodborne pathogens. Such training should include the organization's risk analysis and PPE requirements, a review of the organization's policy and procedures in regard to bloodborne pathogens, and PPE as a part of the annual education program. Documentation that each employee has received the training should be kept in the employee's personnel file.

156. The exposure control plan developed from the risk analysis should be updated annually. This plan should identify the following elements:

    - The location of safety equipment such as PPE, spill kits, and eye wash stations

    - The responsibilities of the safety officer

    - Hazardous chemicals used and their locations

    - Location of safety policies and procedures

- Location of MSDSs for all hazardous material used in the organization
- Instructions for reporting an exposure or injury

157. The exposure control plan should also address each healthcare worker's exposure risk based on job description, the education plan, and vaccination and immunization requirements.

158. The plan to evaluate sharps safety should be addressed in either the exposure control plan or in a separate plan addressing sharps safety.

Safety Compliance

159. For healthcare workers, compliance with safety regulations, standards, and recommendations is not optional. When healthcare workers are not compliance with such safety standards, regulations, and recommendations, they not only put themselves at risk for injury and death, but also put their patients and the organization as a whole at risk.

160. Developing an audit program to ensure that healthcare workers are compliant with organizational policy and procedures, plans, rules, regulations, standards, and recommendations is essential to ensuring that the facility is compliant. Consider developing an audit list that covers at least the following topics:

- PPE attire and safety
- Hand hygiene (washing and wearing of exam gloves and sterile gloves appropriately)
- Safety (sharps safety, patient safety, sterile field)
- Safe medication practices
- Fire
- Electrosurgery safety, to include smoke evacuation
- Time-out (three phases)

Organizational leaders should audit for healthcare worker compliance with safety rules, regulations, standards, and recommendations at least once quarterly. Address issues noted in the audit with the specific healthcare workers immediately.

Section Questions   www

1. Which types of products pose potential chemical hazards in the perioperative environment? [Ref 111]
2. What is the purpose of an MSDS? [Ref 112]
3. Which precautions must be taken when working with potentially hazardous chemicals? [Refs 113–115]
4. How is formaldehyde used in the perioperative setting? [Ref 116]
5. Which precautions will protect perioperative nurses from the adverse effects of formaldehyde? [Ref 117]
6. What is glutaraldehyde? [Ref 118]
7. What are the potential side effects of glutaraldehyde exposure? [Ref 119]
8. Describe the physiological response when an individual has become sensitized to glutaraldehyde. [Ref 120]
9. Which ventilation arrangements will protect the healthcare worker from the adverse effects of glutaraldehyde? [Ref 121]
10. Which additional interventions will protect healthcare workers from the adverse effects of glutaraldehyde? [Refs 122–123]
11. How is methyl methacrylate used in the perioperative setting? [Ref 124]
12. Describe some of the potential side effects of exposure to methyl methacrylate. [Refs 125–128]
13. What is the correct order for mixing the two components of methyl methacrylate? [Ref 129]
14. Which precautions should be taken when mixing methyl methacrylate? [Refs 130–132]
15. Describe the management of a methyl methacrylate spill. [Ref 135]
16. What is another term for surgical smoke? [Ref 136]

(continues)

Section Questions (continued)

17. Describe the hazards associated with exposure to surgical smoke. [Refs 137–139]
18. Describe the recommendations for smoke evacuation. [Ref 141]
19. Which type of reaction to latex is the most hazardous? [Ref 146]
20. What is OSHA's mandate about PPE? [Ref 149]
21. Which items are considered PPE in the perioperative setting? [Ref 153]
22. When is PPE discarded? [Ref 154]
23. List the recommended components of an exposure control plan. [Refs 156–158]
24. Discuss the consequences of failure to comply with safety standards. [Ref 159]
25. List items to include in an audit of safety issues. [Ref 160]

• • • **References**

Accreditation Association for Ambulatory Health Care (AAAHC) (2012). *2012 Accreditation Handbook for Ambulatory Health Care.* Skokie, IL: AAAHC.

Association of periOperative Registered Nurses (AORN) (2012a). *Fire Safety Tool Kit.* Denver, CO: AORN. Available at: www.aorn.org/Secondary.aspx?id=20877#axzz1z8QgEJqQ. Accessed July 2012.

Association of periOperative Registered Nurses (AORN) (2012b). *Perioperative Standards and Recommended Practices.* Denver, CO: AORN.

Association of periOperative Registered Nurses (AORN) (2012c). *Surgical Smoke and Bio-aerosols Position Statement.* Denver, CO: AORN. Available at: www.aorn.org/Clinical_Practice/ToolKits/Surgical_Smoke_Evacuation_ToolKit/Surgical_Smoke_And_Bio-Aerosols_Position_Statement.aspx#axzz1z8QgEJqQ. Accessed July 2012.

Bell J, Collins J, Dalsey E, Sublet V (2010). *Slip, Trip, and Fall Prevention for Healthcare Workers.* Publication Number 2011–123. Atlanta, GA: Centers for Disease Control and Prevention, DHHS (NIOSH). Available at: www.cdc.gov/niosh/docs/2011-123/pdfs/2011-123.pdf. Accessed July 2012.

Bruley M (2012). Interview for *Fire in the OR: hundreds are hurt every year.* Available at: www.msnbc.msn.com/id/26874567/ns/health-health_care/t/fire-or-hundreds-are-hurt-every-year/#.T-3BFpE4R8F. Accessed July 2012.

Bureau of Labor Statistics (BLS) (2011). *Nonfatal occupational injuries and illnesses requiring days away from work.* Available at: www.bls.gov/news.release/osh2.nr0.htm. Accessed July 2012.

Center for Disease Control and Prevention (CDC) (2012). *Defining overweight and obesity.* Atlanta, GA: CDC. Available at: www.cdc.gov/obesity/adult/defining.html. Accessed July 2012.

Emergency Care Research Institute (ECRI) (2012). ECRI Medical Device Safety Reports: *The Patient Is on Fire! A surgical fires primer. Guidance*; 21(1): 19–34. Available at: www.mdsr.ecri.org/summary/detail.aspx?doc_id=8197. Accessed July 2012.

Emergency Care Research Institute (ECRI) (2012). *Surgical Fire Prevention.* Available at: www.ecri.org/surgical_fires. Accessed July 2012.

Environmental Protection Agency (EPA) (1994). *Methyl Methacrylate Fact Sheet.* Washington, DC: EPA. Available at: www.epa.gov/chemfact/methy-fs.txt. Accessed June 2012.

Environmental Protection Agency (EPA) (1998). *Toxicological Review of Methyl Methacrylate.* Washington, DC: EPA. Available at: http://nepis.epa.gov/Exe/ZyPDF.cgi?Dockey=P1006D1N.pdf. Accessed July 2012.

Healthcare Facilities Accreditation Program (HFAP) (2009). *Accreditation Requirements for Healthcare Facilities.* Chicago, IL: HFAP.

National Fire Protection Agency (NFPA) (2012). NFPA 101: 2012 *life safety code.* Quincy, MA: NFPA. Available at: www.nfpa.org/onlinepreview/online_preview_document.asp?id=10112#. Accessed July 2012.

National Institute for Occupational Safety and Health (NIOSH) (2012). *Pocket Guide to Chemical Hazards.* Available at: www.cdc.gov/niosh/npg/npgd0426.html. Accessed July 2012

National Institute for Occupational Safety and Health (NIOSH) (1996). *Control of Smoke from Laser/Electric Surgical Procedures.* Atlanta, GA: NIOSH. Available at: www.cdc.gov/niosh/docs/hazardcontrol/hc11.html. Accessed July 2012.

Occupational Safety and Health Administration (OSHA) (2012a). *Methyl Methacrylate.* Washington, DC: OSHA. Available at: www.osha.gov/dts/sltc/methods/organic/org094/org094.html. Accessed July 2012.

Occupational Safety and Health Administration (OSHA) (2012b). OSHA Technical Manual: Section VII, Chapter 1: *Back Disorders and Injuries*, Section V: *Prevention and Control*. Available at: www.osha.gov/dts/osta/otm/otm_vii/otm_vii_1.html#5. Accessed July 2012.

Occupational Safety and Health Administration (OSHA) (2012c). Standard Number: 1910.1030. *Bloodborne pathogens*. Available at: www.osha.gov/pls/oshaweb/owadisp.show_document?p_table=standards&p_id=10051 Accessed July 2012.

Ogden C, Carroll M, Kit B, Flegal K (2012). National Center for Health Statistics (NCHS) Data Brief #82. *Prevalence of Obesity in the United States, 2009–2010*. Available at: www.cdc.gov/nchs/data/databriefs/db82.pdf. Accessed July 2012.

Premier, Inc. (2012). *Back Injury Prevention: Safe Patient Handling*. Available at: www.premierinc.com/safety/topics/back_injury/. Accessed July 2012.

Samuel F E, Jr. (1991). *Safe Medical Devices Act of 1990*. Health Affairs, 10, (1) 192–195. Available at: http://content.healthaffairs.org/content/10/1/192.full.pdf. Accessed July 2012.

The Joint Commission (TJC) (2012). *2012 Hospital Accreditation Standards*. Oakbrook Terrace, IL: TJC. Available at: www.jcrinc.com/Accreditation-Manuals/HS12/4107/. Accessed July 2012.

The Joint Commission (TJC) (2011). *Sentinel Event Alert: Radiation Risks of Diagnostic Imaging*. Issue 47. Available at: www.jointcommission.org/assets/1/18/SEA_47.pdf. Accessed July 2012.

The Joint Commission (TJC) (2003). *Sentinel Event Alert: Preventing Surgical Fires*. Issue 29. Available at: www.jointcommission.org/assets/1/18/SEA_29.pdf. Accessed July 2012.

Washington State Department of Labor and Industries (WSDLI) (2012). *Helpful Tools for Specific Rules*. Tumwater, WA: WSDLI. Available at: www.lni.wa.gov/Safety/Rules/HelpTools. Accessed July 2012.

Post-Test

Read each question carefully. Each question may have more than one correct answer.

1. Which of the following organizations has primary responsibility for publishing and enforcing workplace safety and health standards?
   a. OSHA
   b. NIOSH
   c. CDC
   d. EPA

2. What are the three basic elements of a safe environment?
   a. Building design protects patient, employees, and visitors.
   b. There is a no-smoking policy.
   c. Equipment is maintained on a regular basis.
   d. People understand their responsibility for minimizing risks in the environment.

3. Which of the following environmental risks is (are) addressed in the TJC's Environment of Care chapter?
   a. Safety and security of the facility
   b. Equipment maintenance and testing
   c. Product failure and recalls
   d. Fire safety

4. Which of the following is the "voice of the marketplace" for setting and assessing compliance with standards?
   a. AAMI
   b. ECRI
   c. EPA
   d. ANSI

5. Which of the following is (are) components of a job safety analysis?
   a. Identification of tasks performed in the workplace
   b. Identification of hazards in the workplace
   c. Selection of a safety officer
   d. Review of conditions in the workplace

6. Seventy-five percent of surgical fires occur
   a. because of pooled prep solution.
   b. because the electrosurgical active electrode is not properly managed.
   c. when lasers ignite oxygen in the endotracheal tube.
   d. on the oxygen-rich environment surrounding the patient's face.

7. The definition of a "sentinel event" is
   a. a mistake that could have been prevented if someone had spoken up.
   b. a situation that should never have happened
   c. an unexpected occurrence involving death or serious physical or psychological injury or the threat thereof.
   d. an unexpected occurrence involving death or serious physical or psychological injury.

8. The fire triangle includes which of the following?
    a. Ignition source
    b. Oxygen
    c. Fire extinguisher
    d. Fuel

9. The most common cause of surgical fires is
    a. a laser unit.
    b. an electrosurgical unit.
    c. vapors from prep solutions.
    d. an uncoupled fiber-optic light cable.

10. Methods of reducing the potential for a surgical fire include
    a. placing the electrosurgical active electrode in a holder when it is not in use.
    b. allowing prep solutions to dry.
    c. tenting the drapes to trap oxygen.
    d. uncoupling fiber-optic cords from the light source when the light is not in use.

11. Which responsibilities for managing a fire does the acronym RACE stand for?
    a. Rescue–alert–communicate–extinguish/evacuate
    b. Report–advise–confine–extinguish/evacuate
    c. Report–alert–communicate–extinguish/evacuate
    d. Rescue–alert–confine–extinguish/evacuate

12. A fire safety plan should include which of the following?
    a. Clear definition of responsibilities
    b. Methods for training staff members
    c. Instruction in the use of fire extinguishers
    d. Scenarios for fire drills

13. The perioperative nurse's responsibilities in case of fire include
    a. turning off emergency shutoff valves.
    b. removing burning material from the patient.
    c. staying with the patient during evacuation.
    d. completing appropriate documentation.

14. In response to an LIM alarm, the perioperative nurse should
    a. plug the last piece of electrical equipment into another outlet.
    b. unplug electrical equipment starting with the device most recently plugged in.
    c. send all electrical equipment to biomedical engineering for testing.
    d. send the electrical device that set off the alarm to biomedical engineering for testing.

15. The Joint Commission has described the dangers of diagnostic imaging as including
    a. cancer.
    b. burns.
    c. allergic reactions.
    d. pneumonia.

16. During fluoroscopy, how many feet away from the X-ray tube should staff remain?
    a. 4 feet
    b. 6 feet
    c. 10 feet
    d. 15 feet

17. Which of the following is (are) correct ways to handle lead shielding devices?
    a. Fold them carefully and store them in a mobile cart.
    b. Hang them on a fixed rack designed for them.
    c. Drape them neatly over the X-ray machine.
    d. Discard them after each procedure.

18. Which of the following is (are) correct statements about dosimeters?
    a. A dosimeter consists of a strip of X-ray film encased in a plastic holder.
    b. Wear the dosimeter in the same place all the time.
    c. Clip the dosimeter to the scrub shirt pocket under the lead apron.
    d. The dosimeter should be read weekly to assess exposure.

19. More than one-third of back injuries suffered by nurses occur when they are
    a. lifting instrument sets.
    b. pushing patients on stretchers.
    c. moving heavy pieces of equipment.
    d. moving a patient.

20. Factors that influence the number of back injuries include
    a. the advancing age of the nursing workforce.
    b. obesity of patients and staff.
    c. sicker, less mobile patients.
    d. lack of exercise.

21. Proper body mechanics for lifting include
    a. bending at the waist.
    b. using the leg muscles to lift.
    c. avoiding reaching for objects above shoulder level.
    d. placing the feet apart to create a wide base of support.

22. How can the scrubbed person maintain good posture?
    a. Sit on a stool when not involved in passing instruments.
    b. Change positions frequently.
    c. Place one foot on a stool.
    d. Lean against the operating-room bed to relieve pressure on the back.

23. What is included in an MSDS?
    a. List of all hazardous chemicals in the workplace.
    b. Description of hazards associated with a chemical
    c. Description of first-aid measures for exposure to a chemical
    d. Contact information for reporting exposure

24. Which precautions should be taken when working with glutaraldehyde?
    a. Nitrile, butyl rubber, or vitorn gloves
    b. Goggles or contact lenses
    c. Polypropylene gown
    d. Shoe covers

25. What is important to know about handling methyl methacrylate?
    a. Exposure can cause skin rash, itching, watering of the eyes, and headaches.
    b. Breathing the fumes causes irritation to the nose and throat.
    c. Pour the powder into the liquid to decrease aerosolization.
    d. Wear two pairs of gloves.

26. How can surgical smoke negatively affect healthcare personnel?
    a. Interferes with the surgeon's vision of the wound
    b. Has mutagenic potential
    c. Causes ocular and upper respiratory tract irritation
    d. Has unpleasant odors

27. Which steps can be taken to evacuate surgical smoke?
    a. Use a central or portable smoke evacuation system.
    b. Use wall suction with a filter for small amounts of plume.
    c. Wear a high-filtration mask and protective eye wear.
    d. Educate staff.

28. How does latex allergy differ from contact dermatitis?
    a. Allergy is less common but more hazardous.
    b. Dermatitis is caused by exposure to chemicals in glove manufacturing.
    c. Allergy is caused by exposure to latex protein.
    d. Latex allergy symptoms resolve when contact is discontinued.

29. Which of the following statements is (are) true of PPE?
    a. PPE is mandatory, not optional.
    b. OSHA requires the hospital to provide appropriate PPE for all employees.
    c. PPE can be reused if not soiled.
    d. PPE includes gloves, masks, face shields, goggles, gowns, caps, and shoe covers.

30. Which of the following statements is (are) true about safety compliance?
    a. Standards and recommendations are optional.
    b. Noncompliance puts both employees and the facility at risk.
    c. An audit program can help to assure that the facility is compliant.
    d. Fire safety and the time-out process should be included in the facility audit.

• •

Competence Checklist: Workplace Safety

Under "Observer's Initials," enter initials upon successful achievement of the competency. Enter N/A if the competency is not appropriate for the institution.

Name _____

	Observer's Initials	Date

1. Maintains active electrode in holster. _____ _____
2. Does not wrap ESU cord around metal instrument. _____ _____
3. Periodically cleans ESU active electrode tip of eschar. _____ _____
4. Moistens gauze, sponges, and other items during surgery. _____ _____
5. Prevents contact of activated fiber-optic cord with drapes and gowns. _____ _____
6. Can state meaning of the acronyms RACE and PASS. _____ _____
7. Checks electrical cords before plugging in equipment. _____ _____
8. Identifies location of O_2 shutoff valves, LIM, fire extinguisher, and evacuation route. _____ _____
9. Can describe action to take if an LIM alarm occurs. _____ _____
10. Wears lead apron and thyroid collar when potential for radiation exposure exists. _____ _____
11. Hangs X-ray gowns on rack when not in use. (Does not fold.) _____ _____
12. Uses correct body mechanics when lifting items and moving patients. _____ _____
13. Places cords and equipment out of the traffic pattern to prevent tripping injury. _____ _____
14. Wears nonskid shoes. _____ _____
15. Can locate MSDS sheets. _____ _____
16. Uses suction bowl (exhaust hood) when mixing methyl methacrylate and wears double gloves. _____ _____
17. Demonstrates proper use of glutaraldehyde. _____ _____
18. Demonstrates proper use of formaldehyde. _____ _____
19. Prepares methyl methacrylate according to the manufacturer's recommendation. _____ _____
20. List signs and symptoms of sensitivity that the staff or patient may experience while using methyl methacrylate. _____ _____
21. Can describe how to clean up a spill if it occurs with halogenated agents. _____ _____
22. Demonstrates proper use of PPE while working in an environment where halogenated agents can escape into the atmosphere. _____ _____
23. Demonstrates the proper precautions to be used when working in an environment using electrocautery and laser equipment that is creating surgical smoke. _____ _____
24. Demonstrates proper use of PPE. _____ _____
25. Demonstrates the three parts of the time-out process in every case with every patient. _____ _____

	Observer's Initials	Date
26. Demonstrates sharps safety practice.	_____	_____
27. Demonstrates safe medication practices.	_____	_____

Observer's Signature   Initials   Date

_____

Orientee's Signature

_____

Appendix:
Answers to Post–Test Questions

Chapter 1

1. C [Ref 1]
2. C [Ref 5]
3. B [Ref 6]
4. B [Ref 10]
5. C [Refs 11–12]
6. A [Ref 12]
7. C [Ref 13]
8. D [Ref 15]
9. A [Ref 16]
10. C [Ref 18]
11. D [Ref 19]
12. B [Ref 20]
13. A [Ref 20a]
14. C [Ref 21]
15. D [Ref 21a]
16. D [Ref 22a]
17. B [Ref 39]
18. B [Ref 25]
19. A, B, C [Ref 29]
20. A, B, C, D [Ref 32]
21. B [Ref 36]
22. A [Ref 37a]

Chapter 2

1. A [Ref 1]
2. C [Refs 6–9]
3. B [Ref 15]
4. D [Ref 17]
5. B [Ref 26]
6. D [Ref 29]
7. A [Ref 34]
8. C [Ref 36]
9. C [Ref 39]
10. D [Ref 40]
11. B [Ref 42]
12. D [Ref 46]
13. C [Refs 49, 56]
14. A [Ref 52]
15. B [Ref 62]
16. D [Ref 64]
17. C [Ref 69]
18. A [Refs 65–67]
19. D [Ref 66]
20. B [Ref 76]

Chapter 3

1. B [Ref Definitions]
2. A, B [Ref Definitions]
3. A, B, C, D [Refs 5–7]
4. C [Ref 9]
5. A [Refs 13, 15]
6. B [Refs 16–17]
7. D [Ref 21]
8. A [Ref 24]
9. C [Ref 27]
10. B [Refs 33–40]
11. A, B, C [Refs 33, 36, 37, 40]
12. C [Refs 42–53]
13. A, B [Refs 46, 48, 50, 52]
14. C [Ref 46]
15. B, D [Refs 62, 64, 71, 73]
16. A, B [Refs 80–93]
17. B [Refs 80–93]
18. A, B [Refs 80–93]
19. C, D [Refs 92–95]
20. C [Ref 103]
21. B, C, D [Refs 97–105]

22. A, B, C, D [Refs 106–112]
23. B, C, D [Refs 106–115]
24. A, B, C, D [Refs 117–126]
25. A, C [Refs 129–136]
26. C [Ref 137]
27. A, C, D [Refs 139–143]
28. A, B [Refs 144–152]
29. A, B, D [Refs 155–159]
30. B [Ref 186]

Chapter 4

1. A, B, C [Ref Definitions]
2. A, C [Ref Definitions]
3. A, C, D [Ref 2–5]
4. C [Ref 6]
5. D [Ref 7]
6. C [Ref 15]
7. D [Ref 10]
8. A, C, D [Refs 6–12]
9. A, B [Refs 12–16]
10. A, C [Ref 17]
11. A, C [Refs 19–22]
12. C [Ref 25]
13. A, B, C, D [Refs 31–32]
14. A, B, D [Refs 35–37]
15. B [Refs 37–38]
16. B, C [Refs 41–42]
17. B [Refs 46–49]
18. B, D [Refs 51, 53]
19. A, B, C, D [Ref 55]
20. B [Refs 58–63]
21. A, B, C [Refs 66–70]
22. A, B, C [Refs 71–73]
23. A, B [Refs 74–76]
24. A, B, D [Refs 77–81]
25. B [Refs 82–84]
26. D [Refs 86, 90]
27. A, B [Refs 94, 96]
28. A, B, D [Refs 97–99]
29. A, C [Ref 100]
30. D [Ref 101]
31. D [Ref 101]
32. A, B [Refs 102–105]

33. B, C [Ref 108]
34. B, C, D [Refs, 114–115, 117, 121]
35. A [Refs 122–123]

Chapter 5

1. B, D [Ref 3]
2. C [Ref 6]
3. A [Ref 11]
4. A [Ref 11]
5. B, D [Ref 17]
6. A, B, C, D [Refs 18, 21, 22]
7. A, B, C, D [Refs 29–35]
8. A, B, C, D [Refs 36–39]
9. A, C, D [Refs 40–41]
10. A [Ref 41–43]
11. B, C [Ref 45]
12. A, C, D [Refs 46–47]
13. A [Ref 48]
14. A, B, D [Ref 50]
15. D [Ref 53]
16. C [Ref 57]
17. B, C [Refs 58–63]
18. A, B, C [Ref 71]
19. B [Ref 72]
20. A, B [Refs 76–79]
21. B, C, D [Refs 82–85]
22. C, D [Ref 92]
23. D [Ref 93]
24. A, D [Refs 101–109]
25. A, B, C, D [Ref 129]
26. A [Ref 161]
27. A, D [Ref 165]
28. D [Ref 171]
29. A, D [Refs 177–179]
30. A, D [Refs 182–186]
31. B, C, D [Refs 187–190]
32. B, D [Refs 194–199]
33. A, B [Refs 196–199]
34. B, D [Refs 206–209]
35. A, B, C [Refs 216–217]
36. B, D [Refs 222–226, 231]
37. C, D [Refs 241–243]
38. B, D, C [Refs 244–247]

39. A, B, C, D [Refs 248–249]
40. A, D [Refs 250–251]

Chapter 6

1. B, D [Ref 1]
2. A, B, C, D [Ref 2]
3. D [Ref 4]
4. C [Refs 12–13]
5. A, B, C [Refs 13–14, 166]
6. B [Refs 31–32]
7. C [Refs 37, 103, 114]
8. A, B [Ref 39]
9. D [Ref 40]
10. A, B, C, D [Ref 41]
11. A, B, C [Ref 48]
12. C [Ref 49]
13. C [Ref 50]
14. A, B, C [Refs 51–52, 68]
15. D [Ref 57]
16. B, C [Refs 60–61]
17. A, B, D [Ref 70]
18. B, C, D [Ref 74]
19. A, B, C, D [Refs 65, 81, 85–87]
20. A, B, C [Ref 92]
21. D [Ref 98]
22. A, B, D [Refs 104–107]
23. B, C, D [Ref 114]
24. C, D [Ref 116]
25. C [Ref 118]
26. A, C [Ref 123]
27. B, C, D [Refs 127–128, 130–131]
28. D [Ref 135]
29. A, B, C [Refs 140–143]
30. A, C, D [Refs 155–156, 158]
31. C [Ref 166]
32. A, B, C, D [Refs 180–181, 186]
33. B [Ref 193]
34. C [Ref 194]
35. A, B, C, D [Ref 196]

Chapter 7

1. C, D [Refs 1–3]
2. C [Ref 5]
3. A, B, C, D [Refs 5–8]
4. A, D [Refs 10–12, 20]
5. A, C, D [Ref 22]
6. A, B, C [Ref 23]
7. A, B [Ref 31]
8. D [Refs 32–36]
9. A, B, D [Refs 40–42]
10. A, C [Refs 20, 29, 63, 74]
11. B, C, D [Ref 46]
12. A, B, C, D [Refs 52–57]
13. A, B, C [Refs 62–66]
14. A, B, C [Refs 62, 65, 69]
15. A, B, C, D [Ref 74]

Chapter 8

1. A, B, C [Refs 1–3]
2. A, B, D [Refs 4–5]
3. A, C, D [Refs 5–6]
4. C, D [Refs 8–13]
5. A, B, C [Refs 14–17]
6. A, B, C, D [Refs 18–21]
7. A, C, D [Refs 21–29]
8. A [Refs 30–33]
9. B, C, D [Refs 40–41]
10. A, C, D [Refs 37–43]
11. A, C, D [Refs 45–48]
12. A [Refs 57–62]
13. A, B, D [Refs 63–78]
14. A, B, C [Refs 79–82]
15. A, D [Refs 83–88]
16. B, C [Refs 89–92]
17. C, D [Refs 99, 102, 108, 110]
18. C, D [Ref 115]
19. B [Ref 115]
20. C [Refs 122–131]

Chapter 9

1. A [Ref 3]
2. C [Ref 19]
3. B [Ref 25]
4. C [Ref 34]
5. B [Ref 36]
6. D [Ref 41]

7. C [Ref 49]
8. B [Ref 51]
9. A [Ref 62]
10. B [Ref 63]
11. C [Refs 74–75]
12. D [Ref 80]
13. A [Ref 83]
14. D [Ref 88]
15. B [Ref 95]
16. A [Ref 99]
17. B [Refs 101–102]
18. C [Ref 111]
19. D [Ref 116]
20. A [Ref 120]

Chapter 10

1. B, C, D [Refs 2–6]
2. A, B, C, D [Refs 6–7]
3. A, B, C, D [Refs 10–14, 21]
4. B [Ref 15]
5. A, B, C, D [Refs 22–23]
6. B, D [Ref 24]
7. A, C, D [Ref 25]
8. A, B, D [Refs 26–31]
9. A, B, C, D [Refs 33–39]
10. B, C, D [Refs 42–45]
11. B, C [Refs 46–55]
12. D [Refs 58–61]
13. A, B, C, D [Refs 66–68]
14. A, B, D [Refs 69–75]
15. A, C, D [Refs 78–79, 82, 85]
16. A, B, C, D [Refs 90–96]
17. A, C [Refs 97–103]
18. C, D [Refs 104–110]
19. A, B, C [Refs 112–117]
20. A, B, C, D [Refs 122–128]

Chapter 11

1. A, B, C [Refs 4–7]
2. D [Ref 8]
3. B [Ref 10]
4. A, B, C, D [Ref 16]
5. A, C, D [Ref 18]

6. B, C, D [Refs 25–32]
7. A, B, C, D [Ref 35]
8. D [Ref 35]
9. A, B, C, D [Ref 38]
10. A, B, D [Ref 44]
11. A, B, C, D [Ref 47]
12. B [Ref 50]
13. A, B, D [Ref 55]
14. B, D [Refs 65–69]
15. B, C, D [Ref 70]
16. C [Ref 73]
17. D [Ref 77]
18. A, B, C, D [Ref 81]
19. A, B, C, D [Ref 86]
20. A, B, D [Refs 92–98]
21. B, C, D [Refs 104–105]
22. B [Ref 109]
23. D [Refs 110–112]
24. A, C, D [Ref 114]
25. A, B, C, D [Ref 116]
26. A, B, C, D [Refs 118–123]
27. A, B [Refs 124–127]
28. A, C [Refs 129–131]
29. A, B, D [Ref 135]
30. A, B, C, D [Refs 142–147]
31. A, B, C, D [Refs 156–159]
32. A, C [Refs 162–166]
33. A, B, D [Refs 168–173]
34. A, B, C, D [Refs 175–178]
35. A, B, C, D [Refs 198–203]
36. C [Ref 205]
37. B, D [Ref 206]
38. A, B, C, D [Ref 209]
39. A, B [Ref 213]
40. A, B, D [Ref 215]
41. A, B, C [Ref 226]
42. B, C, D [Ref 233]
43. A, B, C, D [Ref 237]
44. A, B, C, D [Refs 241–242]
45. C [Ref 245]
46. A, C [Ref 251]
47. D [Ref 266]
48. A, B, D [Ref 270]

49. A, B, C, D [Ref 273]
50. A, B, D [Refs 275–278]
51. A, B, C, D [Refs 285–293]
52. A, C [Refs 305–307]
53. A, B, D [Ref 311]
54. A, B, C, D [Refs 318–319]
55. A, B, C, D [Refs 333–342]

Chapter 12

1. A [Ref 5]
2. A, C, D [Ref 8]
3. A, B, C, D [Refs 9–10]
4. D [Ref 23]
5. A, B, D [Ref 25]
6. D [Ref 30]
7. C [Ref 33]
8. A, B, D [Ref 35]
9. B [Ref 37]
10. A, B [Refs 38–42, 45]
11. D [Ref 50]
12. A, B, C, D [Ref 63]
13. A, B, C, D [Ref 65]
14. B, D [Ref 74]
15. A, B [Ref 79]
16. B [Ref 79]
17. B [Ref 81]
18. A, B [Ref 83]
19. D [Ref 88]
20. A, B, C [Ref 91]
21. B, C, D [Ref 93]
22. B, C [Ref 98]
23. B, C [Ref 111]
24. A, C [Refs 123, 131]
25. A, B, D [Refs 127–132]
26. A, B, C, D [Refs 138–139]
27. A, B, C, D [Ref 141]
28. A, B, C [Ref 146, Figure 12–2]
29. A, B, D [Refs 152–156]
30. B, C, D [Refs 159–160]

Glossary

Active electrode: An accessory used in electrosurgery to deliver current from an electrosurgical generator to a patient for the purpose of hemostasis and/or dissecting tissue during surgery.

Aeration (ethylene oxide aeration): A process utilizing warm air circulating in an enclosed cabinet to remove residual ethylene oxide from sterilized items. The length of the process is determined by the composition of the sterilized items and the amount of residual ethylene oxide. The process generally takes from 8 to 12 hours.

Alcohol-based hand rub: A product containing alcohol intended for application to the hands for the purpose of reducing the number of microorganisms on the hands. Product is available as a rinse, gel, or foam. It is usually formulated to contain between 60% and 95% alcohol and contains emollients. Some alcohol products have been cleared by the FDA for use as a surgical hand antiseptic and may be used in preparation for gowning and gloving for surgery.

Aldrete postanesthesia scoring system: A scoring system used to evaluate the recovery of patients who have received general anesthesia by assessing patient activity, respiration, circulation, and oxygen saturation.

Amnestic/amnesic: An anesthetic agent that causes amnesia.

Anatomical timed scrub: A scrub procedure using a sponge/brush and an antimicrobial surgical scrub agent, whereby a specified amount of time is allocated for scrubbing each surface of the fingers, hands, and portion of the arms with an antimicrobial agent.

Anesthesia assistant: A person with a premedical bachelor degree who has completed a clinical program at the graduate level. An anesthesia assistant must be supervised by an anesthesiologist.

Anesthesia standby: See *Moderate sedation/analgesia.*

Antisaligogue: An agent that diminishes or arrests the flow of saliva (e.g., atropine).

Antiseptic: A germicidal agent used on skin and tissue to destroy and prevent growth of microorganisms.

Anxiolytic: A drug that relieves anxiety.

Asepsis: The absence of pathogenic microorganisms.

Aseptic practice/technique: The practices by which contamination from microorganisms is prevented.

Atraumatic suture: Suture that is attached to the needle during manufacture. The needle and suture are a continuous unit in which needle diameter and suture diameter are matched as closely as possible, thereby creating minimal trauma as the needle and strand are pulled through tissue.

Autoclave: A steam sterilizer.

Back table: Also referred to as an instrument table. A stainless steel table covered with a sterile drape on which sterile surgical instruments are arranged for use during surgery.

Bagging: Manual delivery of anesthetic agents by compressing the reservoir bag on the anesthesia machine.

Barrier (sterile): Material, such as a sterile drape or wrapper, that is used to protect the sterility of items by preventing the entry or migration of microorganisms from an unsterile surface or area. Gowns, drapes, and package wrappers are examples of sterile barriers.

Bier block (intravenous block): A technique in which a local anesthetic agent is injected into a tourniquet-occluded extremity for purposes of analgesia.

Bioburden: A population of viable microorganisms on an item.

Biofilm: A collection of microscopic organisms that exist in a polysaccharide matrix and that adhere to a surface and prevent antimicrobial agents from reaching the cells.

Biological monitor/biological indicator: A sterilization monitor consisting of a known population of spores resistant to measurable and controlled parameters of a sterilization process.

Bonewax: Wax made from beeswax, which is used to stop bleeding from bone. It is used most often in neurosurgery and orthopedic surgery.

Bovie: Dr. William Bovie was instrumental in developing the first spark-gap vacuum tube generator that produced cutting with hemostasis. Modern electrosurgical units are still referred to as "Bovies." The more accurate term is *electrosurgical unit.*

Bowie-Dick test: A test of a steam sterilizer's ability to remove air and noncondensable gases from the chamber.

Capacitive coupling: The transfer of electrical (stray) current from the active electrode into other conductive surgical equipment. Capacitive coupling can cause a burn injury, such as bowel perforation, during laparoscopic surgery that may go unnoticed and lead to peritonitis.

Capillarity: A process that allows tissue fluid to be soaked or absorbed into suture material and carried along the strand.

Capnography: A process of monitoring the inhaled and exhaled concentration or partial pressure of carbon dioxide in respiratory gases.

Cavitation: In fluids, the process in which high-intensity sound waves generate tiny bubbles that expand until they collapse or implode, causing a negative pressure on the surfaces of the instruments that dislodges soil.

Certified registered nurse anesthetist (CRNA): A registered nurse with at least 2 years of anesthesia training after basic nursing school and acute care training.

Chemical indicator: A device used to monitor one or more process parameters in the sterilization cycle. The device responds with a chemical or physical change (usually a color change) to conditions within the sterilization chamber. It is usually supplied as a paper strip, tape, or label that changes color or as a pellet that melts when the parameter has been met. A chemical indicator reading of "acceptable" does not guarantee sterility.

- Class 1 (process indicator): Chemical indicator intended for use with individual units (e.g., packs, containers) to demonstrate that the unit has been exposed to the sterilization process and to distinguish between processed and unprocessed units.
- Class 2 (Bowie-Dick test indicator): Chemical indicator designed for use in a specific test procedure (e.g., the Bowie-Dick test is used to determine whether air removal has been adequate in a steam sterilization process).

- Class 3 (single-parameter indicator): Chemical indicator designed to react to one of the critical parameters of sterilization and to indicate exposure to a sterilization cycle at a stated value of the chosen parameter.
- Class 4 (multi-parameter indicator): Chemical indicator designed to react to two or more of the critical parameters of sterilization and to indicate exposure to a sterilization cycle at stated values of the chosen parameters.
- Class 5 (integrating indicator): Chemical indicator designed to react to all critical parameters over a specified range of sterilization cycles and whose performance has been correlated to the performance of the stated test organism under the labeled conditions (AAMI, 2011, p. 7).
- Class 6 (emulating indicator): Cycle-specific chemical indicator that verifies the presence or the absence or a specific time and temperature during a sterilization cycle.

Circulating nurse: A perioperative nurse who is present during a surgical procedure, is not scrubbed, and is responsible for managing the nursing care of the patient and for coordinating and monitoring other activities during the procedure.

Clean contaminated wound (Class II): A wound in which the gastrointestinal, genitourinary, or respiratory tract is entered under planned, controlled means. No spillage occurs, and no infection is present. Examples of clean contaminated procedures include cholecystectomy, cystoscopy, and colon resection.

Clean wound (Class I): A wound in which the gastrointestinal, genitourinary, or respiratory tract is not entered. No inflammation is encountered, and there is no break in aseptic technique. Examples of clean surgical procedures include hernia repair, carpal tunnel repair, and total joint replacement.

Closed gloving: A method of donning sterile gloves in which the arms are inserted into the gown up to the point where the fingers reach the proximal edge of the gown cuff. Gloving is accomplished without the fingers or hands extending beyond the proximal edge of the gown. Only after the glove is donned are the fingers extended beyond the gown edge and inserted into the finger slots.

Conscious sedation: See *Moderate sedation/analgesia.*

Contaminated: Soiled or potentially soiled with microorganisms. All items opened for surgery, whether or not they were used, are considered to be contaminated.

Contaminated wound (Class III): A wound in which gross contamination is present but obvious infection is not. Included in this category are incisions in which nonpurulent inflammation, gross spillage from the gastrointestinal tract, a traumatic wound, or a major break in aseptic technique is encountered. Examples of contaminated procedures include a gunshot wound, rectal procedures, colon resection with GI spillage, and inflamed but not ruptured appendix.

Cottonoid: A small sponge made of compressed cotton often used in neurosurgery. Cottonoids contain a radiopaque marker and come in a variety of sizes.

Counted stroke scrub: A scrub procedure using a sponge/brush and an antimicrobial surgical scrub agent, whereby a prescribed number of strokes is specified for scrubbing each surface of the fingers, hands, and arms.

Critical item: An item that is introduced beneath a mucous membrane or into a vascular space. Critical items must be sterile.

Decontamination: A process of cleaning, disinfecting, or sterilizing that renders items safe for handling by personnel not wearing personal protective equipment, whereby they are no longer capable of transmitting infectious particles. Decontaminated items are not considered sterile.

Desiccation: An electrosurgical method of coagulation, whereby an active electrode is placed in direct contact with tissue.

Dirty wound (Class IV): A wound in which an old traumatic wound with dead tissue exists or an infectious process is present. Examples of dirty or infected procedures include colon resection for ruptured diverticulitis and amputation of a gangrenous appendage.

Disinfectant: An antimicrobial agent used on inanimate surfaces to destroy microorganisms. The composition and concentration of the disinfectant and the amount of time an item is exposed to it determine the number and types of organisms that will be killed.
- High-level disinfectants kill all bacteria, viruses, fungi, and some spores. They are used only on instruments and medical devices.
- Intermediate-level disinfectants kill vegetative bacteria, mycobacteria, viruses, and fungi. They are used on environmental surfaces.
- Low-level disinfectants that are used on environmental surfaces to kill vegetative forms of bacteria, lipid viruses, and some fungi.

Disinfection: A process that kills all living microorganisms, with the exception of high numbers of spores.

Dispersive electrode: An accessory used in electrosurgery that is in contact with the patient and returns electrosurgical current from the patient to the generator.

Dynamic-air-removal sterilizer: A type of sterilizer that uses a series of steam flush and pressure pulses to remove air from the chamber.

Electrosurgery: A method of hemostasis and cutting that is provided when radiofrequency electrical current is passed through the patient's body. The energy is supplied from an electrosurgical generator, delivered to the patient from an active electrode, and returned to the generator via a dispersive electrode. Electrosurgery is used for purposes of cutting tissue or coagulating bleeding points.

Endogenous source of infection: A source of infection that arises from within the body.

Endotoxin: Part of the outer wall of a gram-negative bacteria.

Esmarch: A long piece of rolled latex used to drain the blood from an extremity. The extremity is elevated and the Esmarch bandage is then applied beginning at the fingers and progressing toward the shoulder.

Ethylene oxide sterilization: A method of sterilization that utilizes ethylene oxide gas as the sterilant. It is used primarily for items that cannot tolerate the heat and moisture of steam sterilization.

Event-related sterility: A sterile item remains sterile until an event happens to render that package unsterile.

Exogenous source of infection: A source of infection from outside the body.

Extended cycle: A sterilization cycle that requires an exposure time greater than the more common cycle of 4 minutes at 270°F to 275°F (132°C to 135°C).

Fasciculation: Skeletal muscle contractions that occur when groups of muscles that are innervated by the same neuron contract simultaneously. The contractions appear as twitching. Fasciculation following administration of depolarizing muscle relaxants progresses in a cephalocaudal sequence.

Flash sterilization: See *Immediate-use steam sterilization.*

Fluid proof: Prevents the penetration of fluids through an intact barrier.

Fluid resistant: Resistant to the penetration of fluids. Over time, fluids will penetrate.

Fulguration: An electrosurgical method of coagulation whereby sparking is used to coagulate large bleeders. The active electrode does not contact tissue. Sparks contact the tissue, causing superficial coagulation followed by deep necrosis. The purpose of this process is to destroy tissue.

Gelatin sponge (Gelfoam): A sponge, resembling Styrofoam, made from purified gelatin solution and used for hemostasis.

Gossypiboma: Surgical complications resulting from the unintentional retention of soft goods. The term "gossypiboma" is derived from the Latin *gossypium* ("cotton wool, cotton").

H_2O_2 gas plasma: A fourth state of matter consisting of a cloud of ions, neutrons, and electrons created by the application of an electric or magnetic field. The plasma phase of the sterilization cycle creates free radicals that are reactive with almost all of the molecules essential for normal metabolism of living cells.

H_2O_2 vapor sterilization: Low-temperature sterilization accomplished by deactivating microorganisms.

Hand-off: The transfer of patient information from one caregiver to another. An example is the transfer of patient information from the preoperative holding area nurse to the circulating nurse.

Hemoclip: See *Ligating clip.*

Immediate-use steam sterilization (IUSS): A steam sterilization process for sterilizing heat- and moisture-stable items that are needed immediately. IUSS is used when there is insufficient time to process an item in the prepackaged method. IUSS-processed items cannot be stored or used at a later time. Previously known as "flash sterilization."

Indicator: See *Chemical indicator.*

Induction: The period from the beginning of anesthesia through loss of consciousness.

Inhalation induction: Induction of anesthesia using only inhalation agents given by mask.

Integrator: A device used to monitor more than one process parameter of the sterilization cycle. An example is a wicking paper that melts and progresses along the paper over time when the desired parameters have been achieved. The results are displayed in a window along the strip that indicates the process is acceptable if the wicking reaches the target area on the strip.

Intraoperative: The period beginning when the patient is transferred to the operating room bed and ending with transfer of the patient to the recovery area.

Intravenous block: See *Bier block.*

Intravenous induction: Induction of anesthesia using intravenous medications to induce a loss of consciousness.

Invasive procedure (as defined by the Centers for Medicare and Medicaid, 2009, p. 2): An operative procedure in which skin or mucous membranes and connective tissue are incised, or an instrument is introduced through a natural body orifice (exclusive of examinations and minor procedures such as drawing blood).

Iodophor: A complex of free iodine combined with detergent that is used to kill microorganisms.

I PASS the BATON: A communication tool (mnemonic) consisting of the following steps: introduction, patient, assessment, situation, safety concerns, background, actions, timing ownership, next.

IV conscious sedation: See *Moderate sedation/ analgesia.*

Kitner: A small roll of heavy cotton tape that is usually clamped to forceps and used for dissection or absorption.

Laminar air flow: A high-powered unidirectional air flow of approximately 100 ft/min; the air passes through a HEPA filter that removes all particles equal to or greater than 0.3 μm, with an efficiency of 99.7%. The intended purpose is to reduce airborne contamination.

Lap pad (tape): A square or rectangular gauze pad used for absorption where moderate or large amounts of blood or fluid are encountered.

Laryngeal mask airway (LMA): A tube with an inflatable cuff that is inserted into the pharynx (unlike an esophageal tube, which is inserted into the larynx). It supports spontaneous and artificial ventilation but does not protect the lungs from aspiration.

Ligating clip: A stainless steel, titanium, or tantalum clip used to permanently clamp a vessel.

Local anesthesia: A form of regional anesthesia in which only a small, localized area is infiltrated with an anesthetic agent.

Local standby: See *Moderate sedation/analgesia.*

Malignant hyperthermia (MH): An emergency complication of general anesthesia that is characterized by a rapid rise in temperature (temperatures as high as 109.4°F [43°C] have been reported), extraordinary oxygen consumption, rapid uncontrolled muscle metabolism, and production of heat and carbon dioxide. Malignant hyperthermia is a crisis, and the patient will most likely die if not treated.

Mayo stand: A stand on top of which fits a removable stainless steel tray. The legs of the stand slide under the operating-room table and the tray extends over the patient. Instruments that are frequently used are placed on the Mayo stand. The scrubbed person hands instruments from the Mayo stand to the surgeon during the procedure.

Memory: A characteristic that causes a material to return to the state in which it was originally folded or placed.

Microfibrillar collagen (Avitene, Instat): A fluffy, white, absorbable material made from purified bovine dermis that is used to provide hemostasis. Its application is topical. It is used for oozing or friable tissue.

Moderate sedation/analgesia: A minimally depressed level of consciousness that allows a surgical patient to retain the ability to independently and continuously maintain a patent airway and respond appropriately to verbal commands and physical stimulation (AORN, 2012, p. 411). Medications are administered intravenously to provide sedation, systemic analgesia, and depression of the autonomic nervous system. This anesthesia technique may not require the presence of an anesthesia care provider. In the absence of an anesthesia care provider, the patient is monitored by the perioperative nurse with demonstrated competency in monitoring patients receiving moderate sedation/analgesia. Also referred to as intravenous (IV) conscious sedation, monitored anesthesia care (MAC), anesthesia standby, and local standby.

Monitored anesthesia care (MAC): Moderate sedation/analgesia that is delivered with an anesthesia provider present.

Muscarinic effect: Bradycardia, reduced stroke volume of the heart, bronchiolar constriction, arteriolar dilatation, increased tone, motility and secretion in the alimentary tract, and increases in salivation and lacrimation in response to an anesthetic agent.

Nursing diagnosis: A clinical judgment about actual or potential individual, family, or community experiences/responses to health problems/life processes. A nursing diagnosis provides the basis for selection of nursing interventions to achieve outcomes for which the nurse has accountability (NANDA, 2012).

Open gloving: A technique for donning sterile gloves. In this procedure, the fingers of the scrubbed person are extended beyond the cuff on the gown sleeve prior to gloving. Scrubbed hands touch only the inside of the gloves.

Oxidized cellulose: A specially treated gauze or cotton that is applied directly to an oozing surface to control bleeding (Oxycel, Surgicel, and Surgicel Nu-Knit).

Passivation: A process used in making surgical instruments. The instrument is immersed in a nitric acid solution that removes carbon steel particles and promotes the formation of a chromium oxide coating on the surface.

Peanut: A very small sponge approximately the size of a peanut that is commonly used for blotting blood. It is also used for dissection.

Peel pack: A see-through pouch made of plastic and paper, or plastic and Tyvek, that is used to contain items during sterilization and to maintain them in a sterile state during storage.

Perfusionist: A member of the surgical team who is a highly skilled technician and is responsible for operating the cardiac bypass equipment during open-heart surgery.

Perioperative: Encompasses the three phases of the surgical experience: preoperative, intraoperative, and postoperative. Perioperative nursing activities are activities that occur in any or all of the three phases.

Perioperative Nursing Data Set (PNDS): A standardized nursing vocabulary developed by the Association of periOperative Registered Nurses (AORN) that may be used to describe perioperative nursing practice. It identifies nursing diagnoses and interventions relative to care of the patient undergoing a surgical or invasive procedure.

Plasma (sterilization): Hydrogen peroxide gas plasma sterilizers use a technology consisting of hydrogen peroxide vapor and low-temperature gas plasma to rapidly sterilize medical devices. Plasma is a state of matter produced through the action of a strong electric or magnetic field. In hydrogen peroxide gas plasma sterilization, a plasma state is created by the action of electrical energy upon hydrogen peroxide vapor. Plasma sterilization is used primarily for sterilization of heat- and moisture-sensitive items.

Pledget: A small piece of felt used as a support under friable tissues.

Plume: Smoke that results from cauterizing tissue—most often from application of electrosurgery.

Pneumatic sequential compression device: A device used to prevent formation of a thrombus or DVT. It consists of a sleeve that is wrapped around the patient's leg; the sleeve automatically inflates and deflates in sequential progression.

Postoperative: The period beginning when the patient is transferred to the recovery room and ending with resolution of surgical sequelae.

Preoperative: The period that begins when the decision to have surgery is made and ends when the patient is transferred to the operating-room bed.

Primary intention: See *Wound healing*.

Prion: An infectious proteinaceous particle that is responsible for causing Creutzfeldt-Jakob disease and other spongiform encephalopathies.

Process challenge device (PCD): A device used to assess the effective performance of a sterilization process by providing a challenge to the process that is equal to or greater than the challenge posed by the most difficult item routinely processed (AAMI, 2011, p. 105).

Prep: See *Surgical prep*.

Rapid-readout biological monitor: An enzyme-based biological indicator that is used to monitor the sterilization process. Enzyme activity correlates to the inactivation of spores; it provides a reading that may be obtained soon after sterilization. A biological monitor is included within the product and may be incubated for an additional reading.

Raytex: A gauze sponge used where a small amount of blood or fluid is encountered. Supplied in $4^3/_4$- or $4^3/_8$-inch size.

Regional anesthesia: Anesthesia that blocks the conduction of pain impulses from a specific region of the body. The patient is awake but does not feel pain during surgery.

Restricted area: An area within the operating-room department where surgical procedures are performed and where sterile supplies are unwrapped. Surgical attire and hats are required apparel in this area. The Association of periOperative Registered Nurses also recommends masks in this area when sterile supplies are open or persons are scrubbed (AORN, 2012, p. 95).

Ring stand: A metal stand with wheels that is draped to become part of the sterile field to hold stainless steel basins for water and saline.

Saturated steam: Steam that contains the greatest amount of water vapor possible.

SBAR: A communication technique that highlights the situation, background, assessment, and recommendations.

Scrub: See *Surgical hand antisepsis*.

Scrubbed person: A person who performs a surgical scrub on his or her arms and hands, dons sterile attire, stands within the sterile field, and provides sterile instruments and other items to the surgical team during surgery. The scrubbed person is a member of the sterile team and is either a nurse or a surgical technician/technologist.

Secondary intention: See *Wound healing*.

Secured airway: An airway with an endotracheal tube equipped with a cuff that prevents gastric contents from entering the trachea.

Sellick maneuver: Manual compression of the esophagus between the cricoid cartilage and the vertebral column, done for the purpose of visualizing the tracheal lumen and preventing regurgitation and aspiration during intubation.

Semi-critical item: An item that makes contact with an intact mucous membrane but is not introduced below the membrane. Semi-critical items may be sterilized but must be at least high-level disinfected when used on patients.

Semi-restricted area: An area within the operating-room department that includes scrub sinks, areas where clean and sterile supplies are stored, areas where instruments are processed, and corridors that lead to the restricted area of the operating room. Surgical attire and hats are required. Traffic is limited to authorized personnel in surgical attire and to patients.

Sequential compression device: See *Pneumatic sequential compression device*.

Shelf life: The amount of time an item may be assumed to be sterile. Shelf life is related to events and not to actual time. The longer an item remains on a shelf, the greater the possibility that an event will occur to cause contamination of the item. If no contamination occurs, the item is considered sterile for an indefinite amount of time.

Single-use device: A device manufactured for one-time use; it is not intended to be reprocessed and reused. Also referred to as a disposable.

Skin prep: See *Surgical prep*.

Spore: An inactive, or dormant but viable, state of a microorganism that is difficult to kill. Sterilization methods are monitored by their ability to kill known populations of highly resistant spores.

Standard precautions: Guidelines recommended by (Siegel et al., 2007, pp. 66–67) the Centers for Disease Control and Prevention for reducing the risk of transmission of bloodborne and other pathogens in hospitals. They are the basic level of infection control precautions that are to be used, at a minimum, in the care of all patients. Under standard precautions, blood, all body fluids, secretions, and excretions except sweat, whether or not they contain visible blood, nonintact skin, and mucous membranes, are considered potentially infectious. Infection prevention practices include hand hygiene, cough etiquette, safe injection practices, and personal protective equipment, such as gown, gloves, mask, eye protection, or face shield when there is the potential for exposure to these patient fluids.

Steam sterilization: A sterilization process that uses steam to kill all forms of microbial life.

Sterile: Free of all viable microorganisms, including spores.

Sterile field: The area immediately surrounding the patient into which only sterile items may be entered. A sterile field is created by placing sterile barriers over nonsterile items. The sterile field includes the area around the site of the incision and may include furniture covered with sterile drapes and personnel attired in sterile gowns and gloves and wearing a head covering and mask.

Sterility assurance level (SAL): The probability of a viable microorganism being present on an item after sterilization. The SAL for medical devices is 10^{-6}, or equal to or less than one chance in 1 million that there is a viable microorganism present on a device after sterilization.

Sterilization: A process that kills all living microorganisms, including spores.

Sterilizer (steam): Any of the following sterilization devices:

- Gravity displacement: A type of steam sterilizer in which steam displaces air through an outlet port by means of gravity.
- Prevacuum: A type of dynamic-air-removal steam sterilizer in which a vacuum is created to remove air at the beginning of the cycle and prior to steam entry into the chamber.
- Pulse pressure: A type of dynamic-air-removal steam sterilizer in which a series of steam flushes and pressure pulses at above-atmospheric pressure remove air from the chamber.

Strike-through: An event that occurs when liquids soak through a barrier from a sterile area to an unsterile area, or from an unsterile area to a sterile area. Strike-through renders items contained within the barrier unsterile.

Styptic: An agent that causes blood vessel constriction. An example is epinephrine.

Superheating: Occurs when fabrics that are dehydrated are subjected to steam sterilization. The temperature of the fabric exceeds the temperature of the steam. Superheating destroys cloth fibers.

Surgical conscience: An inner commitment to strictly adhere to aseptic practice, to report any break in aseptic technique, and to correct any violation, whether or not anyone else is present or observes the violation. A surgical conscience mandates a commitment to aseptic practice at all times.

Surgical counts: The counting of sponges, sharps such as blades and needles, and instruments that are opened and delivered to the field for use during surgery. Counts are performed both prior to incision and before closing; these counts should match. Counting is a safety mechanism intended to decrease the risk that items used during the surgery might be retained in the patient.

Surgical hand antisepsis: Antiseptic hand wash or antiseptic hand rub performed prior to surgery by surgical personnel to eliminate transient microorganisms and reduce resident hand flora. Done in preparation for gowning and gloving.

Surgical hand antiseptic: An antimicrobial product formulated to significantly reduce the number of microorganisms on skin. Products are broad spectrum and should exhibit both persistence and a cumulative effect that prevents or inhibits proliferation or survival of microorganisms. Products used in preparation for gowning and gloving for surgery must be cleared by the FDA for use as a surgical hand antiseptic.

Surgical prep: Preparation of the patient's skin at the incision site and surrounding area. The patient's skin is cleansed with an antimicrobial agent to reduce the number of microorganisms to as low a level as possible and to prevent rebound growth for as long as possible. The prep may or may not include hair removal at the incision site.

Surgical scrub: A process of cleansing the hands and arms for the purpose of removing as many microorganisms as possible from the hands and portion of the arms prior to donning a sterile gown and gloves. See also *Anatomical timed scrub*, *Counted stroke scrub*, and *Surgical hand antisepsis*.

Surgical-site infection (SSI): Any of the following types of infection:

- Superficial incisional: Infection involving only the skin or subcutaneous tissue.
- Deep incisional: Infection involving deep soft tissue, such as fascia or muscle.
- Organ/space: Infection involving the visceral cavity or anatomic structures not opened during the surgery.

Suture: (noun) A strand of material used to tie a blood vessel so as to occlude the lumen or sew tissue together; (verb) to sew tissue using suture material.

Suture ligature: A tie with an attached needle that is used to anchor the tie through the vessel for purposes of hemostasis.

Tape: See *Lap pad.*

Telfa: A nonadherent wound dressing.

Tensile strength: The amount of tension or pull that a suture will withstand when knotted before it breaks. The tension or pull is expressed in pounds. Tensile strength determines the amount of wound support that the suture provides during the healing process.

Terminal sterilization: Sterilization of an item that has been processed and wrapped. Terminal sterilization permits storage of the sterilized item for later use.

Thrombin: An enzyme made from dried beef blood that is used to control capillary bleeding. It is supplied as a white powder and may be mixed with water or saline to form a thrombin solution.

Tie: A strand of material that is tied around a vessel to occlude the lumen for purposes of hemostasis.

Tonsil sponge: Cotton-filled gauze in the shape of a ball with a long attached tape. It is used in the mouth or throat for absorption of blood. The tape extends outside the mouth to permit easy retrieval.

Transmission-based precautions: A method of infection control that is applicable to patients known or suspected to be infected or colonized with highly transmissible or epidemiologically important pathogens for which additional precautions are needed to prevent transmission. There are three types of transmission-based precautions: airborne, droplet, and contact. These are used in addition to standard precautions.

- Airborne precautions: Appropriate for protection against pathogens that are transmitted by the airborne route. Includes use of respiratory protection and special air handling and ventilation.
- Droplet precautions: Appropriate for protection against pathogens transmitted through droplets. Includes wearing a mask within 3 feet of an infected patient and positioning other patients at least 3 feet from infected patients.
- Contact precautions: Appropriate for protection against pathogens that are transmitted by direct or indirect contact. Includes wearing a gown and gloves and cleaning and disinfecting patient equipment (Siegel et al., 2007, pp. 70–71).

Tyvek: Material made from high-density polyethylene fibers.

Universal precautions: A method of infection control that requires the blood and body fluid of all humans (patients and personnel) to be considered infectious and that the same safety precautions be taken whether or not the patient is known to have a bloodborne infectious disease. Universal precautions have been incorporated into standard precautions.

Unrestricted area: An area within the operating-room department where street clothes are permitted. Includes a control point where communication between the semi-restricted and restricted areas is coordinated.

Washer-disinfector/washer-decontaminator: Automated processing units used to decontaminate instruments. Cycles within these machines vary but include washing and rinsing and may include ultrasonic cleaning. A chemical or thermal phase within the cycle destroys specific microorganisms.

Washer-sterilizer: An automated processing unit that washes instruments for the purpose of decontamination. Includes washing, rinsing, and sterilization. Instruments processed in a washer-sterilizer are not ready for patient use and must be subject to an additional sterilization process in a sterilizer.

Webril: A cotton padding used under a cast or tourniquet.

Wet pack: Condensation on the inner or outer surface of a package/device following a terminal sterilization process.

Wound dehiscence: A partial or complete separation of the wound edges after wound closure as a result of failure of the wound to heal or failure of the suture material to secure the wound during healing.

Wound evisceration: The protrusion of the abdominal viscera through the incision as a result of failure of the wound to heal or failure of suture to secure the wound during healing.

Wound healing: The restoration of an injured area.

- Primary intention: Wound healing that occurs by primary union. Wound edges are approximated. Wounds heal by primary intention when minimal tissue damage occurs, aseptic technique is maintained, tissue is handled gently, and all layers of the wound are approximated. Wounds that heal by primary intention heal quickly and result in minimal scarring.

- Secondary intention: Wound healing that occurs by wound contraction. Wound edges are not approximated. The wound is left open and healing occurs from the bottom upward. Granulation tissue forms in the wound and gradually fills in the defect.

- Third (tertiary) intention: Wound healing that occurs when the wound is sutured several days after surgery. Wound suturing is delayed for several days to permit granulation to occur in an area where gross infection or extensive tissue was removed. The wound is closed only if there is no sign of infection.

Wrong-site surgery: Surgery performed on the wrong patient, body part, side, level, or site.

● ● ● **References**

Association for the Advancement of Medical Instrumentation (AAMI) (2011). *Steam Sterilization and Sterility Assurance in Health Care Facilities.* (ANSI/AAMI ST79: 2011). Arlington, VA: AAMI.

Association of periOperative Registered Nurses (AORN) (2012). *Perioperative Standards and Recommended Practices* (pp. 411–420). Denver, CO: AORN.

Centers for Medicare & Medicaid Services (CMS) (2009). National Coverage Determination (NCD) for Surgical or Other Invasive Procedure Performed on the Wrong Body Part (140.7) (p. 2). Baltimore: CMS. Available at www.cms.gov/medicare-coverage-database/details/ncd-details.aspx?NCDId=328&ncdver=1&bc=AgAAQAAAAAAA&. Accessed December 11, 2012.

North American Nursing Diagnosis Association (NANDA) (2012). *International Nursing Diagnosis Glossary of Terms.* Available at: www.nanda.org/Diagnosis Development/DiagnosisSubmission/PreparingYour Submission/GlossaryofTerms.aspx. Accessed July 2012.

Siegel, J. et al. (2007). *2007 Guideline for Isolation Precautions: Preventing Transmission of Infectious Agents in Healthcare Settings.* Atlanta, GA: CDC. Available at www.cdc.gov/hicpac/pdf/isolation/Isolation2007.pdf Accessed October, 2012.

Index

Exhibits, figures, and tables are indicated by exh, f, and t following the page number.